IMAGE RECONSTRUCTION FROM PROJECTIONS

The Fundamentals of Computerized Tomography

This is a volume in

COMPUTER SCIENCE AND APPLIED MATHEMATICS

A Series of Monographs and Textbooks

Editor: WERNER RHEINBOLDT

A complete list of titles in this series appears at the end of this volume.

IMAGE RECONSTRUCTION FROM PROJECTIONS

The Fundamentals of Computerized Tomography

GABOR T. HERMAN

Department of Computer Science
State University of New York at Buffalo
Amherst, New York

1980

ACADEMIC PRESS

A Subsidiary of Harcourt Brace Jovanovich, Publishers

New York   London   Toronto   Sydney   San Francisco

ACADEMIC PRESS, INC.
Orlando, Florida 32887

United Kingdom Edition published by
ACADEMIC PRESS, INC. (LONDON) LTD.
24/28 Oval Road, London NW1 7DX

Library of Congress Cataloging in Publication Data

Herman, Gabor T
    Image reconstruction from projections.

    Includes bibliographies.
    1. Tomography.   2. Imaging systems in medicine.
I. Title.
RC78.7.T6H47   616.07'572   79–6785
ISBN 0–12–342050–4

PRINTED IN THE UNITED STATES OF AMERICA

83   9 8 7 6 5 4 3 2

Contents

5 Data Collection and Reconstruction of the Head Phantom under Various Assumptions

6 Basic Concepts of Reconstruction Algorithms

7 Backprojection

8 Convolution Method for Parallel Beams

9 Other Transform Methods for Parallel Beams

10 Convolution Methods for Divergent Beams

11 The Algebraic Reconstruction Techniques

12 Quadratic Optimization Methods

13 Noniterative Series Expansion Methods

14 Truly Three-Dimensional Reconstruction

15 Three-Dimensional Display of Organs

16 Mathematical Background

References   297

Preface

The problem of image reconstruction from projections has arisen independently in a large number of scientific fields. An important version of the problem in medicine is that of obtaining the density distribution within the human body from multiple x-ray projections. This process is referred to as *computerized tomography;* it has revolutionized diagnostic radiology over the past decade. The 1979 Nobel prize in medicine has been awarded for work on computerized tomography.

This book is devoted to the fundamentals of this field. Its topic is the computational and mathematical procedures underlying the data collection, image reconstruction, and image display in the practice of computerized tomography. It is written from the point of view of the practitioner: points of implementation and application are carefully discussed and illustrated. The major emphasis of the book is on reconstruction methods; these are thoroughly surveyed.

After a summary of diverse application areas (from radio astronomy to electron microscopy) the book discusses in some detail the area of x-ray computerized tomography. This is followed by a classification and thorough discussion of reconstruction algorithms and a treatment of the computational problems associated with the display of the results. While all mathematical concepts and claims are carefully stated, they are mostly left unproved in the main body of the work, to ensure an easy flow of the presentation. Proofs of the most important of these claims are provided in the final chapter.

The book is based on a two-semester introductory graduate course that the author has taught during the past three years in the Department of Computer Science at the State University of New York at Buffalo. The material has been constantly revised to make it as up-to-date as possible in an introductory text. The presently used syllabus for this course follows this preface; there is a nearly complete overlap between syllabus and the contents.

The topic of the book is of potential interest in many fields of medicine, engineering, and science. An attempt has been made to carefully introduce all but the most commonly known notions, so that the book should be useful to readers with diverse backgrounds.

Each chapter ends with a section of Notes and References. These are *not* intended to provide a full history of the topic of the chapter. They always acknowledge the immediate sources on which the chapter is based, sometimes give references to early and current work in the field, but usually do not mention anything between. The reference list at the end of the book is no more than that, and no attempt has been made to turn it into a bibliography of the field.

The author began to work in the field of image reconstruction from projections over ten years ago. At that time there were only a handful of publications on the topic published in journals serving diverse fields, with just about no awareness of other relevant work. Even three years ago, when serious writing of this book began, it seemed feasible that the field could be surveyed thoroughly in less than 400 pages. Research progressed faster than the author could write, and the book is handed over to the reader as an introductory text to what has surely been one of the most explosive and exciting interdisciplinary developments in the history of science.

Syllabus for an Introductory Two-Semester Course on Image Reconstruction

I. DATA COLLECTION

How projection data are obtained in various sciences and medicine, such as electron microscopy, radio astronomy, nuclear medicine, but concentrating on x-ray transmission data. Measurements viewed as line and strip integrals. The nature of noise in experimental measurements: photon noise, scatter, beam hardening, etc. Preprocessing of data to reduce the effect of noise, data fitting, interpolation, and smoothing.

II. RECONSTRUCTION ALGORITHMS

Radon transform, the Radon inversion formula, regularization of the singular integral in the Radon inversion formula, numerical evaluation of the regularized integral. Fourier transforms, the projection theorem, convolution, sampling and aliasing, the discrete Fourier transform, and the fast Fourier transform. Convolution reconstruction methods and Fourier space interpolation reconstruction methods, the effect of filtering and interpolation in such methods.

Basis functions, the mapping of images into finite-dimensional vectors, using series expansion. The reconstruction problem as an optimization problem in finite-dimensional vector spaces, functions to be optimized. Norms, generalized inverses, least squares solutions, maximum entropy solutions, and most likely estimates. Richardson's algorithm and its variants in image reconstruction. Iterative relaxation methods.

Comparative evaluation of various reconstruction methods: accuracy under ideal circumstances, noise magnification, computational costs, and general applicability.

III. Computer Technology

Design and maintenance of a large programming system (SNARK) and data base for image reconstruction. The application of SNARK in designing, implementing, and evaluating reconstruction algorithms.

Display and analysis of reconstructed results: two-dimensional versus three-dimensional display, color versus black and white, dynamic versus stationary. Interpolation in display. Edge and surface detection, the display of three-dimensional surfaces.

IV. Applications

Computed tomography, x-ray scanners, positron scanners, lunar occultations, the structure of symmetric viruses, dynamic analysis, display of cardiac and pulmonary function, etc.

Acknowledgments

The author has the privilege of having been the Director of the Medical Image Processing Group in the Department of Computer Science at the State University of New York at Buffalo since its establishment in 1976. The constant interaction with this outstanding group of individuals has had a major influence on the writing (and repeated rewriting) of the book. Joint papers in the reference list at the end of the book give some indication of specific credit due to individuals on different parts of the book, but all of the following past and present members of the Medical Image Processing Group have contributed to its final appearance: M. D. Altschuler, E. Artzy, Y. Censor, T. Chang, B. S. Dane, P. P. B. Eggermont, W. Falk, G. Frieder, A. Kogan, P. A. Kontio, J. Kostyo, Y. Kuo, A. V. Lakshminarayanan, S. Leibovic, A. Lent, R. M. Lewitt, H. K. Liu, A. Louis, H.-P. Lung, M. R. McKay, W. A. Paddock II, S. W. Rowland, R. G. Simmons, P. Slocum, J. E. Turner, Jr., H. Tuy, J. K. Udupa, M.-M. Yau, G. Yuval, and S. Yussuff. Special thanks for most of the numerous illustrations are due to Reid Simmons (who did all the computer runs to produce the graphic display outputs and plots) and Barbara S. Dane (who was responsible for the hand-drawn figures and the photography, as well as the technical typing). Other colleagues at the State University of New York at Buffalo (both in and outside the Department of Computer Science) have been a great help since 1969, when Dr. Richard Gordon (at that time a member of the Center for Theoretical Biology at Buffalo) introduced the author to the field of image reconstruction from projections.

Another major influence was the author's cooperation with the Biodynamics Research Unit at the Mayo Clinic, Rochester, Minnesota. Scientific cooperation since 1972 (and in particular a nine-month visit during 1975–1976) with members of this illustrious group provided a major motivation for the author's own work.

Cooperation with other research groups in hospitals, universities, and industry has also had its effects. The most significant of these joint efforts was the continual series of combined research projects that the author has undertaken in cooperation with employees of the General Electric Company since 1974.

The author's research work during the writing of this book has been supported by the following grants and contracts: NIH grants HL4664, HL18968, and RR-7; NCI contracts CB53860 and CB84235; and NSF grant MCS7522347.

1

Introduction

In this chapter we discuss a number of the many different scientific areas in which the procedures described in this book are applicable. We also introduce some statistical concepts which are useful for understanding much of the later material.

1.1   IMAGE RECONSTRUCTION FROM PROJECTIONS

The problem of image reconstruction from projections has repeatedly arisen over the last 25 years in a large number of scientific, medical, and technical fields. The range of applicability is staggering. At one end of the scale, data from electron microscopes are used to reconstruct the molecular structure of bacteriophages; while at the other end, data collected by rockets sent outside the earth's atmosphere are used to reconstruct the x-ray structure of supernova remnants. These seemingly different applications, and many others to be mentioned here, have the same mathematical and computational foundations. It is the purpose of this book to discuss these foundations.

Of all the applications, probably the greatest effect on the world at large has been in the area of diagnostic medicine: *computerized tomography* (CT) has revolutionized radiology. Images of cross sections of the human body are produced from data obtained by measuring the attenuation of x rays along a large number of lines through the cross section. Most of this book uses CT as the framework within which the problems and solutions are presented. We therefore say very little about it in this section, but survey some of the numerous other applications.

We start with a simple artificial problem to demonstrate the underlying ideas. While the solution to this problem is of no known practical usefulness, the problem is very similar to a practical problem in astrophysics (to be mentioned in the following), and shares its basic structure with all other applications of image reconstruction from projections.

Suppose we have a rectangular area containing some sources of light. A simple example is a television screen displaying a still picture. Suppose that we also have a "detector" which can measure the *total* intensity of light in the picture. That, of course, would not help us to record the details in the picture. One way of getting at the details is to make a "collimator," by cutting a small square hole into a sheet of nontransparent material. If we put the collimator in front of the picture, the detector measures only the light emanating from the small region behind the square hole. By moving the hole in discrete steps across the picture and measuring the intensity each time, we can build up an image of the picture. The image is made up of small square regions whose brightness is proportional to the average intensity in the original picture in the corresponding region. We can move the collimator so that small square regions are abutting and cover the whole picture. In such a case, the resulting image (referred to as a *digitization* of the picture later in this book) resembles the picture, provided only that the collimator is small enough. This is illustrated in Fig. 1.1.

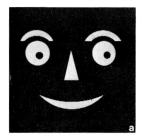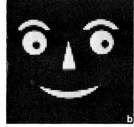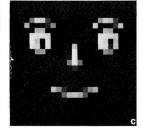

Fig. 1.1. Three different digitizations of the same picture. (a) is a 243 × 243 digitization, (b) an 81 × 81 digitization, and (c) a 27 × 27 digitization.

Suppose now that we lack the capability of cutting a small square hole into our opaque sheet. It may then appear that we can no longer produce an image of our picture. However, image reconstruction from projections comes to our rescue. We now illustrate the processes of "projection taking" and "reconstruction" on our simple problem.

The process of projection taking in this case consists of moving the opaque sheet across the picture in small discrete steps in a fixed direction. After each move, we use our detector to measure the total intensity of light in the uncovered part of the picture. Subtracting from the measured value of total intensity at any time the measured value of total intensity at the previous time, provides us with the total intensity of light in each of a set of parallel

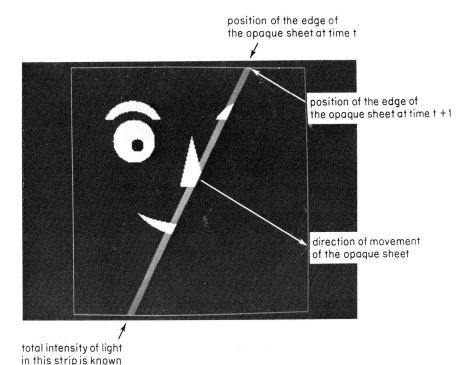

position of the edge of
the opaque sheet at time t

position of the edge of
the opaque sheet at time t + 1

direction of movement
of the opaque sheet

total intensity of light
in this strip is known

Fig. 1.2. The process of projection taking. The line integral of the brightness along the central line of a strip (shown half-illuminated) is estimated by dividing the total brightness in the strip by the width of the strip.

abutting thin strips of known location (see Fig. 1.2). We can now repeat this process with the opaque sheet moving in a different direction. This way we get the total intensity of light in each of another set of parallel abutting thin strips of known location. We estimate the *line integral* of the brightness along the central lines of these strips, by dividing the total brightness in the strip by the width of the strip. Doing this repeatedly (say 90 times, moving the orientation of the opaque sheet by 2° each time), we obtain many such sets of measurements. Each set of estimated line integrals is called a projection (for reasons which become clear later), and the collection of all these estimated line integrals is referred to as *projection data*.

The process of *reconstruction* produces an image of the picture from the projection data of the picture. How this is done is the main topic of this book, and we say no more about it here. In Fig. 1.3 we compare the 81 × 81 digitization of a picture with an 81 × 81 reconstruction from 90 projections with 121 estimated line integrals in each.

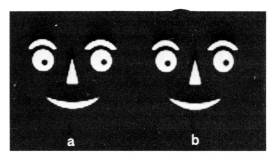

Fig. 1.3. The 81 × 81 digitization of a picture (a) compared to an 81 × 81 reconstruction from 90 projections with 121 measurements in each projection (b).

This example illustrates the informal definition given in the following paragraph. While not all that comes under the heading "image reconstruction from projections" is covered by this informal definition (for example, in Chapter 14 we discuss truly three-dimensional reconstruction), it serves reasonably well to describe our attitude toward image reconstruction throughout most of this book.

Image reconstruction from projections is the process of producing an image of a two-dimensional distribution (usually of some physical property) from estimates of its line integrals along a finite number of lines of known locations.

We now turn to some real life applications. The order in which we take these is according to the size of the object to be reconstructed. The reader is warned that the following is by no means an exhaustive survey of all the application areas of image reconstruction from projections.

Actually, our simple artificial problem has a close analog in *astrophysics*. There are instruments for measuring the brightness distribution of radio sources in the sky which are of too low resolution to provide astrophysicists with the information they seek. However, if the moon moves across the portion of the sky which is of interest, it acts in an analogous fashion to the opaque sheet of our artificial example. The direction of the path of the moon across the sky varies from day to day, providing us with a number of projections, which in this field are referred to as profiles obtained from *lunar occultation* observations. From such observations the two-dimensional brightness distribution of radio sources can be reconstructed.

We discuss a further application in astrophysics in greater detail. Suppose we are interested in reconstructing the x-ray structure of an astronomical object such as a supernova remnant. One way of doing this is to send rockets outside the atmosphere which collect projections of the x-ray surface brightness of the sky. Figure 1.4 shows the instrument that has been used for making such measurements for the Vela supernova remnant. Figure 1.5 shows the

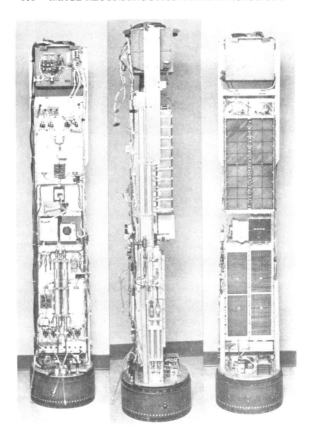

Fig. 1.4. Three views of the payload used to measure projections of the Vela supernova remnant. (Illustration provided by Dr. G. P. Garmire.)

paths of the rocket across the sky. As the rocket travels, it collects data for two projections simultaneously. At each point indicated in Fig. 1.5 data are collected for the estimation of the line integrals of the x-ray brightness along the two lines which make 45° with the path and meet the path at the indicated point. Thus the five paths shown in Fig. 1.5 provide us with ten projections. The reconstructed x-ray brightness map is shown in Fig. 1.6, superimposed on an ultraviolet photograph of the Vela supernova remnant.

Coming nearer to home, reconstruction from projections has been found to be of interest in *solar physics*. The solar corona is a three-dimensional object. There are instruments to measure the total (integrated) electron density along a line of sight. By using such an instrument, we can produce a two-dimensional image in which the brightness of any point is approximately proportional to the total electron density along one of a set of (for all practical

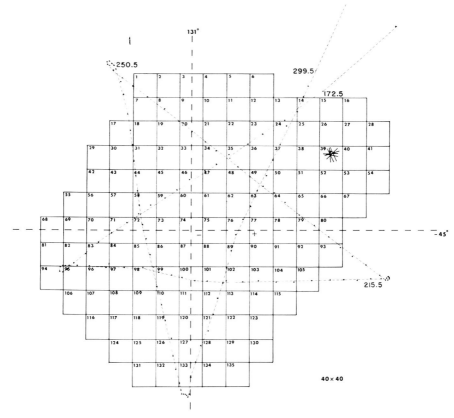

Fig. 1.5. Portion of the sky containing the Vela supernova remnant with a grid of 135 cells superimposed on it. Aim is to reconstruct the x-ray surface brightness in the individual cells. Data are collected by sending a rocket outside the atmosphere, which during its paths (indicated in the figure) simultaneously collects two projections of the x-ray surface brightness. [Reproduced from Moore and Garmire (1975), with permission.]

purposes) parallel lines. Such an image is a two-dimensional projection of the three-dimensional electron density distribution. (Previous examples were basically different: we measured one-dimensional projections of two-dimensional distributions.) As the sun rotates around its axis we get projections from different directions, from which the three-dimensional electron density distribution can be reconstructed. Figure 1.7 shows an estimated electron density distribution on a spherical surface just slightly larger than the limb of the sun. This has been produced from data collected over a period of 14 days, which is a duration of half a solar rotation. Note the zero values between the peaks (solar streamers). The low values were found to correspond

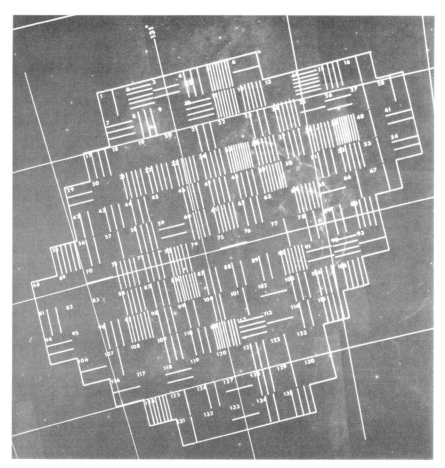

Fig. 1.6. Reconstructed x-ray map superposed on an ultraviolet photograph of the Vela supernova remnant. Each bar in a cell indicates 0.5 standard deviation above background. [Reproduced from Moore and Garmire (1975), with permission.]

to coronal holes. At the edge of the sun these coronal holes cannot be seen in the two-dimensional projection, because they are usually sandwiched between streamers whose projections dominate. The reconstructed coronal electron density can also be used to show the appearance of the sun from directions that cannot be observed from earth. Figure 1.8 shows the appearance of the sun (computer produced based on the three-dimensional reconstruction) from above the north pole of its rotation.

Coming down to earth, we find some large scale applications, such as the estimation of the spatial concentration of certain types of air pollutants.

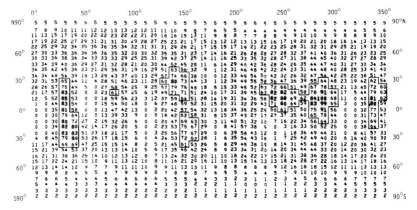

Fig. 1.7. Map of relative electron density of the solar corona at a height of 0.1 solar radii above the visible surface of the sun obtained by reconstruction of line of sight data collected over half solar rotation. (Illustration provided by Dr. M. D. Altschuler.)

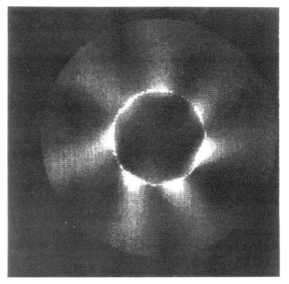

Fig. 1.8. Computer produced picture of the appearance of the sun from above the north pole of its rotation axis. (Illustration provided by Dr. M. D. Altschuler.)

Except for the example given in Fig. 1.9, we forego a discussion of these and concentrate on the most widely used application area: *diagnostic medicine.*

X-ray *transmission computerized tomography* (CT) is discussed in some detail in the succeeding chapters. Here we just indicate its nature using two figures. Figure 1.10 shows an engineering drawing of a typical apparatus

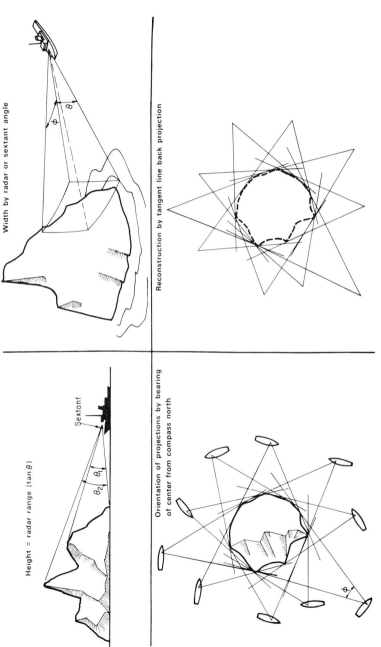

Fig. 1.9. Estimation of iceberg volume from projections. The projections in this example are somewhat different from the other examples in this chapter; essentially they are simple shadows. That is, the "estimated line integrals" in this case can have only two values: one indicating that the line goes through the iceberg and the other indicating that it does not. As the ship moves around the iceberg, its location relative to the iceberg is determined by radar (for measuring distance from the iceberg) and compass (for measuring orientation). The iceberg volume is estimated by the volume of its convex hull; i.e., the convex object which would cast the same shadows in the measured directions that the iceberg casts. Such reconstructions have been used to study the effect of mass and sail area on the movement of icebergs in the North Atlantic. (Illustration provided by Dr. T. F. Budinger.)

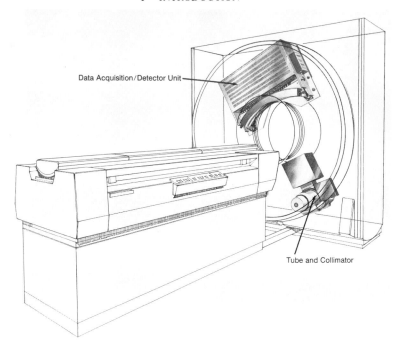

Data Acquisition/Detector Unit

Tube and Collimator

Fig. 1.10 Engineering drawing of a typical CT scanner. (Illustration provided by the General Electric Corporation.)

for data collection in x-ray CT. The tube contains a single x-ray source, the detector unit contains an array of x-ray detectors. Suppose for the moment that the x-ray tube and collimator on the one side and the data acquisition/ detector unit on the other side are stationary, and the patient on the table is moved between them at a steady rate. By shooting a fan beam of x rays through the patient at frequent regular intervals and detecting them on the other side, we can build up a two-dimensional x-ray projection of the patient which is very similar in appearance to the image that is traditionally captured on an x-ray film. Such a projection is shown in Fig. 1.11a. The brightness at a point is indicative of the total attenuation of the x rays from the source to the detector. This mode of operation is *not* CT, it is just an alternative way of taking x-ray images. In the CT mode, the patient is kept stationary, but the tube and the detector unit rotate (together) around the patient. The fan beam of x rays from the source to the detector determines a slice in the patient's body. The location of such a slice is shown by a broken line in Fig. 1.11a. Data are collected for a number of fixed positions of the source and detector; these are referred to as views. For each view, we have a reading by each

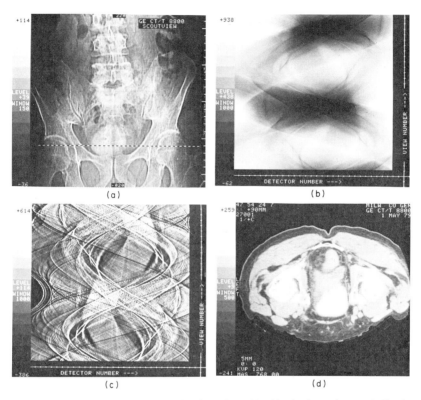

Fig. 1.11. (a) ScoutView (a General Electric trademark) with a horizontal cursor indicating the position where the CT scan (and sinograms) were obtained. (b) Sinogram of the projection data. (c) Sinogram of the convolved data. (d) The CT reconstruction. (Illustration provided by Dr. G. H. Glover.)

of the detectors. All the detector readings for all the views can be represented as a *sinogram*, shown in Fig. 1.11b. The intensities in the sinogram are proportional to the line integrals of the x-ray attenuation coefficient between the corresponding source and the detector positions. From these line integrals, a two-dimensional image of the x-ray attenuation coefficient distribution in the slice of the body can be produced by the techniques of image reconstruction. Such an image is shown in Fig. 1.11d. Inasmuch as different tissues have different x-ray attenuation coefficients, boundaries of organs can be delineated and healthy tissue can be distinguished from tumors. In this way CT produces cross-sectional slices of the human body without surgical intervention. [The picture in Fig. 1.11c is a sinogram of the "convolved projection data," which is to be defined in (1.12) of Chapter 10.]

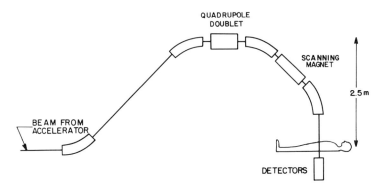

Fig. 1.12. A possible proton beam delivery system. [Reproduced from Hanson (1979), with permission.]

An alternative (not yet in current medical practice) is to use the same basic procedure, but with *protons* instead of x rays. The proposed apparatus is shown in Fig. 1.12. The suggestion of using protons is supported by the claim that similar quality reconstruction can be obtained by much less dose (and hence health hazard) to the patient; see Fig. 1.13.

A modality of data collection with no demonstrated adverse effect on the patient is *ultrasound*. In Fig. 1.14a, we show a photograph of an apparatus used to collect projection data of the female breast. From the physical measurements one obtains estimates of the line integrals of both the acoustic refraction index and of the acoustic attenuation coefficient. Two separate reconstructions can be performed from these: one producing an image of the distribution of the acoustic refraction index in the cross section and the other producing an image of the distribution of acoustic attenuation in the cross section. The two images looked at together give a great deal of information about the nature of the tumors (if any) present in the breast. Two such reconstructions of an excised breast are compared with the corresponding slice of the actual breast in Fig. 1.14d. The rest of Fig. 1.14 contains a block diagram of computer control and data acquisition and a schematic of scan geometry.

Another method of data collection with potential usefulness in diagnostic medicine is provided by *nuclear magnetic resonance*. When an object is placed in a magnetic field gradient, the frequencies of magnetic resonance signals from its nuclei and unpaired electrons depend upon the value of the local applied magnetic field, as well as upon those molecular interactions usually studied by magnetic resonance methods. The integrated signal from the intersection of a surface of constant magnetic field with a three-dimensional object is one point on a one-dimensional projection of a three-dimensional signal. In a uniform linear field gradient, a plot of such signals

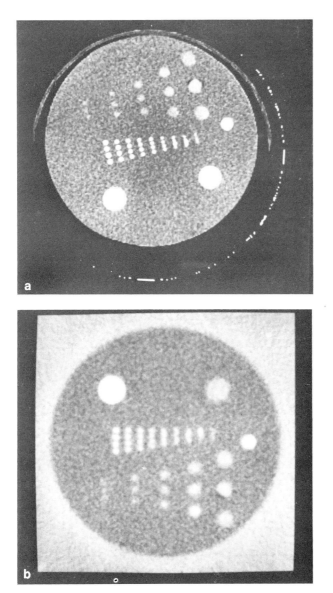

Fig. 1.13. (a) This x-ray CT reconstruction of a phantom needed an average dose of 3.3 rad to be produced. (b) The same phantom reconstructed by proton CT at an average dose of only 0.6 rad. [Reproduced from Hanson (1979), with permission.]

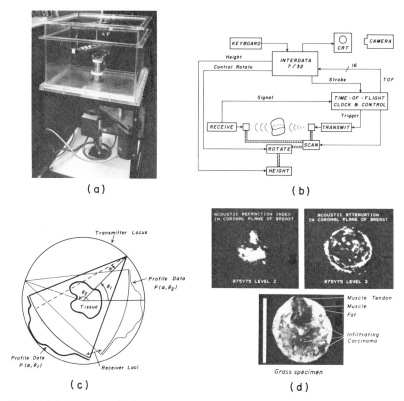

Fig. 1.14. (a) Photograph of apparatus used to collect ultrasonic projection data of cross sections of the female breast. (b) Block diagram of the data acquisition and computer control system. (c) Schematic of scan geometry. Note that, similar to Fig. 1.10, each view consists of data collected along a set of diverging rays. (d) Picture of results in an excised breast with carcinoma. (Illustration provided by Dr. J. F. Greenleaf.)

against frequency is a one-dimensional projection, in a direction perpendicular to the gradient axis, of the total signal intensity. If the direction of the field gradient is varied other projections may be produced, and a two- or three-dimensional image may be reconstructed. For example, an N-shaped water filled cavity inside a 14 mm-diameter plastic disk is shown in Fig. 1.15, together with a few of the nuclear magnetic resonance projections that were taken. The reconstructed image of the test object is shown in Fig. 1.16.

Emission computerized tomography has as its major emphasis the quantitative determination of the moment-to-moment changes in the chemistry and flow physiology of injected or inhaled compounds labeled with radioactive atoms. In this case the distribution to be reconstructed is the distribution of

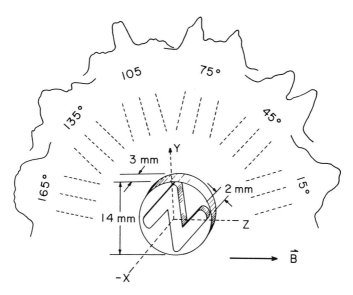

Fig. 1.15. A drawing of the test object used in a nuclear magnetic resonance reconstruction together with copies of typical actual projection data. [Reproduced from Lai, Shook, and Lauterbur (1979), with permission.]

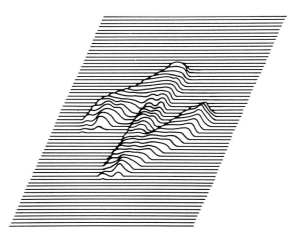

Fig. 1.16. An image of the test object of Fig. 1.15, reconstructed from 180 nuclear magnetic resonance projections. [Reproduced from Lai, Shook, and Lauterbur (1979), with permission.]

radioactivity in the body cross section, and the measurements are used to estimate the total activity along lines of known locations. Figures 1.17 and 1.18 illustrate a device for doing this, the one which is in use at the Donner Laboratory of the University of California, Berkeley. There are a number of such devices in daily medical use all over the world.

Getting away from medicine, we note that image reconstruction from projections has been found useful in *nondestructive testing*. For example, a collection of transmission beam neutron radiographs can be used for the reconstruction (and hence inspection) of fast breeder reactor fuel contained in steel test vehicles. Figure 1.19a shows a 91 pin fuel bundle, which is enclosed in a hexagonal steel ducting (not shown in the figure). The bundle contains three test pins which in the cross section to be reconstructed have voided sections. (This is the defect for which we are looking.) A typical neutron radiograph of this fuel bundle is shown in Fig. 1.19b. From twenty such radiographs the cross section of the fuel bundle has been reconstructed; see Fig. 1.19c.

An application where the "object" to be reconstructed has size of order best measured in centimeters is the determination of three-dimensional

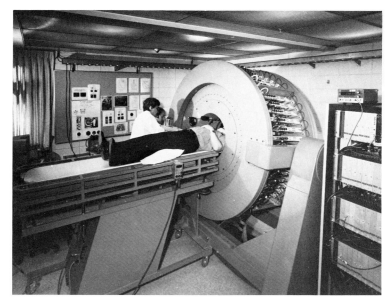

Fig. 1.17. The Donner system for emission computerized tomography uses 280 scintillation detectors surrounding the patient. Data to estimate line integrals of the radioactivity in the patient are simultaneously collected for 240 projections with 105 lines in each. (Illustration provided by Dr. T. F. Budinger.)

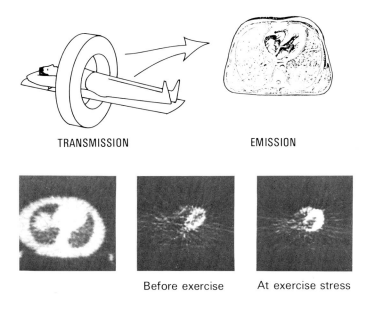

TRANSMISSION   EMISSION

Before exercise   At exercise stress

Ratio of uptake: 1.7

Fig. 1.18. Illustration of the performance of the Donner system in imaging the accumulation of rubidium-82 in the human myocardium. Left lower panel shows a transmission image of the myocardium and dome of the liver. Right two panels show the accumulation of rubidium which reflects coronary blood flow before and at exercise. (Illustration provided by Dr. T. F. Budinger.)

temperature fields by *holographic interferometry*. We do not give an example of this, but move all the way down to the microscopic level.

In Fig. 1.20a we see an *electron micrograph* of a bacteriophage. The bar on the figure represents 1000 Å ($= 10^{-7}$ m). In Fig. 1.20b the boxed area shows a further magnified part of the tail. In Fig. 1.20c we see a diffraction pattern produced by the boxed area. A low resolution model of the structure, based on optical diffraction analysis, shows that the tail is constructed of sections 38 Å thick with three-fold axial rotational symmetry, stacked with a helical screw angle of 41.5°. Assuming that all sections are identical, a single electron micrograph provides us with many projections of the ideal section, making reconstruction possible. Figure 1.20d shows the three-dimensional reconstruction over three sections.

This completes our survey of some of the applications of image reconstruction from projections. Except for some further discussion of x-ray CT, the rest of this book is devoted to the theory, rather than applications, of image reconstruction.

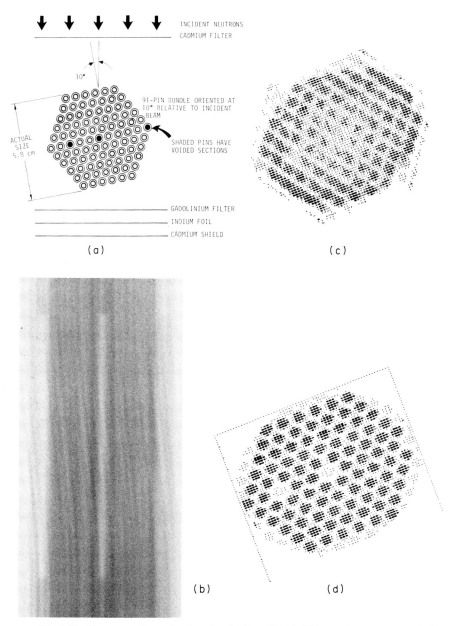

Fig. 1.19. Neutron radiograph of nuclear fuel bundle. (a) Object to be reconstructed. (b) Typical neutron radiograph. (c) Reconstruction from 20 neutron radiographs. (d) Reconstruction from (computer simulated) noise-free data. [Illustration provided by Dr. John P. Barton, IRT Corporation (private communication February 8, 1979).]

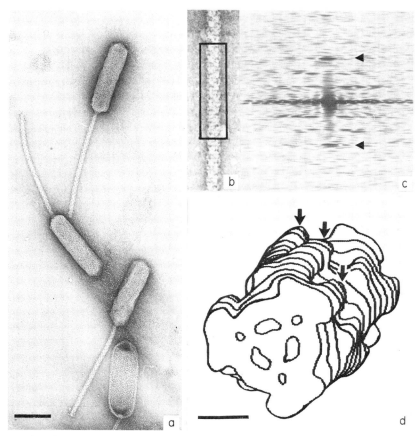

Fig. 1.20. Reconstruction of the tail of the *Caulobacter crescentus* bacteriophage ϕCbK. (a) Electromicrograph of ϕCbK (negatively stained with 1% uranyl acetate). Bar represents 1000 Å. (b) ϕCbK tail. Boxed area is 200 Å × 1000 Å. (c) Diffraction pattern produced by the boxed area. Arrowheads indicate spacing of $\frac{1}{38}$ Å. (d) Three-dimensional reconstruction of ϕCbK tail extending over three axial repeats (114 Å). Bar represents 50 Å. (Illustration provided by Drs. S. Papadopoulos and P. R. Smith.)

1.2   Probability and Random Variables

In order to discuss the processes involved in CT we need to know some of the basic concepts of probability theory. The purpose of this section is to introduce the reader to these concepts. The reader may wish to skim this section at first reading and return to it at times when the notions introduced here are actually used.

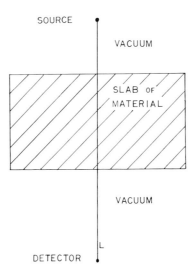

Fig. 1.21. Definition of transmittance.

As an example, consider the situation depicted in Fig. 1.21. There is a box-shaped slab of material. The line L goes through this material. If an x-ray photon enters the slab along the line L through its top face, it will continue to travel along the line L until it is absorbed or scattered. Some photons will be neither absorbed nor scattered before exiting through the bottom face. We shall say such photons are *transmitted* through the slab. The point is that for any individual x-ray photon we cannot be certain whether or not it will be transmitted. All we can say is that, for any fixed energy $\bar{e}$, there is a fixed *probability* ρ that a photon at that energy which enters the slab is transmitted. We call ρ the *transmittance* at energy $\bar{e}$ of the slab along line L, and we define it as follows. The definition is typical of how the "probability" of something happening is defined.

In order to define ρ we carry out a "thought experiment." Such an experiment could be physically carried out if we had at our disposal an infinite amount of time and instruments with unlimited precision. We shoot photons at energy $\bar{e}$ one by one through the slab along the line L, and we test whether they are transmitted. Let $t_1(n)$ denote the number of photons transmitted out of the first n in this experiment. (The subscript 1 refers to the fact that this is the first such thought experiment, in the following we shall discuss whole series of them.) Then ρ is defined as the limit of $t_1(n)/n$ as n tends to infinity, in symbols

$$\rho = \lim_{n \to \infty} (t_1(n)/n). \tag{2.1}$$

That is, the transmittance ρ is a number such that given a positive real number ε, however small, there will always be an integer n_0, such that the difference between ρ and $t_1(n)/n$ is less than ε for all n greater than n_0.

Note that it is not a priori obvious that $t_1(n)/n$ has a limit as n tends to infinity. The claim that it does is based on physical experiments which approximate the thought experiment just described. Note also that it is assumed that the same value of ρ will be provided if the experiment is carried out again. More precisely, let the same thought experiment be carried out the second time, and let $t_2(n)$ denote the number of photons transmitted out of the first n in the second experiment. Then $\rho = \lim_{n \to \infty} (t_2(n)/n)$.

Even though the values of ρ defined by the limits of the two identical thought experiments are the same, it does not mean that we can assume that $t_1(n) = t_2(n)$, for any fixed n. Both $t_1(n)$ and $t_2(n)$ may assume any integer value between zero (no photons are transmitted) and n (all photons are transmitted). However, some of these values are more likely than others. It is reasonable to inquire as to what is the probability $p_n(m)$ that m photons out of n get transmitted.

In order to define $p_n(m)$, we carry out the previously described thought experiment repeatedly up to the point when n photons have entered the slab. Let $t_i(n)$ denote the number of transmitted photons in the ith thought experiment. Let $s(N)$ denote the number of times $t_i(n) = m$, for $1 \le i \le N$. Then we define

$$p_n(m) = \lim_{N \to \infty} (s(N)/N). \tag{2.2}$$

Note that $p_n(m) = 0$ if m is negative or if m is greater than n. Since $p_n(m)$ is supposed to be the probability of m photons being transmitted out of n, this is reassuring. Also it is easy to see by comparing the thought experiments used to define ρ and $p_n(m)$ that $p_1(1) = \rho$. It is somewhat more difficult to show that, in general for $0 \le m \le n$,

$$p_n(m) = \frac{n!}{m!(n - m)!} \, \rho^m (1 - \rho)^{n - m}. \tag{2.3}$$

[$m!$ denotes $m \times (m - 1) \times (m - 2) \times \cdots \times 2 \times 1$, with $0!$ defined to be one.] Equation (2.3) is referred to as the *binomial probability law*.

The set of all possible outcomes of an experiment such as the one just described together with the probability of each outcome is what is called a discrete *random variable*. In this book, we only allow experiments whose outcome is a number, or possibly a column vector of numbers. For example, for a fixed n, the set of all integers m together with the probability $p_n(m)$ is the *binomial random variable* with parameters n and ρ. We call the outcome of a single experiment a *sample* of the random variable. For example, the value of $t_i(n)$, for a fixed i, in the thought experiment just described is a sample of the binomial random variable with parameters n and ρ.

In summary, the number of photons which may be transmitted when n photons enter the slab is a random variable. The actual number of photons transmitted in a single experiment with n photons entering the slab is a sample of the random variable.

Later on we see other examples of random variables. A particularly important one for our purposes is associated with the number of photons emitted by an x-ray source in the direction of a detector during a unit period of time.

Two important properties of a discrete random variable are its *mean* and *variance*. These are defined as follows.

Let X denote the random variable with a set of possible samples S. For x in S, let $p_X(x)$ denote the probability that the outcome of a single experiment will be x. Then the mean μ_X is defined by

$$\mu_X = \sum_{x \in S} x p_X(x), \tag{2.4}$$

and the variance V_X is defined by

$$V_X = \sum_{x \in S} (x - \mu_X)^2 p_X(x). \tag{2.5}$$

Note that the averaged outcome of a very large number of experiments will approximate the mean. Also, the variance will be approximated by taking the average of the square of the distance of the samples from the mean. Thus, the variance is a measure of the spread of the possible outcomes around the mean. For the binomial random variable with parameters n and ρ the mean is $n\rho$ and the variance is $n\rho(1 - \rho)$. The *standard deviation* of a random variable is defined to be the square root of its variance.

We shall say that a random variable *behaves normally* if it has the following properties: the probability that a sample is within one standard deviation of the mean is greater than 0.65, the probability that a sample is within two standard deviations of the mean is greater than 0.95, and the probability that a sample is within three standard deviation of the mean is greater than 0.995. Most random variables that one comes across in CT behave normally.

The importance of the notion of a normally behaving random variable is the following. We often desire to estimate the mean of a random variable from a sample or samples. In 95 cases out of 100 the mean of a normally behaving random variable will be within two standard deviations of a sample. An alternative way of saying this is that we are 95 % *confident* that the mean is within two standard deviations of the sample. If we had a way of estimating the standard deviation (and we often do), then having observed a single sample we can say that we are 95 % confident that the mean lies between two numbers, which are the sample plus/minus twice the standard deviation. Similarly, we can say that we are 99.5 % confident that the mean lies between the sample plus/minus three standard deviations. It can be shown that provided $n\rho(1 - \rho)$ is large (greater than 10), the binomial random variable behaves normally.

Finally we want to discuss functions on random variables. In CT we frequently come across functions whose arguments are samples of random variables. For example, the number of photons counted by a detector during the measurement process is a random variable, which we call D. To remove the effect of the fluctuation in the intensity of the x-ray source the photon count by the detector is usually divided by the photon count by a reference detector, which is also a sample of a random variable, which we call R. The set of all outcomes of the combined experiment of counting photons by the detector, counting photons by the reference detector, and dividing the former by the latter, forms a random variable, which we call N. We assume that the photon count by either detector during the experiment is a positive integer. Let $p_D(x)$ and $p_R(x)$ denote the probabilities that x photons are counted by the detector and the reference detector, respectively. Then the possible outcomes of the combined experiments are the positive rational numbers, and the probability $p_N(q)$ that the outcome of the combined experiment is q is

$$p_N(q) = \sum_{\substack{x, y \\ (x/y) = q}} p_D(x)p_R(y). \tag{2.6}$$

In this case we say that the random variable N is obtained by dividing the random variable D by the random variable R and denote this by $N = D/R$.

Similarly, if X is a random variable with a set S of possible outcomes consisting of positive numbers, then $Y = \ln(X)$ is a random variable whose set of possible outcomes consists of the natural logarithms of elements of S, and is such that for x in S, $p_Y(\ln x) = p_X(x)$.

Further concepts of probability theory will be introduced as and when they are needed.

NOTES AND REFERENCES

A book mainly devoted to the applications of image reconstruction from projections has been edited by Herman (1979c). That book contains state of the art survey articles on using image reconstruction to solve problems of finding the internal structure of the solar corona, the radio brightness of a portion of the sky, the distribution of radionuclides indicating the physiological functioning of the human body, and the dynamic behavior of the beating heart of a patient. Further applications can be found in the *Technical Digest of the Meeting on Image Processing for 2-D and 3-D Reconstruction from Projections* which was held at Stanford, California, in 1975, and was sponsored by the Stanford University Institute for Electronics in Medicine and by the Optical Society of America. A more recent relevant meeting was the Workshop on Physics and Engineering in Computerized Tomography, held at Newport Beach, California, in 1979, whose proceedings have been published in Volume NS-26 of the *IEEE Transactions on Nuclear Science*.

For a description of using lunar occultation observations for the reconstruction of two-dimensional brightness distribution of radio sources, see Taylor (1967). For a general tutorial of image reconstruction in radio astronomy, see Bracewell (1979). Our example regarding the x-ray structure of the Vela supernova remnant is based on Moore and Garmire (1975).

A very thorough survey on the reconstruction of the three-dimensional solar corona is given by Altschuler (1979).

A paper describing the use of reconstruction for estimating the spatial reconstruction of air pollutants is Stuck (1977). For background on iceberg detection, though not on reconstruction, see Budinger (1960).

The first report in the open literature of an apparatus demonstrating the potential of reconstructive tomography in medicine was Oldendorf (1961). The procedure used for doing reconstruction in Oldendorf's paper is essentially the same as the backprojection method (to be discussed in Chapter 7). A more accurate noniterative series expansion method (see Chapter 13) was proposed by Cormack (1963), in a paper also devoted to demonstrating the potential of reconstruction to diagnostic medicine. Another pioneering report in the medical application area is that of Kuhl and Edwards (1963). The first commercially available x-ray CT scanner was designed by Hounsfield (1972, 1973). It was used for scanning the head only. CT body scanning was introduced by Ledley *et al.* (1974). The 1979 Nobel prize in medicine was awarded to G. N. Hounsfield and A. M. Cormack for their pioneering contributions to the development of computerized tomography.

Much of the recent developments in the applications of image reconstruction from projections to medicine can be found in a collection of papers edited by Raviv *et al.* (1979), which includes articles on x-ray, proton, ultrasound, and emission computerized tomography. A progress report on high temporal resolution x-ray CT is given by Wood *et al.* (1979). A brief article (with a long bibliography) on medical imaging by nuclear magnetic resonance is given by Lauterbur (1979). A very comprehensive survey on emission computerized tomography is given by Budinger *et al.* (1979). Work on myocardial uptake of Rubidium-82 has been reported by Budinger *et al.* (1979).

The material on nondestructive testing of fuel bundles is based on a report by Barton (1978).

Methods and experiments on the determination of three-dimensional temperature fields by holographic interferometry are reported by Radulovic and Vest (1976).

The details of the techniques used in producing Fig. 1.20 (as well as references to some of the earlier literature on reconstruction from electro-micrographs) can be found in Smith *et al.* (1976).

Further details on probability and random variables can be found in Parzen (1960), which provides additional material and the original references in this area.

2

An Overview of the Process of CT

In this chapter we describe, in the most general terms, the whole process of x-ray computerized tomography. Our intention is to give a brief overview. Hence, some terms with which the reader may not be familiar are introduced without proper definition. We ask the reader's indulgence; such terms will be carefully defined in subsequent chapters.

2.1 WHAT ARE WE TRYING TO DO?

The aim of CT is to obtain information regarding the nature of material occupying exact positions inside the body.

For example, Fig. 2.1 is a lateral projection of the thorax of a dog. A catheter that has been inserted into the heart is clearly visible, but the exact anatomic position of the catheter cannot be determined from this projection alone. Having reconstructed the internal structure of the thorax from multiple x-ray projections, we can display cross sections of it at arbitrary orientations. Figure 2.2 shows the display of 16 sagittal slices of the thorax of the same dog. The location of the catheter is now precisely determined; it lies in the plane of the sagittal slice which is displayed on the right in the second row.

In addition, the reconstruction enables us to discover and display the precise shape of selected organs. For example, in Fig. 2.3, we display part of the left lung of the dog. This display is obtained by further computer processing of the reconstructed cross sections (see Chapter 15).

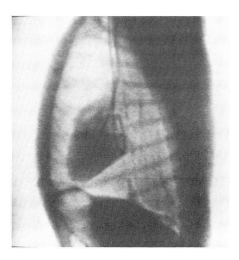

Fig. 2.1. Lateral projection of the thorax of a dead dog. [Reproduced from Robb *et al.* (1976), with permission.]

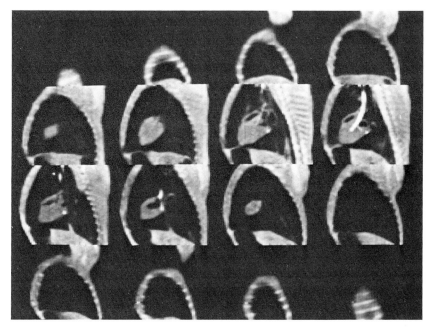

Fig. 2.2. Sixteen sagittal slices of the thorax of the dead dog shown in Fig. 2.1, obtained by computerized tomography. [Reproduced from Robb *et al.* (1976), with permission.]

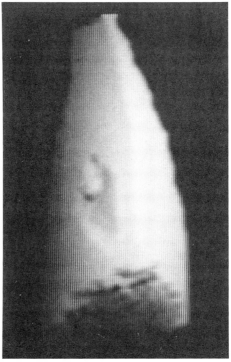

Fig. 2.3. Display of part of the left lung of the dead dog, obtained by computer processing of the reconstructed thorax. The imprints in the lung of the heart and of the major airway above it are clearly visible. [Reproduced from Herman and Liu (1977), with permission.]

2.2   TRADITIONAL TOMOGRAPHY

Prior to the introduction of CT, sectional imaging has been done using various modes of (not computerized) *tomography*. We now describe a mode of tomography (*linear tomography*), illustrated in Fig. 2.4.

If we are interested in a cross section C of a patient, we can obtain a fairly good estimate by the following tomographic method. We place a photographic plate P parallel to the cross section C on one side of the patient, and an x-ray source on the other side. By moving the x-ray source at a fixed speed parallel to C in one direction, and moving P at an appropriate speed in the opposite direction, we can ensure that a point in C always projects onto the same point in P, but a point in the patient above or below C is projected onto different points in P. Thus on the photographic plate the section C will stand out, while the rest of the body will be blurred out.

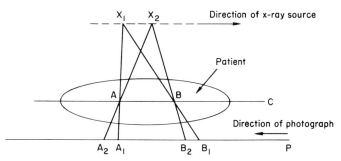

Fig. 2.4. Linear tomography. C, patient cross section; A and B, two points in the cross section C; X_1 and X_2, positions of the x-ray source at times t_1 and t_2; P, the photographic plate; A_1 and A_2, positions of a fixed point on P at times t_1 and t_2; B_1 and B_2, positions of another fixed point on P at times t_1 and t_2. [Reproduced from Gordon and Herman (1974), with permission.]

More closely related to CT is *transaxial tomography*. An example of this is shown in Fig. 2.5. The patient sits in a special rotating chair in an upright position. The x-ray film lies flat on a rotating horizontal table beside the patient. The table is positioned a little below the desired focal plane. X rays are directed obliquely through the patient and onto the film. The x-ray tube remains stationary throughout the exposure. The patient and film both

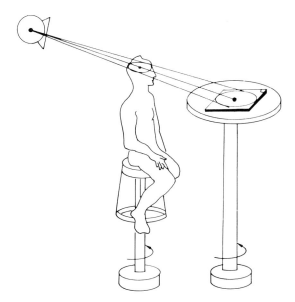

Fig. 2.5. Axial transverse tomography. [Illustration based on Christensen *et al.* (1973), with permission.]

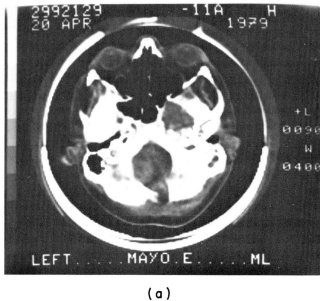

(a)

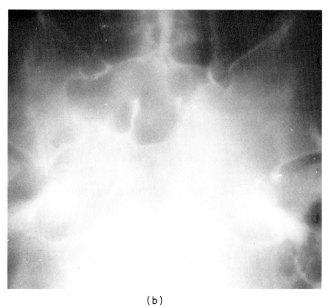

(b)

Fig. 2.6. Scans of a patient who has a large destructive metastatic carcinoma involving the middle fossa on the right, which can be seen on both the CT scan (a) and the conventional tomogram (b). (Illustration provided by Dr. D. F. Reese.)

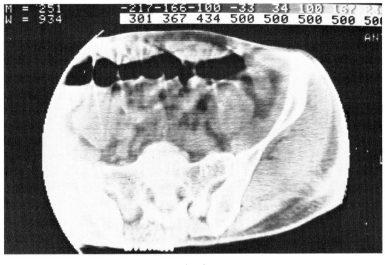

(a)

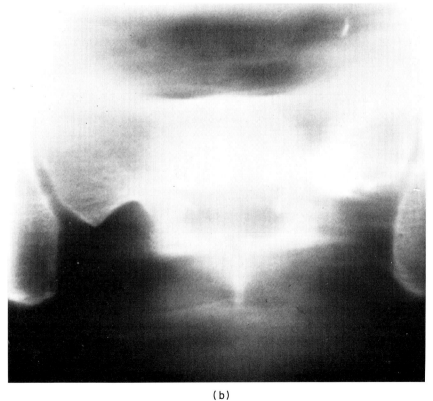

(b)

Fig. 2.7. Images made from CT (a) and transaxial tomography (b) of the first sacral segment on a 35-year-old patient. (Illustration provided by Dr. E. L. Effman.)

rotate in the same direction and at the same velocity. Only those points actually on the focal plane remain in sharp focus throughout a rotation. Points above and below the focal plane are blurred. The section thickness is determined by the angle between the x-ray tube and film. The more obliquely the central ray is directed toward the film the thinner the tomographic section.

In traditional forms of tomography, objects which are out of the focal plane are visible on the image, although in a blurred form. In CT, the images of cross sections are not influenced by the objects outside those sections. Comparison between CT and conventional tomography is provided in Fig. 2.6 (for the head) and in Fig. 2.7 (for the spine).

2.3   DATA COLLECTION FOR CT

A typical method by which data is collected for transverse section imaging in CT is indicated in Fig. 2.8. A large number of measurements are taken.

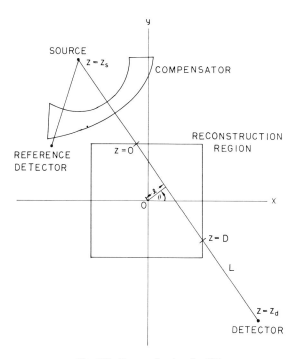

Fig. 2.8. Data collection for CT.

Each of these measurements is related to an x-ray source position combined with an x-ray detector position. Both the source and the detector lie in the plane of the section to be imaged. For each combination of source and detector positions, two physical measurements are taken: a *calibration measurement* and an *actual measurement*. We now explain what these measurements are for a single fixed source and detector position combination.

During the calibration measurement, the object whose cross section we hope to image is not in the path of the x-ray beam from the source to the detector. In fact, it is assumed that the part of the beam which intersects the so-called *reconstruction region* (see Fig. 2.8) traverses through a homogeneous *reference material* such as air or water. The calibration measurement tells us how many out of a large but fixed number of photons that leave the source are counted by the detector. A reference detector serves the purpose of compensating for fluctuations in the strength of the x-ray source. Compensation can be done by dividing the number of photons counted by the detector by the number of photons counted by the reference detector. During the actual measurement, the object of interest is inserted into the reconstruction region, (partially) replacing the reference material. It is an important restriction that the object of interest does *not* occupy any point outside the reconstruction region. On the other hand, we allow the possibility of additional objects occupying fixed positions outside the reconstruction region during both the calibration and the actual measurement. An example of this is the object marked compensator in Fig. 2.8. (It compensates for the thinness of a transverse section of human body near the edges. This makes the number of photons reaching the detector at different positions more uniform and so reduces the range of photon counts which a detector needs to handle.) The actual measurement is defined in the same way as the calibration measurement, except that the cross section to be imaged is now in position. It influences the photon count by the detector, but not the photon count by the reference detector.

In summary, the size of the actual measurement as compared to the size of the calibration measurement depends on the photon absorbing and scattering properties of the object to be reconstructed as compared to those properties of a reference material.

We obtain a calibration measurement and an actual measurement for each of many source and detector position combinations. From these two sets of numbers we wish to produce a third set, namely, the set of CT numbers for the cross section of the object under investigation. These numbers, when coded into gray scale images, give the type of pictures we see in Figs. 2.6 and 2.7. In the next section we discuss the physical interpretation of these numbers and images.

2.4   VOXELS, PIXELS, AND CT NUMBERS

In vacuum all x-ray photons which leave a source in the direction of a detector will reach the detector. When a material is placed between the source and the detector some of the photons which leave the source in the direction of the detector will be removed from the beam (absorbed or scattered). The probability that a photon gets removed depends on the energy of the photon and on the material between the source and the detector.

The *linear attenuation coefficient* $\mu_{\bar{e}}^t$ of a tissue t at energy $\bar{e}$ is defined as follows. Let ρ be the probability that a photon of energy $\bar{e}$, which enters a uniform slab of the tissue t of unit thickness, on a line L perpendicular to the face of the slab, will not be absorbed or scattered in the slab (i.e., ρ is the transmittance at energy $\bar{e}$ of the slab along the line L, see Section 1.2). We define

$$\mu_{\bar{e}}^t = -\ln \rho, \tag{4.1}$$

where ln denotes the natural logarithm. Note that the size of the linear attenuation coefficient is dependent on the unit of length used. As is justified in Section 16.1, the linear attenuation coefficient is measured in units of inverse length. For example, the linear attenuation of water at 73 keV is 0.19 cm^{-1}.

In what follows we shall be working with the *relative linear attenuation* at energy $\bar{e}$. At any point of space, we define the relative linear attenuation to be $\mu_{\bar{e}}^t - \mu_{\bar{e}}^a$, where t is the tissue occupying the point of space during the actual measurement and a is the tissue occupying the point during the calibration measurement. Since we assume that the exterior of the reconstruction region is the same during the two sets of measurements, the relative linear attenuation is zero for all points outside the reconstruction region for all energies. Note also that for all points inside the reconstruction region $\mu_{\bar{e}}^a$ is the same, since the reference material is supposed to be homogeneous during the calibration measurement.

Now suppose that we are interested in a cross-sectional slice of the human body which is, say 1.3 cm thick. We can subdivide this slice into small 1.3 cm long blocks with equal, square shaped cross sections. These blocks are usually referred to as volume elements, or *voxels*, for short. Roughly speaking, a *CT number* is proportional to the average relative linear attenuation in a voxel. Since the relative linear attenuation itself is energy dependent, this definition needs further clarification which is given in the next section. Typically, the background material is assumed to be water (thus the CT number of water is zero), and the scale of CT numbers is adjusted so that the CT number of air is -1000 or possibly -500.

Suppose, for example, that the reconstruction region in Fig. 2.8 is a square 41.6×41.6 cm, and we wish to use voxels which are $1.3 \times 0.13 \times$ 0.13 cm. Then there is a 320×320 array of such voxels which exactly fills the reconstruction region, providing us with a 320×320 array of CT numbers. In displaying the cross section, we display the CT numbers. Ideally, we want to display a 320×320 array of small squares, with the uniform grayness in each one being proportional to the CT number of the voxel in the appropriate position. These small squares are referred to as picture elements, or *pixels*, for short.

2.5   THE PROBLEM OF POLYCHROMATICITY

When an x-ray beam passes through the body, its attenuation at any point depends on the material at that point and on the energy distribution (*spectrum*) of the beam. In CT the spectrum is made up from many energy levels (*polychromatic*) and it changes (*hardens*) as the beam passes through the object. Thus, the attenuation at a point may vary with the direction of the beam passing through it. If we had a spectrum of only one energy level (*monochromatic*), this would not be the case. Each point would have a uniquely assigned attenuation coefficient, and reconstruction of the distribution of these coefficients would be a well-defined aim of computerized tomography.

We would like the following statement to be true: "The CT number assigned to a voxel is a property of the tissue occupying the voxel and does not depend on the location of the voxel in the slice." This is obviously desirable for diagnostic purposes. Also, as we shall see in the following, the truth of the statement is assumed in the development of mathematical procedures for calculating CT numbers.

A suitable definition for CT numbers is one in which a CT number is a multiple of the average relative linear attenuation of a voxel at a specified energy $\bar{e}$. Suppose now that we have a monochromatic x-ray source with photon energy $\bar{e}$. For a fixed position of the source and detector pair, let C_m be the calibration measurement (the count of the number of photons which get from the source to the detector without the object to be reconstructed being between them, divided by the count of the reference detector), and let A_m be the actual measurement (the count of the number of photons which get from the source to the detector with the object of interest in place, divided by the count of the reference detector). We define the *monochromatic ray sum*, m, for this beam by

$$m = -\ln(A_m/C_m), \tag{5.1}$$

and we refer to the set of m's for all source and detector pair positions as the *monochromatic projection data*. Based on the physical and mathematical facts to be discussed, we know that relative linear attenuation inside the slice at the given energy $\bar{e}$ can be accurately estimated from the monochromatic projection data.

In practice, the x-ray beam is polychromatic. Let C_p and A_p denote the calibration and actual measurement, respectively, for a particular source–detector pair position with the polychromatic x-ray beam. We define the *polychromatic ray sum*, p, for this x-ray beam by

$$p = -\ln(A_p/C_p), \tag{5.2}$$

and we refer to the set of p's for all source and detector pair positions as the *polychromatic projection data*.

Our problem is the following. For any source and detector position we can obtain p, but the reconstruction procedure requires m. The question naturally arises: Does p uniquely determine m? Unfortunately, except in unrealistically restrictive cases, the answer is "no."

A more pragmatic question is: Given p, can we approximate m well enough so that it leads to diagnostically useful CT numbers? There the answer appears to be "yes," as is illustrated in the following chapters.

2.6   RECONSTRUCTION ALGORITHMS

We now briefly discuss the major topic of this book: the method for obtaining CT numbers from the monochromatic projection data. In practice, we apply this method using corrected polychromatic projection data in place of the (usually unavailable) monochromatic projection data.

Since we wish to implement our method on a computer, we need precise instructions on how the CT numbers are to be obtained from the monochromatic projection data. A collection of unambiguous instructions which tell us how to get step by step from some given input to the desired output is an *algorithm*. Instructions which a physician writes up for his unskilled laboratory assistants on what tests to perform next on a sample, based on the outcome of previous tests, should (and usually do) form an algorithm. The instructions provided by the Internal Revenue Service on how to fill out a tax return should also form an algorithm; the fact that they do not gives rise to the honorable profession of tax accountancy.

Basically the same procedure would have to be described differently depending on at whom the description is aimed. A computing machine needs a very detailed description (a computer program) in order to perform the same calculations which a mathematician would perform if he were given a few brief formulas.

In order to design an algorithm for obtaining CT numbers from monochromatic projection data, we first replace the problem by a simplified mathematical idealization of it. This has the same standing as the classical assumption one makes in calculating the earth's orbit; namely, that all the mass of the earth is concentrated in a single point at its center. While the assumption is blatantly false, as long as it leads to correct calculations, there is every reason to use it: it makes the theory and the resulting calculations tractable. There is very little we could do in calculating the earth's orbit if we had to know the location of every fly before such a calculation could be carried out.

The simplifying assumptions we make in setting up the theory for reconstruction algorithms are: (1) slices are infinitely thin; (2) for any particular source and detector pair position, all x-ray photons travel in the same straight line (which lies in the infinitely thin slice). A consequence of the first assumption is that the distinction between voxels and pixels disappears. Indeed, since the slice is infinitely thin, it can be thought of as a picture whose grayness at any point (x, y) is proportional to the relative linear attenuation $\mu_{\bar{e}}(x, y)$ at that point. This is the reason why the theory behind reconstruction algorithms is often referred to as "image reconstruction from projections."

Let L be the straight line which is the path of all the x-ray photons for a particular source–detector pair and let m be the corresponding monochromatic ray sum. Based on our definition of a linear attenuation coefficient, it is proved in Section 16.2 that

$$m \simeq \int_0^D \mu_{\bar{e}}(x, y)\, dz. \tag{6.1}$$

In this formula, $\simeq$ denotes "approximately equal," and z is the distance of the point (x, y) on the line L (see Fig. 2.8).

Since $\mu_{\bar{e}}(x, y)$ is 0 for points (x, y) outside the reconstruction region, $\int_0^D \mu_{\bar{e}}(x, y)\, dz$ is the integral of $\mu_{\bar{e}}(x, y)$ along the line L. Thus our problem is to calculate the values of $\mu_{\bar{e}}(x, y)$ from estimates of its integrals along a number of lines, namely from the monochromatic projection data.

In some sense this problem has been solved in 1917 by Radon. Let ℓ denote the distance of the line L from the origin, let θ denote the angle made with the x axis by the perpendicular drawn from the origin to L (see Fig. 2.8), and let $m(\ell, \theta)$ denote the integral of $\mu_{\bar{e}}(x, y)$ along the line L. Radon has proved (see Section 16.3) that

$$\mu_{\bar{e}}(x, y) = -\frac{1}{2\pi^2} \lim_{\varepsilon \to 0} \int_\varepsilon^\infty \frac{1}{q} \int_0^{2\pi} m_1(x \cos\theta + y \sin\theta + q, \theta)\, d\theta\, dq, \tag{6.2}$$

where $m_1(\ell, \theta)$ denotes the partial derivative of $m(\ell, \theta)$ with respect to ℓ. While the exact details of this formula are likely to be obscure to the nonmathematician, its implication should be clear: the distribution of relative linear attenuations in an infinitely thin slice is uniquely determined by the set of *all* its line integrals.

This seems to indicate that the reconstruction problem has been solved since 1917. However, there are some practical difficulties in applying to CT this mathematical solution to the idealized problem:

(a) Radon's formula determines a picture from all its line integrals. In CT we have only a finite set of measurements. Even if these were *exactly* the projections along a number of straight lines, a finite number of them would not be enough to determine the picture uniquely, or even accurately. Based on the finiteness of the data alone one can easily produce objects for which the reconstructions will be very inaccurate (see Section 16.4).

(b) The measurements in computed tomography can only be used to estimate the line integrals. Inaccuracies in these estimates are due to the width of the x-ray beam, scatter, hardening of the beam, photon statistics, detector inaccuracies, etc. Radon's inversion formula is sensitive to these inaccuracies.

(c) Radon gave a mathematical formula; we need an *efficient* algorithm to evaluate it. This is not necessarily trivial to obtain.

There has been a very great deal of activity in recent years to find algorithms which are fast when implemented on a computer and which produce acceptable reconstructions in spite of the finite and inaccurate nature of the data. Much of this book is devoted to this topic.

NOTES AND REFERENCES

The mathematical and computational procedures underlying CT as described in this chapter are summarized in Fig. 2.9. Most of this material is based on Herman (1978) and Herman (1979a).

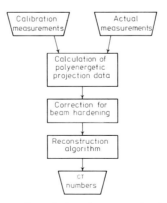

Fig. 2.9. Outline of the mathematical and computational procedures underlying CT. [Reproduced from Herman (1979a), with permission. Copyright by the Institute of Physics.]

The discussion of traditional tomography is based on Gordon and Herman (1974). A recent article is by Strohbehn *et al.* (1979). These papers contain further references.

For a more detailed discussion on the nature of algorithms see, e.g., the relevant entries in Ralston and Meek (1976).

The Radon transform was introduced by Radon (1917), who has derived the inversion formula on which (6.2) is based.

3

Physical Problems Associated
with Data Collection in CT

The main topic of this book is a discussion of the algorithms by which the distribution of the relative linear attenuation at a fixed energy $\bar{e}$, namely $\mu_{\bar{e}}(x, y)$, is calculated from estimates of its line integrals along a finite number of lines. The measurements in CT are taken in order to estimate these line integrals. In this chapter we discuss the physical limitations and problems that arise in estimating the line integrals from the calibration and actual measurements. Except for the problems of photon statistics and beam hardening, our discussion will be limited to a summary of the problems with some indications on how their effects may be reduced. We also discuss the different scanner configurations that are used in computerized tomography. In Chapter 5 we illustrate the effects on the quality of the reconstruction of the different sources of error in the data collection.

3.1 PHOTON STATISTICS

A very basic limitation to the accuracy of measurements taken in CT is the statistical nature of the process of x-ray photon production, photon interaction with matter; and photon detection. We discuss these processes one by one.

Consider the experiment in which we count all the photons emitted in a unit period of time by a stable x-ray source in the direction of a detector. Such an experiment gives rise to a discrete random variable, which we denote by Y (see Section 1.2). The possible outcomes of the experiment are non-negative integers (the photon counts). In this book we accept without further discussion the physical result that there exists a fixed real number λ such that

$$P_Y(y) = \exp(-\lambda)\lambda^y/y!. \tag{1.1}$$

[Notation: The symbol exp denotes the exponential function; thus $\exp(\ln(x))$ $= \ln(\exp(x)) = x$.] In Fig. 3.1 we show the values of $P_Y(y)$ for $y = 0, \ldots, 50$ when (a) $\lambda = 5$ and (b) $\lambda = 25$.

Equation (1.1) is referred to as the *Poisson probability law*, and a random variable Y satisfying it is called the *Poisson random variable* with parameter λ. We note three important properties of such a random variable:

(a) its mean is λ,
(b) its standard deviation is $\sqrt{\lambda}$,
(c) it behaves normally provided λ is large (greater than 100).

This has important practical implications. Suppose, for example, that we are interested in estimating λ, the average number of photons emitted per unit time by a stable x-ray source in the direction of a detector. If we have a way of counting all the photons reaching the detector, we may estimate λ by the count of the number of photons during a particular period of unit time (i.e., by a sample of the random variable). If the true value of λ is 10,000, then there is at most a 1 in 20 chance that we make an error 200 (two standard deviations) or more using this approach. Alternatively, we may count the number of photons for 100 units of time, and divide the count by 100 to give us an estimate of λ. The total number of photons during this longer period is on average 1,000,000, and in 19 cases out of 20, the actual count will be between 998,000 and 1,002,000. So in 19 cases out of 20, the estimate of λ will be between 9,980 and 10,020; i.e., the error is 20 or less. By increasing the time period used for counting photons by a factor of 100 we have reduced the size of the likely error in our estimate by a factor of 10. We observe a similar phenomenon in the following when we discuss how the accuracy of the calibration and actual measurements in CT is dependent on the total number of x-ray photons used.

Now we look at the statistical nature of the interactions of x-ray photons with matter. Suppose that a photon leaves the source in direction of the detector along a line L (see Fig. 2.8). Then there is a fixed probability ρ that the photon will get as far as the detector without being absorbed or scattered. This probability depends on the energy of the photon and the material intersected by the line L between the source and the detector. We call ρ the *transmittance* along L of the material between the source and the detector at that particular energy. If everything between the source and the detector remains stationary for a period of time and during this time 10,000 photons of the same energy leave the source in direction of the detector along the line

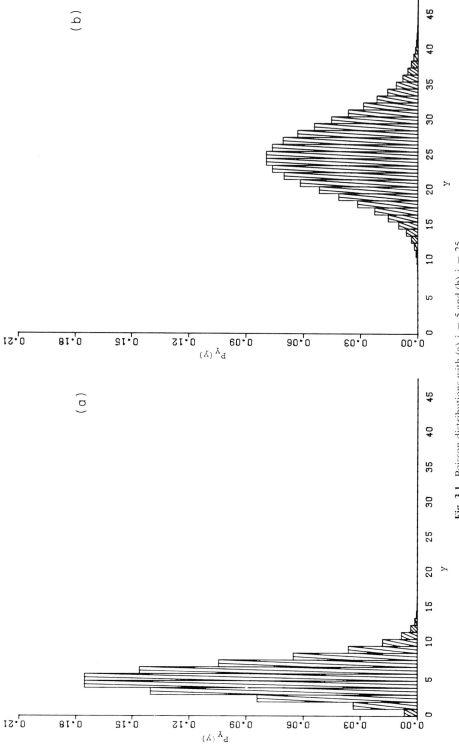

Fig. 3.1. Poisson distributions with (a) $\lambda = 5$ and (b) $\lambda = 25$.

L, then the number of photons reaching the detector will be approximately, but almost never exactly, $10{,}000\rho$. The rest of the photons will be absorbed or scattered.

A photon which reaches the detector is not necessarily counted. For each energy, there is a fixed probability σ that a photon which reaches the detector is counted by the detector. We call σ the *efficiency* of the detector at that particular energy. Continuing with the case discussed in the previous paragraph, the number of photons out of the original 10,000 which will not be absorbed or scattered and will be counted is approximately, but almost never exactly, $10{,}000\rho\sigma$.

The following important statement is proved in Section 16.5.

Let λ denote the average of the number of photons at energy $\bar{e}$ which are emitted in one unit of time by a stable x-ray source along a line L in the direction of a detector. Let ρ denote the transmittance along L of the material between the source and detector at energy $\bar{e}$. Let σ denote the efficiency of the detector at energy $\bar{e}$. Then the number of photons which

(a) are at energy $\bar{e}$,
(b) reach the detector without having been absorbed or scattered,
(c) are counted by the detector in one unit of time,

is a sample of a Poisson random variable with parameter $\lambda\rho\sigma$.

We are now in position to discuss what is being measured during the data collection phase of CT, as described in Section 2.3. For the purpose of this discussion we assume that the x-ray beam is monochromatic, the x-ray source and detectors are negligible in size (hence all photons from the source to the detector travel in the same straight line), and that a photon which has been absorbed or scattered along this line never reaches the detector. In subsequent sections we talk about the errors introduced by the physical unattainability of these assumptions.

Suppose that a monochromatic x-ray source of energy $\bar{e}$ is such that the fraction of emitted photons which leave in the direction of the reference detector is ϕ_r and the fraction of emitted photons which leave in the direction of the actual detector is ϕ_d (see Fig. 2.8). Suppose that the averages of the total number of photons emitted during the periods of the calibration and actual measurements are λ_c and λ_a, respectively. Let ρ_r be the transmittance at energy $\bar{e}$ of the material between the source and the reference detector, and let ρ_c and ρ_a be the transmittances at energy $\bar{e}$ of the material between the source and the detector (see Fig. 2.8) during the calibration and the actual measurement, respectively. Let σ_r, respectively σ_d, be the efficiency at energy $\bar{e}$ of the reference detector, respectively, of the detector. By the discussion just given we may conclude that the numbers of photons counted by the reference detector and the detector during the calibration measurement are samples of Poisson random variables with means $\phi_r \lambda_c \rho_r \sigma_r$ and $\phi_d \lambda_c \rho_c \sigma_d$, respectively. Hence

$$C_m \simeq \phi_d \lambda_c \rho_c \sigma_d / \phi_r \lambda_c \rho_r \sigma_r. \tag{1.2}$$

Also, the numbers of photons counted by the reference detector and the detector during the actual measurement are samples of Poisson random variables with means $\phi_r \lambda_a \rho_r \sigma_r$ and $\phi_d \lambda_a \rho_a \sigma_d$, respectively. Hence

$$A_m \simeq \phi_d \lambda_a \rho_a \sigma_d / \phi_r \lambda_a \rho_r \sigma_r. \tag{1.3}$$

Combining (1.2) and (1.3) with (5.1) of Chapter 2, we get that

$$m \simeq -\ln(\rho_a/\rho_c). \tag{1.4}$$

In Section 16.2 we show that

$$-\ln \frac{\rho_a}{\rho_c} = \int_0^D \mu_{\bar{e}}(x, y) \, dz. \tag{1.5}$$

This is why the monochromatic ray sum m can be used as an estimator to $\int_0^D \mu_{\bar{e}}(x, y) \, dz$ in an algorithm which calculates $\mu_{\bar{e}}(x, y)$ at individual points from the line integrals of $\mu_{\bar{e}}(x, y)$ (see Section 2.6).

The important question is: How accurate an estimator is m of $-\ln(\rho_a/\rho_c)$? It is shown in Section 16.5 that under the assumptions discussed previously m is a sample of a random variable M such that

$$|\mu_M + \ln(\rho_a/\rho_c)| < S, \tag{1.6}$$

and

$$V_M \simeq S, \tag{1.7}$$

where

$$S = (\phi_d \lambda_c \rho_c \sigma_d)^{-1} + (\phi_r \lambda_c \rho_r \sigma_r)^{-1} + (\phi_d \lambda_a \rho_a \sigma_d)^{-1} + (\phi_r \lambda_a \rho_r \sigma_r)^{-1}. \tag{1.8}$$

If we can make this quantity S very small we ensure accurate estimation of $-\ln(\rho_a/\rho_c)$ by m.

Note that one way of making S very small is to make the number of photons leaving the source (λ_c and λ_a) large. Except for the problem of possibly saturating the counting capability of the detectors there is no difficulty in making λ_c very large, and thereby making the first two terms in S negligibly small. In such a case we see that S becomes inversely proportional to λ_a. Unfortunately, one cannot make the number of photons leaving the source during the actual measurement arbitrarily large, since this would result in an unacceptable radiation dose to the patient and may slow the process of projection taking so that errors due to motion become important (see the following). Note, however, that by ensuring that the transmittance ρ_r between the source and the reference detector is relatively large (near 1), we can possibly make the last term in equation (1.8) also negligibly small. This leaves us with

$$S \simeq 1/\phi_d \lambda_a \rho_a \sigma_d, \tag{1.9}$$

which shows in particular that the error in our estimation of $-\ln(\rho_a/\rho_c)$ depends on the transmittance ρ_a during the actual measurement; lesser transmittance results in greater error.

As can be seen from the preceding, a certain amount of error in the measurements due to the statistical nature of the processes of x-ray photon production, photon interaction with matter, and photon detection is unavoidable. The properties of the error, considered as a random variable, are clearly understood. As we shall see, some reconstruction algorithms attempt to make use of these properties. Since the errors in the measurements affect the outcome of the reconstruction process, it is important to understand both the nature of these errors and the way in which the results produced by a given reconstruction algorithm are influenced by such errors.

3.2 BEAM HARDENING

The x-ray beam used in CT consists of photons at different energies. (Such x rays are called polychromatic.) Because the attenuation at a fixed point is generally greater for photons of lower energy, the energy distribution spectrum of the x-ray beam changes (hardens) as it passes through the object. X-ray beams reaching a particular point inside the body from different directions are likely to have different spectra (having passed through different materials before reaching the point in question) and thus will be attenuated differently at that point. This makes it difficult to assign a single value for the attenuation coefficient at a point in the body.

A possible solution to this difficulty is to assign to the point the attenuation coefficient of photons at a particular energy. If we used x-ray beams consisting of photons only at that single energy (such x rays are called monochromatic), beams from different directions would be attenuated in the same way at a fixed point. Reconstruction of such attenuation coefficients is a well-defined aim of computed tomography.

In this section we discuss mathematical formulas which describe the nature of polychromatic ray sums and methods which may be used to find the corresponding monochromatic ray sums.

In particular, it is shown in Section 16.6 that the polychromatic ray sum p approximates an integral of the form

$$p \simeq -\ln \int_0^E \tau_e \exp\left[- \int_0^D (\mu_e(z) - \mu_e^a)\, dz \right] de. \tag{2.1}$$

We now give a detailed explanation of the meaning of the symbols in (2.1).

It is assumed that the source emits a polychromatic x-ray beam with photons at energies between 0 and E. We use τ_e to denote the probability that a photon counted during the calibration measurement is at energy e. Here we have adopted the somewhat nonstandard notation of using τ_e to denote the value of a function of energy at the energy e. We refer to this function as the *detected spectrum during the calibration measurement*.

The symbols D and z have the same meaning as in the last chapter (see Fig. 2.8). $\mu_e(z)$ is a function of two variables (the energy e and the distance z), whose value is the linear attenuation coefficient at energy e at the point z on the line L during the actual measurement. On the other hand, μ_e^a is a function of one variable only (the energy e), whose value is the linear attenuation of the reference material a at energy e. Thus, $\int_0^D (\mu_e(z) - \mu_e^a)\, dz$ is the integral of the relative linear attenuation at energy e along the line L.

Note, in particular, that the polychromatic ray sum depends only on the relative linear attenuations (at all energies between 0 and E) and on the detected spectrum during the calibration measurement.

Rewriting (6.1) of Chapter 2 in the same notation we get

$$m \simeq \int_0^D (\mu_{\bar e}(z) - \mu_{\bar e}^a)\, dz. \tag{2.2}$$

Recall now that CT numbers are multiples of relative linear attenuations at a fixed energy $\bar e$; and that they are to be obtained from estimates of the monochromatic projection data which are themselves calculated from the experimentally obtained polychromatic projection data. The method of estimating the monochromatic projection data from the polychromatic projection data is the topic of the rest of this section.

We start with a theoretical discussion of a special situation.

Suppose that during the actual measurement there are only two types of material, a and b, in the reconstruction region (a is the reference material). Consider a fixed source–detector pair, and assume that the total length of the line L which goes through material b is B. From (2.1) and (2.2) we get

$$p \simeq -\ln \int_0^E \tau_e \exp[-B(\mu_e^b - \mu_e^a)]\, de \tag{2.3}$$

and

$$m \simeq B(\mu_{\bar e}^b - \mu_{\bar e}^a). \tag{2.4}$$

Combining (2.3) and (2.4) we get

$$p \simeq -\ln \int_0^E \tau_e \exp\left[-\frac{\mu_e^b - \mu_e^a}{\mu_{\bar e}^b - \mu_{\bar e}^a}\, m\right] de. \tag{2.5}$$

The important thing to observe in (2.5) is that, provided either $\mu_e^b > \mu_e^a$ for all energies between 0 and E or $\mu_e^b < \mu_e^a$ for all energies between 0 and E, its right-hand side is a monotonically increasing function of m. (Note that τ_e is positive for all e.) Hence, given any value of p, there will be only one value of m which will make the two sides of (2.5) equal. In practice we can use the plot of the right-hand side of (2.5) to correct for beam hardening; we simply find the value of m for which the value of the right-hand side is the experimentally obtained polychromatic ray sum p.

Equation (2.5) was obtained under a rather restrictive assumption: there are only two different types of material in the reconstruction region. If the organ we are looking at is a head inserted into a water bag, this assumption is not too badly violated, since the contents of the head are bone and material whose x-ray attenuation properties are not too dissimilar to water. Thus (2.5) may be used for correcting for beam hardening in such a situation, but in general it is not as good as some other methods to be discussed in the following.

While the precise method based on (2.5) must be considered to be unreliable because of the too restrictive nature of the underlying assumptions, the general approach suggested by it is very attractive: specify a function $f(p)$ of the polychromatic ray sum p such that if we use $f(p)$ as our estimate of the monochromatic ray sum m, then we get reasonably good reconstructions of the relative linear attenuations at the fixed energy $\bar{e}$.

Natural candidates for such a function are polynomials, i.e., functions of the form

$$f(p) = a_n p^n + a_{n-1} p^{n-1} + \cdots + a_2 p^2 + a_1 p + a_0, \qquad (2.6)$$

where n (the order of the polynomial) is a fixed integer and $a_0, a_1, a_2, \ldots,$ a_{n-1}, a_n are fixed coefficients which need to be determined so that $f(p)$ provides an acceptable estimate of m for our purpose. There are two computational advantages of polynomial approximations to others (e.g., approximation by combination of exponentials): the coefficients are easy to calculate and, once they are calculated, (2.6) is easy to evaluate, especially since a low value of n (less than 5) usually suffices (see Section 5.4).

In certain cases there is no single function f such that replacement of m by $f(p)$ in (6.2) of Chapter 2 would lead to acceptable reconstructions. One is then forced to use either multiple correcting functions specific to the source–detector pair positions or an iterative correction procedure, where the correcting function f for the next iteration is based on a reconstruction during the previous iteration (see Section 5.4).

3.3 OTHER SOURCES OF ERROR

If we wish to base our reconstruction algorithm on (6.2) of Chapter 2, then we have to know the values of $m(l, \theta)$ [the line integral of $\mu_{\bar{e}}(x, y)$ along L, see Figure 2.8] for certain l and θ (i.e., for certain lines L). Photon statistics and beam hardening are two reasons why physical measurements can provide us only with approximations of $m(l, \theta)$. In this section we briefly discuss further reasons.

One source of error is that both the x-ray source (more precisely the focal spot of the x-ray source) and the detector have a certain size, and thus the photons which are counted do not all travel along the same line, but rather they travel along one of a bundle of lines forming a rather complicated shape.

One consequence of the nonnegligible size of the focal spot and detector is the so-called *partial volume effect*, which we now explain on a simple two-dimensional example. Suppose we have a point monochromatic x-ray source P and a line segment detector D; see Fig. 3.2. Suppose that the linear

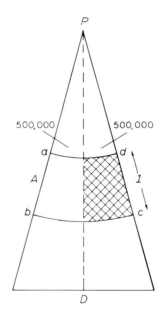

Fig. 3.2. Illustration of the partial volume effect.

attenuation coefficient (see Section 2.4) is everywhere zero except in that half of the area A which is cross-hatched in Fig. 3.2, where its value is two. It is assumed that length of intersection with A of any line from P to D is unity. Suppose also that the reference material has linear attenuation coefficient zero (vacuum) and that the number of photons read by the reference detector during both calibration and actual measurement is 1000. Hence the number of photons which leave the source in direction of the detector is about the same during calibration and actual measurement. Suppose this number is 1,000,000. Thus the calibration measurement is $C_m \simeq 1000$. Breaking the x-ray beam into two equal halves as shown in Fig. 3.2 we see that approximately 500,000 photons will enter both halves of A. In the left half, where the linear attenuation coefficient is zero and hence transmittance is one, all 500,000 photons reach the detector. In the right half, where the linear attenuation is two, and hence transmittance is $e^{-2} \simeq 0.135$, the number of photons which reach the detector is about 68,000. Hence the total number of detected photons is about 568,000 and the actual measurement is $A_m \simeq 568$. Using (5.1) of Chapter 2 we get $m \simeq 0.566$. This is an estimate [see (6.1) in Chapter 2] of the average of the line integral of the relative linear attenuation between the source and points on the detector. However, it is easy to see that the true value of this average is 1.0. The reason for this rather large error (43.4%) in the estimation of the average is that the beam is only partially blocked by attenuating material and the processes of taking exponentials and logarithms give unproportionately great importance to the unblocked portion of the beam.

In principle, one can reduce the size of the source and the detector by putting lead shielding with long narrow pinholes in front of both of them, but this would have two undesirable consequences. One is that the error due to photon statistics would considerably increase, because the value of ϕ_d in (1.9) would become very small. The second consequence arises when we search for possibly small features in large organs (such as tumors in the lung) by taking cross-sectional slices. If the physical slices are thin, we have to use many slices to ensure that we do not miss what we are looking for. This results in longer time to be spent by the computer which provides the reconstructions and possibly by the radiologist who needs to examine them.

We have just given one example of a phenomenon which is rather common in CT. Methods which can be used to combat error due to one physical phenomenon result in increasing the error due to another one. A further example of this is the way one handles *motion artifacts*.

It is an underlying assumption in CT that the $m(l, \theta)$, which we try to measure, are integrals along different lines of the same function $\mu_{\bar{e}}(x, y)$. However, this assumption is violated if the different lines L go through a moving organ, such as the lung or the heart, and if the actual measurements are taken at different times for different L, since the function $\mu_{\bar{e}}(x, y)$ changes as the organ moves. One way of combating this is to use multiple arrays of detectors and possibly even multiple sources (more about this in the next section), so that all the measurements can be taken within a small period of time during which organ motion is insignificant. However, this results in increase of error due to detection of *scattered* photons, a phenomenon which we now discuss.

Note that in Section 3.1, we have assumed that the detector counts a photon only if it has left the source in the direction of the detector and has reached the detector without having been absorbed or scattered. If there is a single source and a single detector, this is a reasonable assumption, since a scattered photon can reach the detector only if it has been scattered in a direction very nearly the same as its original direction or if it has been multiply scattered away from and then back towards the detector. These events are sufficiently unlikely, so that the error due to scatter in a single source single detector case is rather small. However, if we have an array of detectors, a photon scattered out of its path towards one detector may very well reach another detector and be counted by it. Since the ratio of scattered photons to unscattered photons which reach a detector is dependent on the object to be reconstructed (and in a rather complicated way), the error introduced by scatter can not be completely removed from the measurements prior to reconstruction. Collimation, which absorbs photons coming towards a detector from directions other than the source, can reduce the number of scattered photons which are counted by the detector.

Finally, we discuss some errors which are due to the machine used for collecting the data not functioning exactly as intended.

It is important that the source and the detectors do not change their behavior between the calibration measurement and the actual measurement. For example, in our derivation in Section 3.1 we have assumed that the efficiency σ_d of the detector is the same during the calibration and the actual measurement. Change in detector efficiency would make (1.4) invalid.

Detector efficiency is assumed to be independent of the number of photons the detector has to count. This may be difficult to achieve in practice, since detectors can be saturated by too many photons getting to them. One way of combating this is by insertion of a compensator (see Fig. 2.8) which ensures that even along lines which either miss or hardly touch the object to be reconstructed, the total attenuation is significant enough for the detector not to get saturated. Alternatively, one can achieve this by using water as the reference material into which one inserts the object to be reconstructed during the actual measurement. One reason for preferring the former of these two methods is that it requires less radiation dose to achieve the same photon statistics. This is due to the absorption of photons by the water between the patient's body and the detector.

Mechanical stability is also of importance; the lines along which data are collected should be the same lines which the algorithms assumes as the lines of data collection.

There are other possible sources of errors in data collection, but their discussion is beyond the scope of this book.

3.4   SCANNING MODES

Figure 3.3 shows five basic designs that are being used by devices used for data collection in CT. While various variants of these scanning modes exist, we restrict our attention to these five basic modes. We discuss some of the advantages and disadvantages of each from the point of view of their proneness to the errors we have discussed in the previous section.

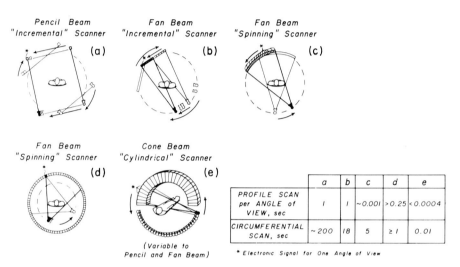

		a	b	c	d	e
		PROFILE SCAN per ANGLE of VIEW, sec	I	I	~0.001	>0.25	<0.0004
		CIRCUMFERENTIAL SCAN, sec	~200	18	5	≥ I	0.01

(Variable to Pencil and Fan Beam)

* Electronic Signal for One Angle of View

Fig. 3.3. Scanning modes in CT. (a) Single source, single detector, translate–rotate. (b) Single source, multiple detector, translate–rotate. (c) Single source, multiple detector, rotate only; see also Fig. 1.10. (d) Single rotating source, stationary detector ring. (e) Multiple source, multiple-planar detector. [Illustration provided by Drs. E. L. Ritman and E. H. Wood, reproduced from Wood (1977), with permission.]

In the first scanning mode (Fig. 3.3a) there is a single x-ray source and a single detector. There are two motions involved. First, both the detector and the source are moved in parallel in a direction perpendicular to the line connecting the source to the detector. During this time projection data are collected for one set of parallel rays. Second, the apparatus is rotated by a small amount (typically 1°). By repetition of these two motions, data are collected for a large number (typically 180) of sets of parallel rays.

There are a number of attractive features of this method of data collection. There is very little noise due to scatter. The detector can be calibrated at the beginning of each of the parallel scans, since we can ensure that the first ray of a scan misses the reconstruction region. The source detector combination can be moved in small steps, ensuring that enough data are collected for re-construction. (There will be more about this in later chapters.) An un-desirable feature of this method of data collection is the time it takes; typically several minutes. Such a scanning mode is inappropriate for imaging organs which cannot stay stationary for more than a few seconds, such as the lung.

The second scanning mode (Fig. 3.3b) has been introduced to speed up the data collection process without losing most of the desirable features of the first scanning mode. Instead of one detector, an array of detectors is used (typically 30). As the source and detector array move in parallel, data are collected for several sets of parallel rays. When the apparatus is rotated, the rotation can be by a much larger angle than in the first scanning mode (typically 10°), and yet the total number of sets of parallel rays is usually increased. Such scanners have been built which collect all their data in slightly over 10 sec, an acceptable breath holding period for most patients. Apart from increase in cost, the only obvious disadvantage of this scanning mode over the first one is the increased effect of scatter.

The third scanning mode (Fig. 3.3c) involves only one motion. A single x-ray source is faced by a large enough array of detectors so that the angle subtended by the detector array at the source encloses the whole reconstruc-tion region. The source/detector-array combination rotates around the patient. The data are collected for a large number of sets of rays (typically 500 sets with about the same number of rays in each); in each set the rays diverge from the source position to the detectors in the array. All data for one set are collected simultaneously. The complete data collection can be achieved in a matter of few seconds (typically five or less). One potential problem with this arrangement is that calibration has to be done before the patient is inserted for possibly a whole series of scans, since in all positions of the apparatus the line between the source and the central detectors goes through the patient. Very stable detectors seem to have overcome this difficulty. Also, the detectors have to be narrow so that sufficient amount of data are collected for the reconstruction.

An alternative fast method of data collection, with only one motion, is the fourth scanning mode (Fig. 3.3d). A stationary array of detectors has the x-ray source move inside it in a circle. The line from one of the detectors to the source forms a diverging set of rays as the source moves. Calibration of the detector for this set of rays is possible while the line from the detector to the source is outside the reconstruction region. The number of detectors has to be large compared to the previous scanning mode, unless one is willing to have radiation which goes through the body but ends up between detectors. The latter is undesirable, since the body is subjected to potentially harmful radiation which does not contribute any diagnostic information. Also, it is more difficult to reduce scatter by collimation than in the previous scanning mode since the direction from detector to source changes as the source moves.

None of these scanning modes is appropriate for precise imaging of a rapidly moving organ such as the heart. Not only is the speed of data collection far too slow (the heart goes through a whole cycle in about one second), but also it is difficult to achieve a slice-to-slice coherence if the data are collected at different times for each cross-sectional slice. The fifth scanning mode (Fig. 3.3e) has been designed to overcome these difficulties. An array of x-ray sources (typically 28) is arranged in a semicircle. They can be electronically switched on and off. They project the body onto a curved fluorescent screen, so that when an x-ray source is switched on a large part of the body (say the whole thorax) is imaged simultaneously, providing us with projection data for a cone beam of rays diverging from the source. It is possible to complete the data collection in as little as one-hundredth of a second, removing any possibility of organ motion interfering with the reconstruction process. Note that this method of data collection is essentially different from the other four, inasmuch as a series of two-dimensional projections of a three-dimensional object is collected rather than a series of one-dimensional projections of a two-dimensional object. While this arrangement solves the problems which motivated its introduction, it has its own special difficulties. For example, the number of projections that can be taken is severely limited both by the cost and the size of the x-ray tubes, and the error due to scatter is unavoidably much more significant than in the previous scanning modes.

There are many existing and possible variants of these scanning modes, and many more advantages and disadvantages to each than we have space to mention. However, the configurations discussed here include all the basic arrangements that we need to consider when discussing reconstruction algorithms.

Notes and References

Justification for using the Poisson probability law to describe photon generation can be found in standard books, such as Evans (1955). More detailed discussion of the nature of Poisson random variables is also a standard topic; see, e.g., Parzen (1960).

The material on beam hardening is based on Herman (1979a), which gives many other references. An example of an iterative beam hardening correction procedure is given by Joseph and Spital (1978). We return to this topic in Section 5.4. An alternative to correcting for beam hardening is to attempt to make use of the nature of the x-ray spectrum. An example of such an approach is given by Macovski *et al.* (1976).

The shape of the x-ray beam in CT, and what one might do about the errors introduced by it, is discussed by Bracewell (1977). A discussion of the partial volume effect has been given by Glover and Pelc (1979). The nature of scatter and correction for it is dealt with by Stonestrom and Macovski (1976). Errors in reconstruction due to various forms of machine malfunctioning are discussed by Shepp and Stein (1977).

The first commercially available CT scanner was manufactured by EMI Ltd; see Hounsfield (1973). This machine was of the type shown in Fig. 3.3a. A machine of the type shown in Fig. 3.3c has been reported on by Edelheit *et al.* (1977). A machine of the type shown in Fig. 3.3e is the *dynamic spatial reconstructor* reported on by Ritman *et al.* (1978). A table of the physical characteristics of the early commercial scanners is given by Brooks and DiChiro (1976).

4

Computer Simulation
of Data Collection in CT

While the aim of CT is the reconstruction of real objects from their actual x-ray projections, the theoretical development of CT owes a lot to reconstruction of mathematically described objects (*phantoms*) from computer simulated projection data. The basic reason for this is that computer simulation enables us to investigate individually various phenomena which can not be separated physically. For example, x-ray data always contain noise due to both photon statistics and scatter, but simulation can indicate the specific separate effects of noise and scatter.

As can be seen from the previous chapter, a program capable of realistic simulation of data collection using different scanning modes has to be fairly complex. Nevertheless, a number of such programs have been written in recent years. In producing many of the figures for this book we have made repeated use of one of them. This program is part of a programming system called SNARK 77. (The name originates from the Lewis Carroll nonsense poem entitled "The Hunting of the Snark.") SNARK 77 provides a uniform framework in which to implement reconstruction algorithms and evaluate their performance. All reconstruction algorithms discussed in this book, as well as a number of others are incorporated in it. In this chapter we discuss the way SNARK 77 creates test data for use by reconstruction algorithms.

4.1   PICTURES AND DIGITIZATION

It is useful at this stage to make precise a number of concepts we need in the rest of this chapter and elsewhere in the book.

When we talk about a *picture*, we assume that it has two components:

(i) the *picture region* which is a square whose center is at the origin of the coordinate system;

(ii) a *picture function* of two variables whose value is zero outside the picture region.

Sometimes, when this leads to no confusion, we call the function in (ii) the "picture." However, identical functions may give rise to different pictures if the picture regions are different.

We shall often refer to the value of the picture at the point (x, y) as the *density* at (x, y).

An *n*-element *grid* subdivides the picture region into n^2 equal squares. Each of these smaller squares is called a *pixel* (short for picture element).

An $n \times n$ *digitized picture* is one whose value in the interior of any pixel of an *n*-element grid is uniform.

The $n \times n$ *digitization* of a picture is an $n \times n$ digitized picture such that the integral of the original picture over any pixel of an *n*-element grid is equal to the integral of the digitization over the same pixel. (See Fig. 1.1.)

In CT the picture region is the reconstruction region and the density of the picture at the point (x, y) is the relative linear attenuation at some fixed energy of the tissue at the point (x, y).

4.2   CREATION OF A PHANTOM

We now describe how a test phantom is created in SNARK 77. A test phantom is nothing but a picture on which we wish to test reconstruction algorithms or data collection methods.

The phantom is put together by superimposing a number of *elemental objects*, placed at desired positions, at desired orientations and of desired size and density. The density of the elemental objects may be negative. The density of the picture at any point is then defined as the sum of the densities associated with all the elemental objects within which the point lies.

To obtain an estimate of the density within a pixel, the user specifies a number K, which has the effect that the density within a pixel is determined by averaging the value of the density at $K \times K$ uniformly spaced points within the pixel. Thus, the density assigned to a pixel can be expressed by the sum

$$\frac{1}{K^2} \sum_{k=1}^{K^2} \sum_{j=1}^{J} \delta_{k,j} \, d_j, \tag{2.1}$$

where J is the number of elemental objects in the phantom, d_j is the density of the jth elemental object, $\delta_{k,j} = 1$ if the kth of the $K \times K$ points in the pixel

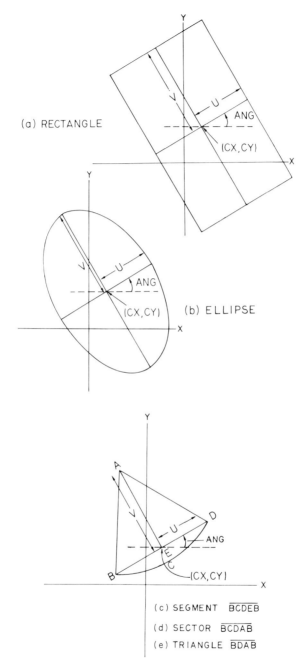

Fig. 4.1. Elemental objects. In SNARK 77, an elemental object consists of both the boundary and the interior of the rectangle, ellipse, triangle, or segment or sector of a circle, respectively.

is in the jth elemental object, and $\delta_{k,j} = 0$ otherwise. Note that the digitized picture produced by this method is only an approximation to the digitization of the phantom.

An elemental object in SNARK77 may be an ellipse, a rectangle, an isosceles triangle, or a segment or a sector of a circle. The location of an elemental object is described by five variables CX, CY, U, V, and ANG. For each type of elemental object the explanation of these variables is given by Fig. 4.1. The boundary of an elemental object is considered to be part of the object.

Note that in practice there is often an "effective energy" of polychromatic radiation (see Section 16.6). In such cases it is desirable to compare reconstructions from polychromatic projection data with a monoenergetic phantom at the effective energy.

4.3   A HEAD PHANTOM

The most important application to date of image reconstruction from projections has been in the area of diagnostic radiology. The region of the body for which such procedures have been most widely and successfully used is the head. For this reason, all ideas and methods introduced in this book are demonstrated on a typical cross section of the human head, containing tumors, a blood clot, ventricles and, of course, the skull enclosing the brain.

The purpose of this book is to introduce methods of image reconstruction from projections and to illustrate how they perform under different circumstances. Since we want to be able to precisely control the circumstances and to compare the results of the reconstruction with a known original, rather than using an actual cross section of a human head, we use a mathematically defined head phantom. In the rest of this section we describe precisely how we have arrived at the head phantom which will be used repeatedly throughout the book.

For general shape and dimensions we have observed a cross section of a human head which has been reconstructed by CT (see Fig. 4.2). Based on this cross section we have described a skull enclosing the brain with ventricles, two tumors, and a hematoma (blood clot) using five ellipses, eight segments of circles, and two triangles. The tumors were placed so that they are vertically above the blood clot in the display. This facilitates reporting on our results as will be seen later on. The positioning of these ellipses, segments, and triangles is shown in Fig. 4.3.

We assume that the reference material is air whose linear attenuation coefficient can be taken to be zero for all energies. Hence the density of the

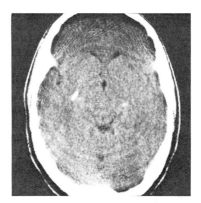

Fig. 4.2. Central part of a CT produced reconstruction of a cross section of the head of a human patient. This served as a basis for our standard head phantom.

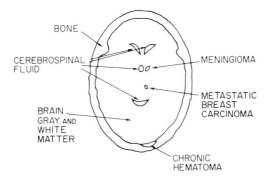

Fig. 4.3. Outlines of the different parts of the standard head phantom, with tissue type indicated for each area.

phantom at a point (x, y) is the linear attenuation coefficient at some fixed energy of the tissue at (x, y). Table 4.1 gives the linear attenuation coefficients of the various tissues in our head phantom at different energies.

Table 4.2 gives a precise mathematical description of the location and densities of the elemental objects in Fig. 4.3, assuming 60 keV photons.

We used SNARK77 to obtain the density in each of 115×115 pixels of size 0.1504 cm with $K = 7$. The resulting array of numbers is represented in Fig. 4.4. The nature of this display deserves careful discussion.

The densities given to the elemental objects were such that the resulting values are the linear attenuation coefficients at 60 keV of the appropriate tissue types measured in centimeters^{-1}. Thus the values range between zero (background, can be thought of as air) and 0.416 (bone of the skull). However, the interesting part of the picture is the interior of the skull. The values there

TABLE 4.1

LINEAR ATTENUATION COEFFICIENTS (cm^{-1}) AS A FUNCTION OF PHOTON ENERGY FOR TISSUES
WHICH OCCUR IN OUR HEAD PHANTOM

Energy (keV)	Bone	Brain (gray and white matter)	Metastatic breast carcinoma	Meningioma	Chronic hematoma	Cerebrospinal fluid
41	0.999	0.265	0.288	0.269	0.266	0.260
52	0.595	0.226	0.241	0.227	0.228	0.222
60	0.416	0.210	0.220	0.213	0.212	0.207
84	0.265	0.183	0.190	0.187	0.184	0.181
100	0.208	0.174	0.179	0.176	0.175	0.171

range from 0.207 (cerebrospinal fluid) to 0.220 (metastic breast tumor). The
small differences between tissues inside the skull would not be noticeable if
we used black to display zero, white to display 0.5 and corresponding
grayness for values in between. In order to see clearly the features in the
interior of the skull, we use intensity zero (black) to represent the value
0.1945 (or anything less) and the intensity 255 (white) to represent the value

TABLE 4.2

DESCRIPTION OF ELEMENTAL OBJECTS USED TO PRODUCE FIG. 4.4[a]

No.	Type	CX	CY	U	V	ANG	Density
1	Ellipse	0.000	0.00	8.625	6.4687	90.00	0.416
2	Ellipse	0.000	0.00	7.875	5.7187	90.00	−0.206
3	Ellipse	0.000	1.50	0.375	0.3000	90.00	−0.003
4	Ellipse	0.675	−0.75	0.225	0.1500	140.00	0.010
5	Ellipse	0.750	1.50	0.375	0.2250	50.00	0.003
6	Segment	1.375	−7.50	1.100	0.6250	19.20	−0.204
7	Segment	1.375	−7.50	1.100	4.3200	19.21	0.204
8	Segment	0.000	−2.25	1.125	0.3750	0.00	−0.003
9	Segment	0.000	−2.25	1.125	3.0000	0.00	0.003
10	Segment	−1.000	3.75	1.000	0.5000	135.00	−0.003
11	Segment	−1.000	3.75	1.000	3.0000	135.00	0.003
12	Segment	1.000	3.75	1.000	0.5000	225.00	−0.003
13	Segment	1.000	3.75	1.000	3.0000	225.00	0.003
14	Triangle	5.025	3.75	1.125	0.5000	110.75	0.206
15	Triangle	−5.025	3.75	1.125	0.9000	−110.75	0.206

[a] Tissue types are: bone in air (object 1), brain in bone (object 2), cerebrospinal fluid
in brain (objects 3, 8, 10, 12), carcinoma in brain (object 4), meningioma in brain (object
5), hematoma in bone (object 6), bone in hematoma (object 7), brain in cerebrospinal fluid
(objects 9, 11, 13), bone in brain (objects 14, 15).

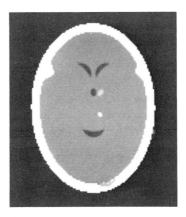

Fig. 4.4. The standard head phantom.

0.22 (or anything more). This way a change in value by 0.001 corresponds to a change in intensity of ten, which is visible. We used this method to produce Fig. 4.4 and *all the reconstructions of the head phantom* which are used as illustrations in this book. (In some cases, where this range is inappropriate, display of an additional range is also given.)

4.4   CREATION OF THE RAY SUMS

The simulation of the data collection in SNARK77 is based on (5.2) in Chapter 2:

$$p = -\ln(A_p/C_p). \tag{4.1}$$

We first discuss how the calibration measurement, C_p, is calculated. C_p is given by

$$C_p = C_0/C_r, \tag{4.2}$$

where C_0 is the number of photons counted by the detector under consideration and C_r is the number of photons counted during the same period by a reference detector. As it has been discussed in Section 3.1 both C_0 and C_r are samples of Poisson random variables. In SNARK77 it is assumed that C_0 and C_r are samples of the same random variable (with a user provided mean), and so the expected value of C_p is one. In fact, if the user of the programming system requests the simulation of the physically unattainable case of no error due to photon statistics, the value of C_p is taken to be exactly one. Otherwise, a random number generator is used to produce C_0 and C_r.

A subtle point is that, except in the case of the fifth scanning mode (Fig. 3.3e), C_p is not to be calculated separately for each source–detector pair. This is because of the way calibration is done in the different scanning modes (see Section 3.4). In the first two scanning modes (Fig. 3.3a and b), C_p is the same for all source–detector pair positions which are used to obtain data for one set of parallel rays. Similarly, in the fourth scanning mode (Fig. 3.3d), C_p is the same for all rays which diverge from the same detector as the source moves. The situation with the third scanning model is essentially different: C_p is the same for all rays which connect the source to a particular detector as the apparatus moves. All these rays are tangential to the same circle, and this may cause a ringlike feature to appear on the reconstruction if an error has been made during the calibration measurement.

We now turn to how the actual measurement, A_p, is calculated. A_p is given by

$$A_p = A_0/A_r, \tag{4.3}$$

where A_0 is the number of photons counted by the detector under consideration and A_r is the number of photons counted by the reference detector. Again A_r is taken to be a sample of a Poisson random variable with a user provided mean, λ, say.

The calculation of A_0 is more complex since it is during this calculation that SNARK77 introduces polychromaticity, the shape of the x-ray beam, and scatter.

In order to understand this clearly, we have to go back to the way we create a phantom (Section 4.2). The phantom is put together from a number of elemental objects each with an associated density. Since the phantom represents the distribution of relative linear attenuation at a fixed energy, we need only one density associated with each elemental object. If we want to represent the relative linear attenuation at a different energy, we need to use different densities for the elemental objects. In order to describe the interaction of a polychromatic x-ray beam with the phantom, densities for all energies in the beam need to be given.

SNARK77 solves this problem as follows. It assumes that the x-ray spectrum is discrete; i.e., it consists of photons which are of one of a finite number of different energies. For each energy the user has to specify the percentage of photons at that energy (based on the detected spectrum during the calibration measurement, see Section 3.2) and the density at that energy of all the elemental objects. (In general, the user also needs to specify the absorption properties of the reference material at the different energies, but since in our example the reference material is air, we shall not dwell on the details of this point.)

Since the density (in our case: relative linear attenuation at a fixed energy) at a point is the sum of the densities of all the elemental objects within which the point lies, the integral of the density along a line L is the sum over all elemental objects of the products of the length of intersection of L with the elemental object and the density in the elemental object.

Assume for now that we have a point source, a point detector, with a line L between them, and no scatter. Then (2.1) of Chapter 3 combined with (4.1) and (4.3) in this section yield

$$A_0 \simeq \lambda \int_0^E \tau_e \exp\left[- \int_0^D (\mu_e(z) - \mu_e^a)\, dz \right] de, \qquad (4.4)$$

where we have made use of the assumptions that the expected values of C_p and A_r are 1 and λ, respectively. In SNARK77, the expression on the right-hand side of (4.4) is evaluated as follows.

Let I be the number of discrete energy levels and J be the number of elemental objects. Let $d_{j,i}$ be the density of the jth elemental object at energy level i, let ℓ_j be the length of intersection of the line L with the jth elemental object (ℓ_j may be 0), and let t_i be the probability that a photon counted during the calibration measurement is at energy level i (these probabilities are user specified). Then A_0 is taken to be a sample of a Poisson random variable with mean

$$\lambda \sum_{i=1}^I t_i \exp\left[- \sum_{j=1}^J \ell_j d_{j,i} \right]. \qquad (4.5)$$

If the user wishes to simulate the physically unattainable case of no photon statistics, SNARK77 sets A_0 equal to the value provided by (4.5).

To simulate the shape of the x-ray beam, SNARK77 calculates A_0 as the weighted average of the values of (4.5) for a number of different lines between the source and the detector.

To simulate scatter, SNARK77 replaces the value A_0 for a detector position by a weighted average of the values of A_0 for that detector position and the neighboring detector positions. The scatter contribution of a detector position to another one is assumed to depend only on the distance between the two detector positions. Mathematically, we express this by saying that the values A_0 with scatter taken into consideration are obtained by *convolution* of the values of A_0 without scatter and a fixed *scatter function*. (The notion of convolution, which is essential for some of the reconstruction algorithms, is explained in Section 8.1.) This model for the scattering process is a very much simplified version of what really happens; scatter simulated by SNARK77 resembles true physical scatter only in its gross characteristics.

In the next chapter we give examples of how SNARK77 simulates the different processes just described and of the effects of these processes on the quality of the reconstruction.

NOTES AND REFERENCES

SNARK77 is described in detail in Herman and Rowland (1978).

The linear attenuation coefficients of the various tissue types (except for bone) at the different energies were estimated from the values published by Phelps *et al.* (1975). Values for bone were estimated based on the assumption that it is a mixture of calcium and fat. Head phantoms, which are less realistic than the one discussed in Section 4.2, have been proposed by Herman and Rowland (1973) and Shepp and Logan (1974).

5

Data Collection and Reconstruction
of the Head Phantom
under Various Assumptions

In this chapter we give examples of simulating various errors and modes of data collection in CT. In each case we show the result of a reconstruction from the simulated data and compare it to the test phantom.

5.1 METHODS OF PICTURE COMPARISON

A reconstruction is a digitized picture. In case it is a reconstruction from simulated projection data of a test phantom, we can judge the quality of the reconstruction by comparing it to the digitization of the test phantom. Naturally, both the picture region and the grid must be the same size for the reconstruction and the digitized phantom. This section is devoted to a discussion of how one illustrates and measures the resemblance between the reconstruction and the phantom.

Visual evaluation is of course the most straightforward way. One may display both the phantom and the reconstruction and observe whether all features in which one is interested in the phantom are reproduced in the reconstruction and whether any spurious features have been introduced by the reconstruction process. A difficulty with such a qualitative evaluation is its subjectiveness, people will often disagree on which of two pictures resembles a third one more closely.

A more quantitative way of evaluating pictures is the following. Select a column of pixels, which is such that it goes through a number of interesting features in the original. For example, in our digitized head phantom (described in Section 4.3) the 63rd of the 115 columns goes through the ventricles, both tumors, and the hematoma. In Fig. 5.1 we indicate this column. One way to

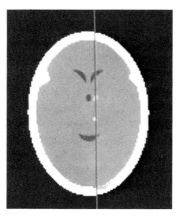

Fig. 5.1. Head phantom with the 63rd of the 115 columns indicated by a vertical line. The values along this column are plotted for all the reconstructions shown in this book.

evaluate the quality of reconstruction is to compare the graphs of the 115 pixel densities for this column in the original and the reconstruction. This will be done for all reconstructions of the head phantom that we report on in this book.

It also appears desirable to use a single value which measures the closeness of the reconstruction to the original. We now describe, and later on we use, three different methods of doing this. The reader must however be warned that a single number, or even collection of a few numbers, cannot possibly take care of all the ways in which two pictures may differ from each other. Rank ordering reconstructions based on a single measure of closeness to the original can be very misleading.

In this book, we report on three *picture distance measures.* In our definition of these measure we use $t_{u,v}$ and $r_{u,v}$ to denote the densities of the vth pixel of the uth row of the digitized test phantom and the reconstruction, respectively, and $\bar{t}$ to denote the average of the densities in the digitized test phantom. We assume that both pictures are $\ell \times \ell$ and use $[\ell/2]$ to denote the largest integer not greater than $\ell/2$. The measures defined in equations (1.1)–(1.5) are variants of often-used measures in the reconstruction literature.

$$d = \left(\sum_{u=1}^{\ell} \sum_{v=1}^{\ell} (t_{u,v} - r_{u,v})^2 \bigg/ \sum_{u=1}^{\ell} \sum_{v=1}^{\ell} (t_{u,v} - \bar{t})^2 \right)^{1/2}, \qquad (1.1)$$

$$r = \sum_{u=1}^{\ell} \sum_{v=1}^{\ell} |t_{u,v} - r_{u,v}| \bigg/ \sum_{u=1}^{\ell} \sum_{v=1}^{\ell} |t_{u,v}|, \qquad (1.2)$$

$$e = \max_{\substack{1 \le i \le [\ell/2] \\ 1 \le j \le [\ell/2]}} |T_{i,j} - R_{i,j}|, \qquad (1.3)$$

where

$$T_{i,j} = \tfrac{1}{4}(t_{2i,2j} + t_{2i+1,2j} + t_{2i,2j+1} + t_{2i+1,2j+1}), \qquad (1.4)$$

$$R_{i,j} = \tfrac{1}{4}(r_{2i,2j} + r_{2i+1,2j} + r_{2i,2j+1} + r_{2i+1,2j+1}). \qquad (1.5)$$

These three measures emphasize different aspects of picture quality. The first one, d, is a *normalized root mean squared distance measure*. A large difference in a few places causes the value of d to be large. Note that the value of d is 1 if the reconstruction is a uniformly dense picture with the correct average density. The second one, r, is a *normalized mean absolute distance measure*. As opposed to d, it emphasizes the importance of a lot of small errors rather than of a few large errors. Note that the value of r is 1 if the reconstruction is a uniformly dense picture with zero density. The third measure, e, is a *worst case distance measure*. Its value is the largest density difference between the $[\ell/2] \times [\ell/2]$ digitizations of the test phantom and the reconstruction. In the definition of e we use a rougher digitization than what is used for the reconstruction, since the size of the smallest feature in our phantom is several pixels and in practice we would use the average density in these pixels to estimate the relative linear attenuation of the tissue or tumor in which we are interested. The measure e provides us with the guaranteed reliability of such an estimate. All three measures are given for all reconstructions we report on in this book.

The real measure of the appropriateness of a reconstruction procedure is its performance in the clinical diagnostic situation. Unfortunately, this measure is difficult to quantify. One approach is by the use of *receiver operating characteristic* (ROC) curves, a topic beyond the scope of this book.

5.2   RECONSTRUCTION FROM PERFECT DATA

We now describe the basic geometry of data collection which we use throughout this book, except in those cases where the point to be illustrated needs a different geometry.

Our basic geometry is based on the third scanning mode in Section 3.4, the fan beam spinning scanner shown in Fig. 3.3c.

Schematically, the method of data collection is shown in Fig. 5.2. The source and the detector strip are on either side of the object to be reconstructed and they move in unison around a common center rotation denoted by 0 in Fig. 5.2. The data collection (actual measurement) takes place in M distinct steps. The source and detector strip are rotated between two steps of the data collection by a small angle, but are assumed to be stationary while the measurement is taken. The M distinct positions of the source during the M steps of the data collection are indicated by the points $S_0, \ldots, S_{M-1}$ in Fig. 5.2. In simulating this geometry of data collection, we assume that the source is a point source.

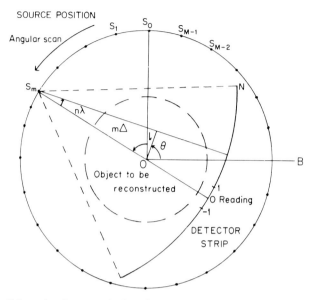

Fig. 5.2. Schematic of our standard method of data collection (divergent beam). Physical methods of data collection shown in Figs. 1.10 and 1.14 are special cases of this.

The detector strip consists of $2N + 1$ detectors, spaced equally on an arc whose center is the source position. The line from the source to the center of rotation goes through the center of the central detector. In this section we assume that each of the detectors are point detectors, the effect of using detectors which have nonnegligible widths will be shown in Section 5.5.

The object to be reconstructed is a picture such that its picture region is enclosed by the broken circle shown in Fig. 5.2. We assume that the origin of the coordinate system which is used to define the picture is the center of rotation, 0, of the apparatus.

In this section we assume that we have perfect data, i.e., that we know exactly the integrals of the picture to be reconstructed along the $M(2N + 1)$ lines which connect the source to the $2N + 1$ detectors for each of the M source positions.

The algorithm we use for reconstruction from these data is a "divergent beam convolution algorithm." The nature of these algorithms is explained in Section 10.1. So that the effects of the different problems associated with data collection are clearly seen, we use exactly the same reconstruction algorithm in all cases where it is applicable. (The only exceptions will be where the data are assumed to be collected along sets of parallel lines.) The exact parameters used in this algorithm are given in Section 10.6, after the explanation of the nature of a divergent beam convolution algorithm.

Specifically, unless otherwise stated, we use in this book the following geometry of data collection. (We refer to this as the *standard geometry* of data collection.) The number of source positions, M, is 288. The source positions are equally spaced around a circle of radius 78 cm. A consequence of this is that the angle $m\Delta$ shown in Fig. 5.2 is $1.25m$ degrees. The distance of the source from the detector strip is 110.735 cm. There are 165 detectors, and the distance between two detectors along the arc of the detector strip is 0.21336 cm.

The reconstruction algorithm estimates a digitization of the original from the projection data. Figure 5.3 shows both the 115×115 digitization of the head phantom (same as Fig. 4.4) and the reconstruction from perfect projection data for the geometry described previously. Figure 5.4 shows the

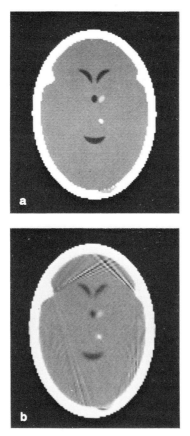

Fig. 5.3. (a) Head phantom. (b) Reconstruction of the head phantom from "perfect" data collected for the standard geometry.

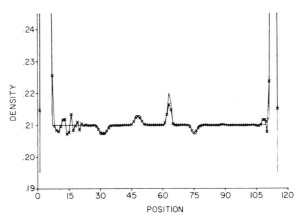

Fig. 5.4. Line plots of the 63rd column of phantom and reconstruction from perfect data using standard geometry. (Reconstruction plot is labeled by ×'s.)

values of the original and the reconstruction along the 63rd column. The values of the picture distance measures for this reconstruction are

$$d = 0.0900, \qquad r = 0.0379, \qquad e = 0.0517. \qquad (2.1)$$

Note that even though the data are perfect, the reconstruction is not. This is because a picture is not uniquely determined by its integrals along a finite number of lines (see Section 16.4). The best that a reconstruction algorithm can do is to *estimate* the picture from its projection data.

In order to show how the quality of the reconstruction is affected by the number of samples of its line integrals, we carried out six further experiments with perfect data; three with fewer samples and three with more samples than our standard geometry. Table 5.1 shows the effect of the number

TABLE 5.1

PICTURE DISTANCE MEASURES FOR RECONSTRUCTIONS FROM PERFECT DATA
WITH DIFFERING NUMBER OF SOURCE POSITIONS AND DETECTOR SPACING

No. source positions	Detector spacing	No. detectors	d	r	e
144	0.42672	83	0.1947	0.0858	0.1142
288	0.42672	83	0.1942	0.0847	0.1170
144	0.21336	165	0.0974	0.0471	0.0527
288	0.21336	165	0.0900	0.0379	0.0517
576	0.21336	165	0.0899	0.0374	0.0515
288	0.10668	329	0.0415	0.0222	0.0254
576	0.10668	329	0.0328	0.0154	0.0247

of source positions and of the detector spacing on the picture distance measures. (The length of the arc between the first and the last detector is kept constant.) The reconstructions are shown in Fig. 5.5 with plots of the 63rd column in Fig. 5.6.

5.3   EFFECTS OF PHOTON STATISTICS

The projection data for the reconstructions shown in this section have been generated according to the principles explained in Section 4.4, under the assumptions of a point source, point detector, monochromatic x rays, and no scatter. For any source–detector pair the monochromatic ray sum is calculated as

$$m = -\ln \frac{A_0/A_r}{C_0/C_r}, \qquad (3.1)$$

where A_0, A_r, C_0, C_r are samples of Poisson random variables with means λ_a, λ, λ_c, λ_c, respectively. Here, λ_a is related to λ by the equation

$$\lambda_a = \lambda \exp\left[-\sum_{j=1}^{J} \ell_j d_j \right], \qquad (3.2)$$

where d_j is the density of the jth elemental object at the fixed monochromatic energy level. This equation is an immediate consequence of (4.5) of Chapter 4 in case the number of energy levels, I, is one.

What we are interested in is the effect of the choice of λ and λ_c on the quality of the reconstruction. We also look at the effect of the scanning mode when there are errors in the calibration measurement (see the discussions in Sections 3.4 and 4.4). In addition to the third scanning mode, we look at our standard geometry with the fourth scanning mode. Altogether four experiments have been carried out to investigate the effects of photon statistics.

In the experiment which is most realistic from the point of view of present day CT scanners, we used $\lambda = 10^6$ and $\lambda_c = 288 \times 10^6$. This means that we assume that during the actual measurement approximately a million photons are counted by the reference detector and that about the same number of photons would be counted by the detector if the object to be reconstructed were removed from the reconstruction region. For our phantom, this results in the values of λ_a being between 40,000 and 1,000,000, depending on how much and what type of tissue the ray in question goes through. Thus, the standard deviation of the random variable of which the photon counts are samples is always less than 0.5% of the mean. The figure for λ_c has been arrived at by considering the standard practice of calibrating the CT scanner

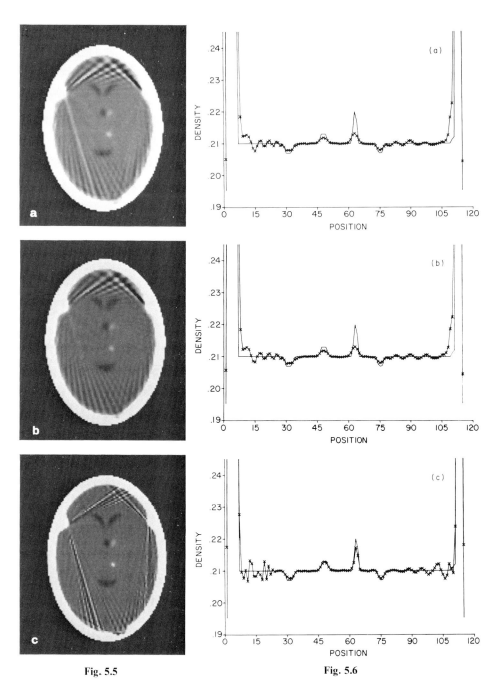

Fig. 5.5   Fig. 5.6

Fig. 5.5. Reconstructions of the head phantom from perfect data with number of source positions and detector spacing as follows. (a) 144 and 0.42672. (b) 288 and 0.42672. (c) 144 and 0.21336. (d) 576 and 0.21136. (e) 288 and 0.10668. (f) 576 and 0.10668.

Fig. 5.6. Line plots of the 63rd columns of reconstruction shown in Fig. 5.5.

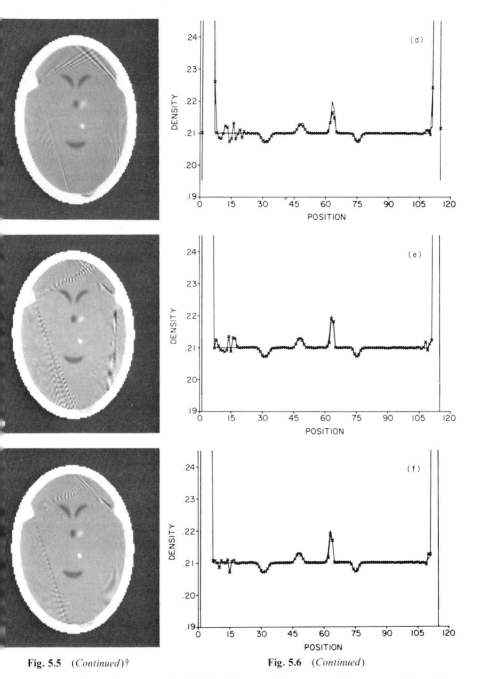

Fig. 5.5 (*Continued*)†   **Fig. 5.6** (*Continued*)

†*Note*: A certain amount of variability of the overall darkness of the contents of the skull has been introduced by the photographing process. For example, in Fig. 5.5c the brain appears to be darker than in Fig. 5.5f. This does not represent a true overall difference between the CT numbers, as can be seen by looking at Figs. 5.6c and f. These (and all other) photographs of reconstructions should be used for observing only the variations in intensity, the absolute values should be determined from the plots.

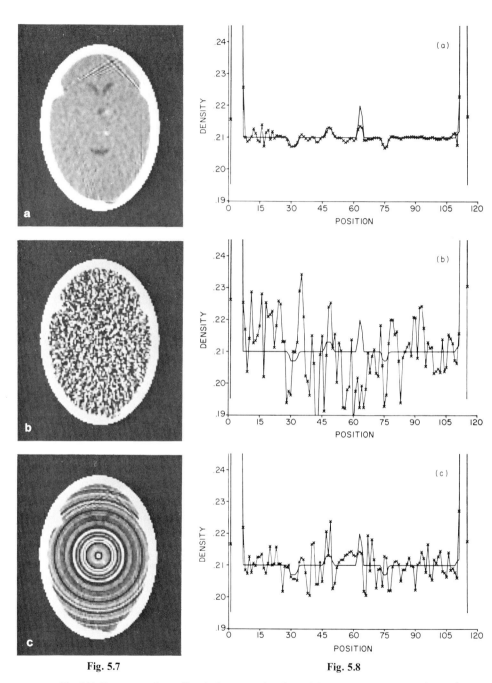

Fig. 5.7   Fig. 5.8

Fig. 5.7. Reconstructions of head phantom using data with photon noise only. (a) $\lambda = 10^6$ and $\lambda_c = 288 \times 10^6$. (b) $\lambda = 10^4$ and $\lambda_c = 288 \times 10^6$. (c) $\lambda = 10^6$ and $\lambda_c = 10^4$. (d) $\lambda = 10^6$ and $\lambda_c = 10^4$. The third scanning mode was used in (a), (b), and (c), and the fourth scanning mode was used in (d).

Fig. 5.8. Line plots of the 63rd columns of the reconstructions shown in Fig. 5.7.

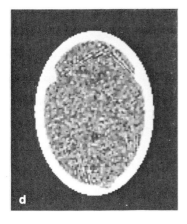

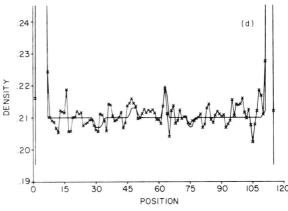

Fig. 5.7   (*Continued*)   Fig. 5.8   (*Continued*)

by going through a complete scan of some reference material. Since in our standard geometry we assume 288 views, we get $\lambda_c = 288\lambda$.

In our other experiments we have taken smaller values of λ and λ_c than customary, in order to emphasize the effects of low photon counts. Table 5.2 reports on the picture distance measures. The reconstructions are shown in Fig. 5.7 with plots of the 63rd column in Fig. 5.8.

TABLE 5.2

Picture Distance Measures for Different Photon Statistics
and Scanning Modes[a]

λ	λ_c	Scanning mode	d	r	e
∞	∞	3 or 4	0.0900	0.0379	0.0517
10^6	288×10^6	3	0.0904	0.0387	0.0506
10^4	288×10^6	3	0.1079	0.0666	0.0472
10^6	10^4	3	0.0945	0.0481	0.0494
10^6	10^4	4	0.0920	0.0437	0.0524

[a] The first line reports on perfect data, it is the same as the fourth line in Table 5.1.

These results demonstrate the following.

For accurate reconstruction it is important to have a sufficient number of photons, i.e., to keep λ and λ_c high. Unfortunately, to reduce the potentially harmful x-ray dose to the patient it is important to keep λ low. The resolution of this dilemma (reconstruction efficacy versus radiation damage) is one of the most important practical problems in CT.

Errors in calibration are unlikely to come from photon limitations, since there is no damage to patients during the calibration process. However, inaccuracy in calibration may occur for other reasons, e.g., lack of stability in the detector. The effects of such inaccuracies can be simulated by low values of λ_c. As can be seen, using the third scanning mode, this leads to very noticeable ringlike artifacts on the reconstruction (Fig. 5.7c), while the fourth scanning mode is not so seriously affected. This has been one of the major motivations for introducing the fourth scanning mode. However, improvements in detection technology and the development of computer algorithms for ring removal resulted in CT devices, using the third scanning mode, which produce pictures without the ring artifact (see Fig. 1.11).

5.4   EFFECTS OF BEAM HARDENING

To illustrate the effects of beam hardening, we have collected polychromatic projection data of the head phantom using (4.5) of Chapter 4. The number of discrete energy levels, I, is five and the t_i's (the probability that a photon counted during the calibration measurement is at energy level i) are provided by Table 5.3. In the real x-ray situation the spectrum is continuous; Table 5.3 gives a discrete approximation of a continuous spectrum typical of what is used in CT.

In applying (4.5) of Chapter 4, Table 4.2 has been used for the size and location of the elemental objects, with the $d_{j,i}$'s (the density of the jth elemental object at energy i) calculated using the information in Table 4.1. In calculating the polychromatic projection data, a point source, a point detector, and no scatter and no photon statistics have been assumed.

TABLE 5.3

SPECTRUM (t_i) OF THE POLYCHROMATIC X-RAY BEAM USED IN THE EXPERIMENTS AND LINEAR ATTENUATION COEFFICIENTS (μ_i) OF METASTATIC BREAST CARCINOMA AT THE ENERGY LEVELS OF THE DISCRETE SPECTRUM

i	Energy level (keV)	t_i	μ_i (cm^{-1})
1	41	0.1	0.288
2	52	0.3	0.241
3	60	0.3	0.220
4	84	0.2	0.190
5	100	0.1	0.179

We are interested in how well the phantom (based on linear attenuation coefficients at 60 keV) reconstructs from the polychromatic projection data, and in the improvement in the quality of reconstruction that can be achieved using the correction techniques (see Section 3.2).

Figure 5.9a shows the reconstruction from the polychromatic data with the plot along the 63rd column in Fig. 5.10a. The reader should observe the "cupping" of the reconstructed linear attenuation coefficients inside the skull. This is a characteristic beam hardening artifact for head reconstructions.

We now look at a simple correction method which assumes that there are only two types of material in the reconstruction region. Clearly, one of these should be air, since it occupies a very large part of the reconstruction region. The attenuation properties of the other material should be similar to the properties of the brain, but possibly a bit more attenuating in view of the fact that x rays will go through bone as well as brain. Among the tissues listed in Table 4.1, metastatic breast carcinoma is the one which appears most appropriate; its linear attenuation coefficient, μ_i, at energy level i is listed in Table 5.3. Translating (2.5) of Chapter 3 into our discrete spectrum with material a as air and material b as metastatic breast carcinoma we get the following relationship between the polychromatic ray sum p and the monochromatic ray sum m.

$$p \simeq -\ln \sum_{i=1}^{5} t_i \exp\left(-\frac{\mu_i}{\mu_3} m\right) \tag{4.1}$$

(see Table 5.3 for values of t_i and μ_i).

The polynomial

$$q'(p) = -0.000088p^3 + 0.009429p^2 + 0.986407p - 0.000022 \tag{4.2}$$

is a "solution" to (4.1) in the following sense. By looking at the monochromatic projection data for our head phantom, we have observed that the value of m for any ray is between 0 and 4. Let

$$m_j = 0.0001 \times j, \tag{4.3}$$

and

$$p_j = -\ln \sum_{i=1}^{5} t_i \exp\left(-\frac{\mu_i}{\mu_3} m_j\right). \tag{4.4}$$

In other words, p_j is the value of the right-hand side of (4.1) when m_j is substituted for m. We have calculated m_j and p_j for $j = 0, 1, \ldots, 39,999$ (i.e., for $m_j = 0, 0.0001, \ldots, 3.9999$) and found that

$$\sqrt{\frac{\sum_{j=0}^{39,999} (m_j - q'(p_j))^2}{40,000}} = 0.000060. \tag{4.5}$$

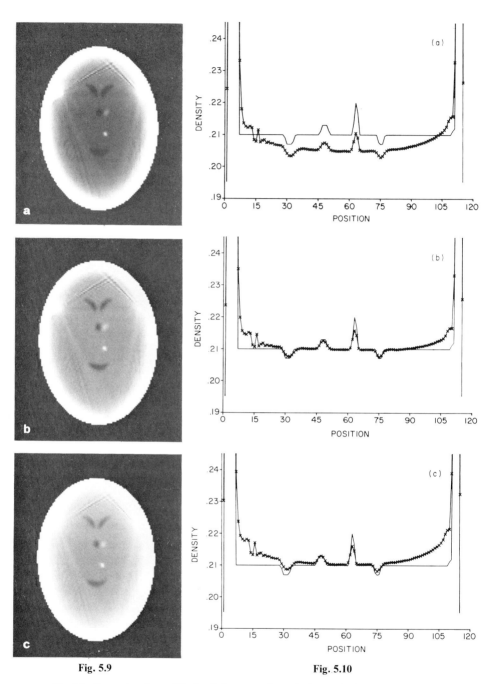

Fig. 5.9   Fig. 5.10

Fig. 5.9. Reconstructions of the head phantom using polychromatic data. (a) No correction.
(b) Correction using (4.2). (c) Correction using (4.7). (d) Correction using (4.9), first iteration.
(e) Correction using (4.9), second iteration. (f) Monochromatic reconstruction (same as Fig.
5.3b).

Fig. 5.10. Line plots of the 63rd columns of the reconstructions shown in Fig. 5.9.

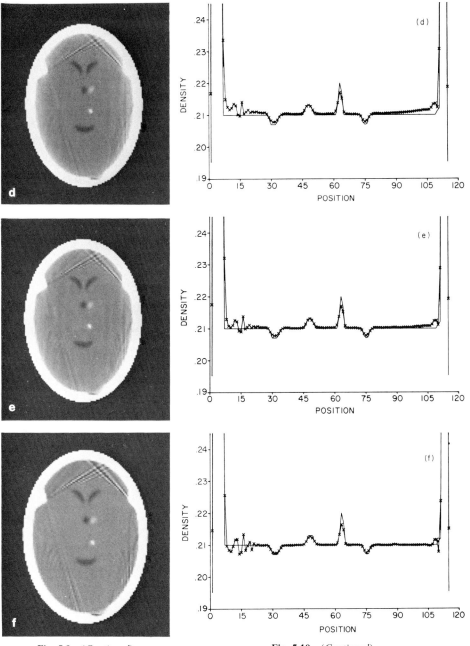

Fig. 5.9 (*Continued*)   **Fig. 5.10** (*Continued*)

This means that for the range of m_j's that we are interested in, the root mean squared distance between the true value of m_j and the value estimated by (4.2) is only 0.00006. It is in this sense that (4.2) is a "solution" of (4.1).

This leads to the following beam hardening correction method. For a ray with polychromatic ray sum p, we estimate the monochromatic ray sum to be $q'(p)$. If the assumption embodied in (4.1), namely that the only materials in the reconstruction region are air and metastatic breast carcinoma, were correct, this would be a very good correction method.

Note, by the way, that (4.5) supports our claim in Section 3.2 that a low order polynomial correction function is likely to be sufficient. We have shown that for objects consisting of air and a limited amount of metastatic breast a cubic correction [$n = 3$ in (2.6) of Chapter 3] works excellently.

Figure 5.9b shows the reconstruction from the corrected polychromatic projection data using (4.2), with the plot along the 63rd column in Fig. 5.10b. The fact that this reconstruction is not as good as the reconstruction from monochromatic projection data (Figs. 5.3b and 5.4) is due to the inaccuracy of the assumption of only two materials in the reconstruction region.

If we wish to measure how well correction for beam hardening based on (4.2) succeeds, we should look at the actual ray sums for our phantom. There are 288 source positions and 165 detectors, providing us with a total of 47,520 rays. Let us order these rays in some fashion and let m_j^t and p_j^t denote the monochromatic and polychromatic ray sums for the jth ray ($1 \le j \le 47,520$). A measure of the success of the correction is indicated by the fact that

$$\sqrt{\frac{\sum_{j=1}^{47,520} (m_j^t - q'(p_j^t))^2}{47,520}} = 0.050593. \tag{4.6}$$

Note that the right-hand side of (4.6) is considerably larger than the right-hand side of (4.5). What we would like to do is to find a polynomial q, such that if q is used in place of q' in (4.6) the right-hand side would become nearly as small as can be for any polynomial function in place of q. We find that the polynomial

$$q(p) = 1.0265p \tag{4.7}$$

serves this purpose. In fact,

$$\sqrt{\frac{\sum_{j=1}^{47,520} (m_j^t - q(p_j^t))^2}{47,520}} = 0.0385; \tag{4.8}$$

a result superior to that indicated in (4.6).

It is interesting to note that the $q(p)$ in (4.7) is a first order polynomial. In fact, for this data set, one can not do much better with higher order polynomials. The best that can be achieved with a fifth order polynomial is that the right-hand side of (4.8) reduces to 0.0381. It must be emphasized that this is a property of the cross section under consideration. For a different part of the body, and even for more bony cross sections of the head, higher order polynomials have been found more appropriate.

Figure 5.9c shows the reconstruction from the corrected polychromatic projection data using (4.7), with the plot along the 63rd column in Fig. 5.10c. In this reconstruction the CT numbers very nearly reflect the actual tissue linear attenuation coefficients in the central region. However it is impossible for a linear polynomial to correct for the cupping, as it can only "lift" the CT numbers equally in all pixels. A cursory comparison of the uncorrected and polynomial corrected reconstructions might lead one to prefer the un-corrected on its visual qualities. This anomaly is due to the choice of window used to display the figures.

Given that the polynomial correction failed to correct for cupping, the task is to find an improved correction method. We now illustrate an iterative procedure.

If one could obtain estimates m' and p' of the monochromatic and poly-chromatic ray sums such that $m' - q(p')$ closely resembles $m - q(p)$, where q is the correcting polynomial, then one could obtain an approximation to the monochromatic ray sum by

$$m \simeq m' - q(p') + q(p). \tag{4.9}$$

An approach is outlined in the following.

Represent the reconstruction, which is a digitized picture, by a J-di-mensional vector x, where J is the number of pixels, and the jth component, x_j, of x is the estimate of the relative linear attenuation in the jth pixel at energy $\bar{e}$. We estimate m' and p' based on x.

Let r be the J-dimensional vector whose jth component, r_j, is the length of intersection of the ray with the jth pixel. Then we define the *pseudo mono-chromatic ray sum, m',* by

$$m' = \sum_{j=1}^{J} r_j x_j. \tag{4.10}$$

Let, for $1 \leq i \leq I$ and $1 \leq j \leq J$, $\mu_{i,j}$ denote the average relative linear attenuation at the ith energy level in the jth pixel. Suppose that we can produce, based on physical information, I functions g_i such that, for $1 \leq i \leq I$,

$$g_i(x_j) \simeq \mu_{i,j}. \tag{4.11}$$

Using t_i to denote the probability that a photon counted during the calibra-tion measurement is at energy level i, we define the *pseudo polychromatic ray sum, p',* by

$$p' = -\ln \sum_{i=1}^{I} t_i \exp\left[-\sum_{j=1}^{J} r_j g_i(x_j) \right]. \tag{4.12}$$

By comparing (4.10) with (6.1) of Chapter 2 and (4.12) with (2.1) of Chapter 3, we see that if x provides a good approximation to the digitization of the picture to be reconstructed, then (4.9) is likely to be valid. The right-hand side of (4.9) provides us with a new estimate of the monochromatic projection data, which then can be used as an input to the reconstruction algorithm. Figure 5.9d shows the reconstruction produced from such an input, with the plots along the 63rd column in Fig. 5.10d. Both the picture and the plot reveal how well this single iteration works. The central area, which was already well corrected, is largely unaffected, but much of the cupping is eliminated and the skull/brain border is much better defined. Most noticeable is that the hematoma is again visible in the picture. This reconstruction compares quite favorably to the monochromatic reconstruction (Fig. 5.9f) toward which we are trying to correct.

However with better pictures comes a price, and this step has a heavy price. Whereas the polynomial correction involved only a few multiplications per ray sum, even for higher order polynomials, the pseudo ray sum calculation involves making many multiplications per ray sum, determining ray–pixel intersections, and exponentiation. The corresponding times for the polynomial correction of the projection data and generating the projection data for the iterative step are 50 and 1000 sec, respectively. Even though these programs did not use specialized reconstruction software, so that commercially much lower times should be expected, they do give some indication of the magnitude of difference in the expense of the two correction methods.

Given that the new reconstruction (Fig. 5.9d) is better than the old one (Fig. 5.9c), one would expect that recalculating m' and p' from the new reconstruction and using (4.9) one would get an even better reconstruction. Such a reconstruction is shown in Fig. 5.9e, with the plots of the 63rd column

TABLE 5.4

PICTURE DISTANCE MEASURES FOR MONOCHROMATIC,
POLYCHROMATIC, AND CORRECTED POLYCHROMATIC
PROJECTION DATA

Data	d	r	e
Polychromatic projection data	0.1448	0.0723	0.0830
Correction using (4.2)	0.1388	0.0665	0.0777
Correction using (4.7)	0.1314	0.0683	0.0736
Correction using (4.9)			
First iteration	0.1082	0.0525	0.0542
Second iteration	0.1041	0.0486	0.0553
Monochromatic projection data	0.0900	0.0379	0.0517

in Fig. 5.10e. There is only a slight improvement over the previous recon-struction. In view of the cost, further iterations of the process are not worth-while.

Table 5.4 reports on the picture distance measures for the reconstructions.

5.5   THE EFFECTS OF DETECTOR WIDTH AND SCATTER

As has been discussed in Section 3.3, there are a number of other reasons, besides photon statistics and beam hardening, why physical measurements can only provide us with approximations of the line integrals of the relative linear attenuation. In this section we show the effects of two of these: the width of the detectors and the scattering of photons.

The mathematics of reconstruction, at least as embodied in (6.2) of Chapter 2, assumes the availability of line integrals of the relative linear attenuations. The nonnegligible size of the focal spot of the x-ray source and of the detector gives rise to the partial volume effect, discussed in Section 3.3. We have simulated this effect for our head phantom and standard geometry, assuming a point source but a wide detector. In fact, we have assumed that each one of our detectors are 0.21336 cm wide; i.e., that there is no gap between adjacent detectors on the detector strip (see Fig. 5.2). This makes the width of the detectors as large as they can possibly be for the assumed mode of data collection.

As mentioned in Chapter 4, SNARK77 simulates such a situation by calculating A_0 as the weighted average of (4.5) of Chapter 4 for a number of lines between the point source and the detector. In our simulation we placed five points on the detector (one-fifth of the detector width apart from each other), and gave equal weights to the lines between the source and each of the five points. We assumed no photon statistics, monochromatic x rays, and no scatter.

Reconstruction from the data so obtained is shown in Fig. 5.11, with line plots for the 63rd column in Fig. 5.12. The values of the picture distance measures for this reconstruction are

$$d = 0.0987, \qquad r = 0.0341, \qquad e = 0.0596. \qquad (5.1)$$

It may appear surprising to the uninitiated that this reconstruction compares very well with the reconstruction from perfect data; c.f. (2.1) and (5.1). That this is reasonable will become clearer from our discussion of the implementation of reconstruction algorithms. For now the following summary explanation has to suffice. The estimation of the partial derivative $m_1(\ell, \theta)$ in the Radon inversion formula, (6.2) of Chapter 2, is difficult from the discrete samples of $m(\ell, \theta)$ if the value changes significantly from one

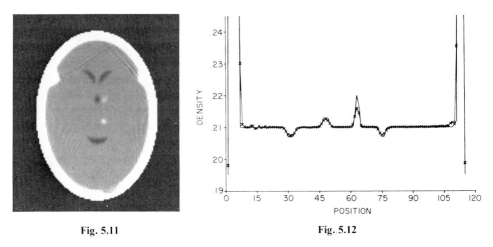

Fig. 5.11   Fig. 5.12

Fig. 5.11. Reconstruction of the head phantom from data collected with a nonpoint detector.

Fig. 5.12. Line plot of the 63rd column of the reconstruction shown in Fig. 5.11.

sample to the next. The finite detector width "smooths" the discrete data, and thereby improves our ability to estimate $m_1(\ell, \theta)$. This, to some extent, counteracts the partial volume effect.

The same argument applies to a limited amount of scatter. To illustrate this we consider two different situations, one with high scatter and one with low scatter. In the high scatter case we assume that 50% of the photons counted by a detector have been scattered; in the low scatter case we put the same figure at 5%. In either case, we assume that of the counted scattered photons 44% were moving (prior to scatter) in the direction of the detector which eventually counted them, 48% were moving in the direction of one of the two immediately neighboring detectors, and 8% were moving in the direction of one of the two detectors on the opposite sides of the immediate neighbors. This assumption reflects the fact that a scattered photon is most likely to move in a direction similar to its direction prior to scatter. The given percentages are average values. The actual numbers for any detector depend on the object to be reconstructed, in the manner indicated in Section 4.4.

The case of 50% of the counted photons being scattered is extreme, but not impossible, for a scanner of the type we are discussing (third scanning mode). However, careful engineering design, combined with mathematical correction (intended to eliminate the effect of scatter) applied to the raw photon counts, probably makes the 5% figure more realistic. (At the time of writing this book, very little data exist in the open literature regarding this matter.)

Using the scatter model of SNARK77 we have simulated projection data for both low and high scatter, with no other sources of error. Figure 5.13 shows the reconstructions and Fig. 5.14 shows line plots of the 63rd column.

The associated picture distance measures are shown in Table 5.5.

As can be seen, the reconstruction obtained from data with low scatter compares well with reconstructions from perfect data, but high scatter has a significant blurring effect on the reconstruction.

We do not give examples of the effects of other important sources of error discussed in Section 3.3.

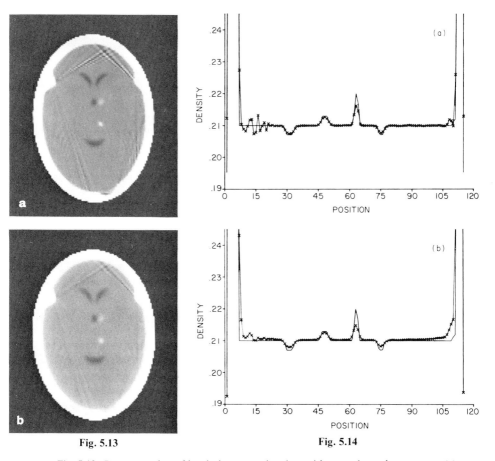

Fig. 5.13   Fig. 5.14

Fig. 5.13. Reconstruction of head phantom using data with error due only to scatter. (a) 5% of the counted photons have been scattered. (b) 50% of the counted photons have been scattered.

Fig. 5.14. Line plots of the 63rd columns of the reconstructions in Fig. 5.13.

TABLE 5.5

THE EFFECT OF SCATTERING ON THE PICTURE
DISTANCE MEASURES

% counted photons scattered	d	r	e
0	0.0900	0.0379	0.0517
5	0.0942	0.0390	0.0548
50	0.1404	0.0526	0.0873

5.6   SIMULATION OF DIFFERENT SCANNING MODES

When data are collected by an actual CT scanner all the different sources of error that we have discussed in the last three sections are present simultaneously. In testing reconstruction algorithms we want realistic projection data. We now define the *standard projection data*, which will be used for most of the remaining experiments in this book.

The data are collected for the head phantom with standard geometry as described in Section 5.2. For photon statistics we choose $\lambda = 10^6$ and $\lambda_c = 288 \times 10^6$ (see Section 5.3). The spectrum of the polychromatic x-ray beam is given by Table 5.3. The focal spot of the x-ray source is assumed to be a point, but the detectors are assumed to have width of 0.21336 (i.e., there are no gaps between the detectors). It is assumed that 5 % of the photons counted during the actual measurement are photons which have been scattered, and that the nature of the scatter is as described in Section 5.4. The data so obtained are corrected using (4.9) twice, to provide us with an estimate of the monochromatic projection data. The outcome of this correction is what we refer to as the standard projection data.

Figure 5.15a shows the reconstruction from the standard projection data using the divergent beam convolution algorithm used for all earlier experiments in this chapter. Figure 5.16a shows the line plot for the 63rd column.

The two basic modes of data collection for cross-sectional reconstruction are the parallel beam (Figs. 3.3a and b) and the divergent beam (Figs. 3.3c and d). While many reconstruction algorithms are applicable to both basic methods of data collection, some are restricted to only one of them. We therefore wish to define the *standard parallel projection data*, which is used for illustrating the reconstruction algorithms which assume parallel x-ray beams. We attempt to make the standard parallel projection data have characteristics similar to the standard (divergent) projection data, so that reconstructions from the two data sets will be comparable.

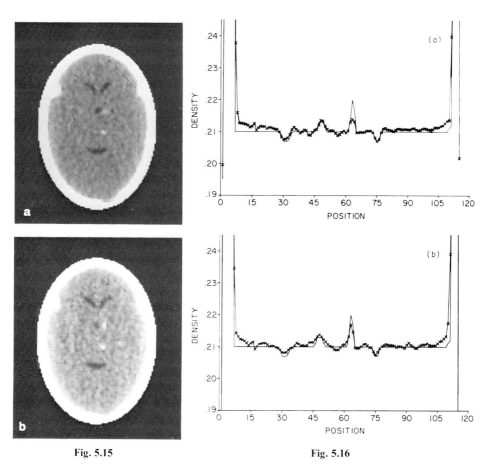

Fig. 5.15   **Fig. 5.16**

Fig. 5.15. Reconstructions from realistic projection data. (a) Standard (divergent) projection data. (b) Standard parallel projection data.

Fig. 5.16. Line plots of the 63rd columns of the reconstructions in Fig. 5.15.

In the standard projection data we have assumed that the 288 source positions are equally spaced around the circumference of a circle (see Fig. 5.2); i.e., that the apparatus makes a full 360° rotation in 1.25° steps (see Fig. 3.3c). Observing Figure 3.3a, we see that, at least in principle, there is no need to rotate the incremental scanner by more than 180° around the patient, since additional rotation would only collect ray sums along the same rays. Hence in the standard parallel projection data, we assume 144 incremental rotations with 1.25° between them. The distance between the parallel rays in a single set of parallel rays has been chosen to be 0.1504 cm, which is about the distance between points on two neighboring diverging rays near the center of rotation in the standard (divergent) geometry. This distance also happens to equal the length of the side of a pixel in the head phantom. In any single set of parallel rays there are 165 rays covering the reconstruction region. Thus the total number of rays is half as much as in the standard geometry.

The data are collected for the head phantom. In order to keep the total exposure of the patient to x rays the same as in the standard data set, for photon statistics we choose $\lambda = 2 \times 10^6$ and $\lambda_c = 288 \times 10^6$ (see Section 5.3). So the numbers of photons used in obtaining the standard divergent and parallel data are the same. The spectrum of the polychromatic x-ray beam is given by Table 5.3. Both the focal spot of the x-ray source and the detectors are assumed to have width of 0.1504 cm (i.e., the strips between successive positions of the source and detector are abutting). It is assumed that 5% of the photons counted during actual measurement are photons which have been scattered, and that the nature of scatter is as described in Section 5.4. (This means that our parallel data reflect the nature of the second scanning mode, see Fig. 3.3b, rather than the first one, where there is no scatter from adjacent detector positions, see Fig. 3.3a. We do this since the second scanning mode is what is now much more customary, mainly because of its greater speed. This also makes our two data sets more similar. As we have seen in Section 5.4, such low level of scatter makes very little difference to the reconstruction.) The data so obtained are corrected using (4.9) twice to provide us with an estimate of the monochromatic projection data. The outcome of this correction is what we refer to as the standard parallel projection data.

Figure 5.15b shows the reconstruction from the standard parallel projection data using the parallel beam convolution algorithm (see Chapter 8). Figure 5.16b shows the line plot for the 63rd column. Note that while the two reconstructions differ in some details, the overall quality appears to be the same, as is further borne out by Table 5.6.

TABLE 5.6

PICTURE DISTANCE MEASURES FOR THE DIVERGENT AND
PARALLEL MODES OF DATA COLLECTION

Reconstruction from	d	r	e
Standard divergent projection data	0.1159	0.0465	0.0674
Standard parallel projection data	0.1175	0.0470	0.0657

Notes and References

The use of line plots to compare phantoms with reconstructions was introduced into the reconstruction literature by Shepp and Logan (1974). Variants of the three picture distance measures in Section 5.1 have been used by a large number of research workers, their first combined appearance is in Herman (1972), which discusses these and other measures and gives references to earlier work on picture comparison. For a discussion of receiver operating characteristics (ROC) curves see, for example, Metz *et al.* (1976).

The basic geometry of our data collection is similar to that of the five-second fan beam CT scanner described by Chen *et al.* (1976).

The method by which the polynomial "solution" (4.2) to the equation (4.1) was obtained is described by Herman (1977a). Much of the material in Section 5.4 closely follows Herman and Simmons (1979). Technical details can be found in Herman (1979b).

6

Basic Concepts of Reconstruction Algorithms

With this chapter we begin our systematic study of reconstruction algorithms. We introduce the notation which is used in the rest of the book. We categorize reconstruction methods into two basic groups: transform methods and series expansion methods. We explain the basic nature of the algorithms in the two groups and indicate what we consider the desirable characteristics of reconstruction algorithms.

6.1 PROBLEM STATEMENT

Until now we have always used the rectangular (Cartesian) coordinates for describing a function of two variables. Thus, we have used $\mu_e(x, y)$ to denote the relative linear attenuation at the point (x, y), where (x, y) was in reference to a rectangular coordinate system, see Fig. 2.8. However, in the more mathematical work that follows it is more convenient to use polar coordinates (r, ϕ), which are related to the rectangular coordinates (x, y) by the formulas $r = \sqrt{x^2 + y^2}$, $\phi = \tan^{-1}(y/x)$, $x = r \cos \phi$, $y = r \sin \phi$. We use the phrase a *function of two polar variables* to describe a function f whose values $f(r, \phi)$ represent the value of some physical parameter (such as relative linear attenuation) at the geometrical point whose polar coordinates are (r, ϕ). The mathematically distinguishing feature of a function of two polar variables f is that $f(0, \phi_1) = f(0, \phi_2)$, for all values of ϕ_1 and ϕ_2. This reflects the fact that the physical parameter represented by f can only have one value at the origin. Furthermore, we do not restrict the domain of the polar variables, that is, we allow r and ϕ to have any real value; hence, a function f of two polar variables must also satisfy the condition $f(r, \phi) = f(-r, \phi + \pi)$.

In Section 4.1 we have defined a picture as a function of two variables whose value is zero outside the picture region, which is a square (of size $\sqrt{2}E \times \sqrt{2}E$, say) whose center is at the origin of the coordinate system. In what follows, we use f to denote the function of two polar variables r and ϕ, which is used to define the picture to be reconstructed. We know that

$$f(r, \phi) = 0 \quad \text{if} \quad |r \cos \phi| \geq E/\sqrt{2} \quad \text{or} \quad |r \sin \phi| \geq E/\sqrt{2}. \quad (1.1)$$

($|x|$ denotes the absolute value of x; it is x if $x \geq 0$ and it is $-x$ if $x < 0$.) In particular, $f(r, \phi) = 0$ if $r \geq E$.

A possible physical interpretation of the picture function f is that the picture region is the reconstruction region of Fig. 2.8 and $f(r, \phi)$ is the relative linear attenuation at the point (r, ϕ). However, the remaining discussion is independent of such an interpretation. Reconstruction algorithms are applicable whatever physical property $f(r, \phi)$ is supposed to represent (see Section 1.1).

One important difference between studying f simply as a function and studying it as a representation of the distribution of some physical property is the way mathematics is handled. Reconstruction algorithms are often based on powerful theorems of mathematics. These are often of the form: "If f has the property that..., then ...." We shall not hesitate to use the conclusion of such a theorem, whenever the validity of the premise appears to be reasonable on physical grounds.

In particular, we shall not hesitate to assume, whenever needed, that pictures satisfy certain integrability conditions. (We use integrals without precise definition. While just about all that we say is valid for any standard definition of integral; those who wish to make our approach mathematically watertight should use integrals in the sense of Lebesgue.) One of our assumptions is that any picture function f is *square integrable*; i.e., that

$$\int_0^{2\pi} \int_0^E (f(r, \phi))^2 r \, dr \, d\phi \quad (1.2)$$

exists. (Existence here means that the integral can be evaluated. Its value is a real number.) This assumption allows us to define the *distance* $d(f_1, f_2)$ between two picture functions f_1 and f_2 by

$$d(f_1, f_2) = \int_0^{2\pi} \int_0^E (f_1(r, \phi) - f_2(r, \phi))^2 r \, dr \, d\phi, \quad (1.3)$$

since it can be proved that if f_1 and f_2 are such that (1.2) exists when f_1 or f_2 are substituted for f, then (1.3) also exists. Clearly, (1.3) is related to the squared distance measure defined by (1.1) of Chapter 5.

We now define the *Radon transform* of a function f of two polar variables. First we introduce a notational convention which is used throughout the book. The Radon transform is an example of an *operator*; when acting on a function it produces another function. We use capital script letters to denote operators; for example, we use $\mathscr{R}$ to denote the Radon transform. If f is a function, the function which is its Radon transform is denoted by $\mathscr{R}f$. The value of $\mathscr{R}f$ at the point (ℓ, θ) in its domain is denoted by $[\mathscr{R}f](\ell, \theta)$.

The Radon transform of f is defined for real number pairs (ℓ, θ) as follows:

$$[\mathscr{R}f](\ell, \theta) = \int_{-\infty}^{\infty} f(\sqrt{\ell^2 + z^2}, \theta + \tan^{-1}(z/\ell))\, dz, \qquad \text{if} \quad \ell \neq 0,$$

$$[\mathscr{R}f](0, \theta) = \int_{-\infty}^{\infty} f(z, \theta + \pi/2)\, dz. \tag{1.4}$$

Observing Fig. 2.8, we see that $[\mathscr{R}f](\ell, \theta)$ is the line integral of f along the line L. (Note that the dummy variable z in (1.4) does not exactly match the variable z as indicated in Figure 2.8. In (1.4) $z = 0$ corresponds to the point where the perpendicular dropped on L from the origin meets L.) The existence of the Radon transform for any ℓ and θ is another one of our integrability assumptions.

Observe that

$$[\mathscr{R}f](\ell, \theta) = [\mathscr{R}f](-\ell, \theta + \pi) = [\mathscr{R}f](\ell, \theta + 2\pi) \tag{1.5}$$

and that

$$[\mathscr{R}f](\ell, \theta) = 0 \qquad \text{if} \quad |\ell| \geq E. \tag{1.6}$$

The last equation follows from (1.1). In view of these equations, the function $\mathscr{R}f$ is completely determined by its values at the points (ℓ, θ) with $-E < \ell < E$ and $0 \leq \theta < \pi$.

There is an important difference between the domains of the functions f and $\mathscr{R}f$. The picture function f is defined for pairs of real numbers (r, ϕ), which represent the polar coordinates of points in the plane. Hence the value of $f(0, \phi)$ is the same for all values of ϕ, since $(0, \phi)$ always represents the origin. This is not the case for $\mathscr{R}f$. Its value for the pair $(0, \theta)$ is the line integral of f along a line through the origin making an angle θ with the positive y axis. Hence, unless f is circularly symmetric about the origin, $[\mathscr{R}f](0, \theta)$ depends on θ. The pair of real numbers (ℓ, θ) in the domain of $\mathscr{R}f$ is not to be interpreted as polar coordinates of a point in the plane.

Roughly speaking, the operator $\mathscr{R}$ associates with a function f over the (r, ϕ) space another function $\mathscr{R}f$ over the (ℓ, θ) space. We can think of a single point in the (ℓ, θ) space as corresponding to a line L (at a distance ℓ from the origin making an angle θ with the positive y axis) in the (r, ϕ) space, since $[\mathscr{R}f](\ell, \theta)$ is the integral of f along L.

To further emphasize the relationship between the two spaces consider Fig. 6.1. It shows the loci in the (ℓ, θ) space of the points corresponding to two

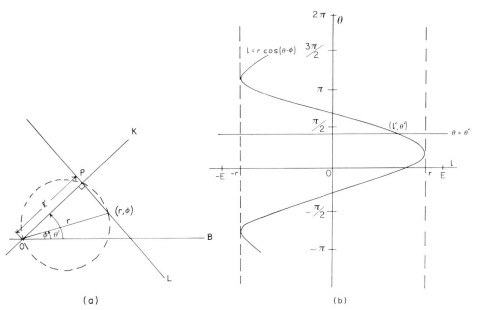

Fig. 6.1. The relationship between the (r, ϕ) space and the (ℓ, θ) space. (a) In the (r, ϕ) space K is a half-line through the origin O making and angle θ' with the baseline B. The point (r, ϕ) is considered given and L is the line through (r, ϕ) perpendicular to K. L meets K at P which is at a distance ℓ' from O. (b) In the (ℓ, θ) space, the points, which correspond to the lines perpendicular to K in (r, ϕ) space, lie on the straight line $\theta = \theta'$. The points, which correspond to the lines through (r, ϕ) in (r, ϕ) space, lie on the sinusoidal $\ell = r \cos(\theta - \phi)$. The point corresponding to L, namely (ℓ', θ'), is the intersection of these two curves. [Reproduced from Herman (1980), with permission.]

sets of lines in the (r, ϕ) space: (i) a set of parallel lines, (ii) a set of lines going through a fixed point.

Consider first the line K which makes an angle θ' with the x axis in Fig. 6.1a. Any line perpendicular to K makes an angle θ' with the positive y axis. Hence the locus of the set of points in the (ℓ, θ) space which corresponds to lines perpendicular to K is the straight line $\theta = \theta'$; see Fig. 6.1b.

Consider next the point (r, ϕ) in Fig. 6.1a. If a line going through this point makes an angle θ with the positive y axis, then its distance ℓ from the origin is

$$\ell = r \cos(\theta - \phi). \tag{1.7}$$

Hence the locus of the set of points in (ℓ, θ) space which correspond to lines through the point (r, ϕ) is the curve whose equation is (1.7), see Fig. 6.1b.

The point in (ℓ, θ) space which corresponds to the line L which is both perpendicular to K (and so makes an angle θ' with the positive y axis) and goes through the point (r, ϕ) is the point $(r \cos(\theta' - \phi), \theta')$.

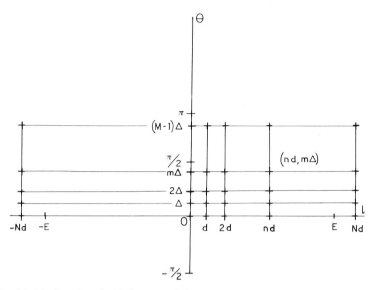

Fig. 6.2. The locations in (ℓ, θ) space of the points which correspond to lines for which measurements have been collected in the parallel mode of data collection. It is assumed that a single source and a single detector move parallel to each other in $2N + 1$ steps of size d, with $Nd > E$, the radius of the circular region containing the object to be reconstructed. After the data have been collected for these $2N + 1$ rays (one view), the whole apparatus is rotated by an angle of Δ, and the data are again collected for the $2N + 1$ rays of the next view. This is repeated M times, where $M\Delta$ is π. Thus, for a complete set of views the apparatus rotates around in a semicircle. A typical point in (ℓ, θ) space is $(nd, m\Delta)$, which lies at the intersection of the two straight lines $\ell = nd$ and $\theta = m\Delta$. [Reproduced from Herman (1980), with permission.]

The input data to a reconstruction algorithm are estimates (based on physical measurements) of the values of $[\mathscr{R}f](\ell, \theta)$ for a finite number of pairs (ℓ, θ); its output is an estimate, in some sense, of f. The main purpose of this chapter is to make this brief description precise.

Suppose that estimates of $[\mathscr{R}f](\ell, \theta)$ are known for I pairs: (ℓ_1, θ_1), $(\ell_2, \theta_2), \ldots, (\ell_I, \theta_I)$. For $1 \leq i \leq I$, we define $\mathscr{R}_i f$ by

$$\mathscr{R}_i f = [\mathscr{R}f](\ell_i, \theta_i). \tag{1.8}$$

$\mathscr{R}_i$ is an example of a *functional*; when acting on a function, it produces a real number. In what follows we use, unless otherwise stated, y_i to denote the available estimate of $\mathscr{R}_i f$ and we use y to denote the I-dimensional column vector whose ith element is y_i. We refer to the vector y as the *measurement vector*.

When designing a reconstruction algorithm we assume that the method of data collection, and hence the set $\{(\ell_1, \theta_1), \ldots, (\ell_I, \theta_I)\}$, is fixed and known. Roughly stated the problem is

given the data y, **estimate** the picture f.

In the next two sections we discuss the basic approaches used for estimating f. We shall usually use f^* to denote the estimate of the picture f.

$\mathscr{R}_i f$ is the value of $\mathscr{R}f$ at the point (ℓ_i, θ_i) in the (ℓ, θ) space. Any geometry of data collection provides us with a finite set of points (ℓ_i, θ_i) at which an estimate of $\mathscr{R}_i f$ is known. For example, in the first and second scanning mode of Chapter 3 (parallel modes of data collection, see Figs. 3.3a and b), the arrangement of points (ℓ_i, θ_i) at which an estimate of $\mathscr{R}_i f$ is known forms a rectangular grid of the type shown in Fig. 6.2. The corresponding arrangements for the divergent modes of data collection (Figs. 3.3c and d) are more complicated; they are discussed in Chapter 10.

6.2 TRANSFORM METHODS

One way of defining the estimate f^* of f is to give a formula which expresses the value of $f^*(r, \phi)$ in terms of $r, \phi, y_1, \ldots, y_I$. Such a formula may be a "discretized" version of a Radon inversion formula, which expresses f in terms of its Radon transform $\mathscr{R}f$. We refer to reconstruction methods based on such an approach as *transform methods*. In the rest of this section we give a more detailed explanation of what has been said previously.

The Radon transform associates with a function f of two polar variables another function $\mathscr{R}f$ of two variables. What we are looking for is an operator, $\mathscr{R}^{-1}$, which is such that $\mathscr{R}^{-1}\mathscr{R}f$ is f (i.e., $\mathscr{R}^{-1}$ associates with the function $\mathscr{R}f$ the function f). Just as (1.4) describes how the value of $\mathscr{R}f$ is defined at any real number pair, (ℓ, θ), based on the values f assumes at points in its domain, we need a formula which for functions p of two real variables defines $\mathscr{R}^{-1}p$ at points (r, ϕ). Such a formula is the following.

$$[\mathscr{R}^{-1}p](r, \phi) = \frac{1}{2\pi^2} \int_0^\pi \int_{-E}^E \frac{1}{r\cos(\theta - \phi) - \ell} p_1(\ell, \theta)\, d\ell\, d\theta, \quad (2.1)$$

where $p_1(\ell, \theta)$ denotes the partial derivative of $p(\ell, \theta)$ with respect to ℓ. [See also (6.2) of Chapter 2.] We prove in Section 16.3 that for any picture function f of two polar variables (satisfying some physically reasonable conditions), $\mathscr{R}^{-1}\mathscr{R}f = f$, in the sense that for all points (r, ϕ),

$$[\mathscr{R}^{-1}\mathscr{R}f](r, \phi) = f(r, \phi). \quad (2.2)$$

In order to understand the nature of the operator $\mathscr{R}^{-1}$, we express it as a sequence of simpler operators.

We use $\mathscr{D}_Y$ to denote partial differentiation with respect to the first variable of a function of two real variables. Thus, for any function p of two real variables and for any real number pair (ℓ, θ),

$$[\mathscr{D}_Y p](\ell, \theta) = \lim_{\Delta\ell \to 0} \frac{p(\ell + \Delta\ell, \theta) - p(\ell, \theta)}{\Delta\ell}, \quad (2.3)$$

assuming of course that the limit on the right-hand side exists.

In our application, the function p which is operated on by $\mathcal{D}_Y$ is the Radon transform of a picture. It is quite easy to describe pictures f such that $\mathcal{D}_Y \mathcal{R} f$ is not defined for all (ℓ, θ). An example is the picture which has value one everywhere inside the picture region. There are mathematically rigorous ways of extending the definition $\mathcal{D}_Y$ so that it makes sense even in such cases. Here we simply assume that for any picture f that we may wish to reconstruct, the right-hand side of (2.3) is defined for $p = \mathcal{R} f$.

The next operator we wish to define is the *Hilbert transform* $\mathcal{H}_Y q$ *with respect to the first variable* of a function q of two variables. For any real number pair (ℓ', θ), we define

$$[\mathcal{H}_Y q](\ell', \theta) = -\frac{1}{\pi} \int_{-\infty}^{\infty} \frac{q(\ell, \theta)}{\ell' - \ell} \, d\ell. \qquad (2.4)$$

Note that this is an *improper integral* since its integrand diverges at $\ell = \ell'$. It is to be evaluated in the Cauchy principle value sense; i.e.,

$$[\mathcal{H}_Y q](\ell', \theta) = -\frac{1}{\pi} \lim_{\varepsilon \to 0} \left\{ \int_{-\infty}^{\ell' - \varepsilon} \frac{q(\ell, \theta)}{\ell' - \ell} \, d\ell + \int_{\ell' + \varepsilon}^{\infty} \frac{q(\ell, \theta)}{\ell' - \ell} \, d\ell \right\}. \qquad (2.5)$$

In our application, q is $\mathcal{D}_Y \mathcal{R} f$ for some picture f. We again assume that for pictures that we wish to reconstruct the limit on the right-hand side of (2.5) exists.

Finally, we introduce an important operator called *backprojection*. Given a function t of two variables, $\mathcal{B} t$ is another function of two polar variables, whose value at any point (r, ϕ) is defined by

$$[\mathcal{B} t](r, \phi) = \int_0^{\pi} t(r \cos(\theta - \phi), \theta) \, d\theta. \qquad (2.6)$$

Observing Fig. 6.1b, we see that the value at point (r, ϕ) of the backprojection of a function t is obtained by integrating t on a segment of the curve (from $\theta = 0$ to $\theta = \pi$) whose equation is (1.7).

The reason for the name backprojection is the following.

Look at the line K in Fig. 6.1a. It makes an angle θ' with the positive x axis. The "projection" of a function of two variables onto the line K is the function of one variable obtained from the line integrals of f along lines perpendicular to K. In other words, it is $[\mathcal{R} f](\ell, \theta')$, considered as a function of ℓ alone. The line L which goes through a point (r, ϕ) and is perpendicular to K meets the line K at a point P which is at a distance $\ell' = r \cos(\theta' - \phi)$ from the origin.

Now consider the reverse process. Rather than producing $\mathcal{R} f$ from f by integrating (projecting) along lines such as L, produce from a given function t of two variables another function $\mathcal{B} t$ by spreading (backprojecting) the values of t along such lines. For a *fixed* θ' (determining the line K), the contribution of t to $\mathscr{B}t$ is the same for all points (r, ϕ) lying on the same line L perpendicular to K; and the value of this contribution is proportional to $t(\ell', \theta')$, where ℓ' is the distance of L from the origin. More precisely, given a point (r, ϕ), we evaluate the value of $\mathscr{B}t$ at (r, ϕ) by summing up (integrating) as θ' varies the values of $t(\ell', \theta')$ for the ℓ' which is the distance of the line L from the origin. Since L goes through (r, ϕ) and K goes through the origin, the locus of the point P where these perpendicular lines meet as θ' varies is the circle with its diameter from the origin to the point (r, ϕ).

Combining (2.3), (2.4), and (2.6) we get that for a function p of two variables and for any point (r, ϕ),

$$[\mathscr{B}\mathscr{H}_Y \mathscr{D}_Y p](r, \phi) = -\frac{1}{\pi} \int_0^\pi \int_{-\infty}^\infty \frac{p_1(\ell, \theta)}{r \cos(\theta - \phi) - \ell} \, d\ell \, d\theta. \qquad (2.7)$$

The identity, except for a multiplicative constant, of the right-hand sides of (2.1) and (2.7) can be concisely described by stating the operator equation:

$$\mathscr{R}^{-1} = -\frac{1}{2\pi} \mathscr{B}\mathscr{H}_Y \mathscr{D}_Y. \qquad (2.8)$$

In words, the inverse Radon transform of a function p of two variables can be obtained by the following sequence of operations:

(i)   partial differentiate p, with respect to its first variable to obtain a function q,
(ii)   Hilbert transform q with respect to its first variable to obtain a function t,
(iii)   backproject t, and
(iv)   multiply the value of the resulting function by $-(1/2\pi)$. This is sometimes called *normalization*.

Such a process assumes that the exact value of $p(\ell, \theta)$ is known for all l and θ and that the required operations can be carried out precisely. Neither of these assumptions is satisfied when we wish to use a computer to estimate a function from its experimentally obtained projection data. Transform methods for image reconstruction are based on (2.8), or on alternative expressions for the inverse Radon transform $\mathscr{R}^{-1}$, but they have to perform on finite and imperfect data using the not unlimited capabilities of computers. How this is done is explained in the following chapters. The essence of what needs to be done is to find *numerical procedures* (i.e., ones that can be implemented on a digital computer), which estimate the value of a double integral, such as appears on the right-hand side of (2.1), from given values of $p(\ell_i, \theta_i)$, $1 \le i \le I$.

6.3   SERIES EXPANSION METHODS

In the approach to the image reconstruction problem which was summarized in the last section the techniques of mathematical analysis are used to find an inverse to the Radon transform. The inverse transform is described in terms of operators on functions defined over the whole continuum of real numbers. For implementation of the inverse Radon transform on a computer we have to replace these continuous operators by discrete ones which operate on functions with a finite number of arguments. This is done at the very end of the derivation of the reconstruction algorithm.

The series expansion approach is basically different. The problem itself is discretized at the very beginning: estimating the function is translated into finding a finite set of numbers. This is done as follows.

It is assumed that we fix a set of J *basis pictures* $\{b_1, \ldots, b_J\}$, whose linear combinations give us adequate approximation to any picture f we may wish to reconstruct.

An example of such an approach is the $n \times n$ digitization discussed in Section 4.1. In that case $J = n^2$. We number the pixels from 1 to J, and define

$$b_j(r, \phi) = \begin{cases} 1 & \text{if} \quad (r, \phi) \text{ is inside the } j\text{th pixel,} \\ 0 & \text{otherwise.} \end{cases} \tag{3.1}$$

Then the $n \times n$ digitization of the picture f is the picture $\hat{f}$ defined by

$$\hat{f}(r, \phi) = \sum_{j=1}^{J} x_j b_j(r, \phi), \tag{3.2}$$

where x_j is the average value of f inside the jth pixel. (A shorthand notation we use for equations of this type is $\hat{f} = \sum_{j=1}^{J} x_j b_j$.)

There are other ways of choosing the basis pictures; some of these are discussed later on. Once the basis pictures are fixed, any picture $\hat{f}$ which can be represented as linear combinations of the basis pictures $\{b_j\}$ is uniquely determined by the choice of the coefficients x_j, $1 \leq j \leq J$, as shown in (3.2). We use x to denote the column vector whose jth component is x_j, and we refer to x as the *image vector*.

This approach restricts the general problem of "estimating a picture f," to the more specific problem of "finding an image vector x" such that $\hat{f}$ defined by (3.2) is as near to f as possible using the given basis pictures. To make this precise we need a definition of "nearness" between two pictures. Such a definition has been provided by (1.3).

It follows from standard results of mathematical analysis that, irrespective of how the basis pictures are chosen, for any picture f there is one and only one picture $\hat{f}$ with the following properties:

(i) $\hat{f}$ is a linear combination of the basis pictures,
(ii) if $\hat{\hat{f}}$ is a linear combination of the basis pictures, then

$$d(f, \hat{f}) \leq d(f, \hat{\hat{f}}). \tag{3.3}$$

Furthermore, if the basis pictures are chosen so that they are linearly independent (i.e., none of them can be expressed as a linear combination of the others), then there is a unique image vector x which gives rise to the $\hat{f}$ defined in (3.2).

For example, if the basis pictures are defined by (3.1), then the $n \times n$ digitization of f is the $\hat{f}$ satisfying (i) and (ii), and the associated image vector x is unique.

Ideally, the series expansion approach should aim at finding the image vector which gives rise to the $\hat{f}$ nearest to f. However, since our data do not uniquely determine f, usually we try to find an image vector x which satisfies a less efficacious, but achievable, optimization criterion. Such criteria are discussed in the next section.

In order to show how the image reconstruction problem translates into a discrete problem using the series expansion approach we need to observe two properties of the functionals $\mathscr{R}_i$ defined by (1.8).

The first property is that they are *linear*. This means that for all pictures f_1 and f_2, for all real numbers c_1 and c_2 and for $1 \leq i \leq I$,

$$\mathscr{R}_i(c_1 f_1 + c_2 f_2) = c_1 \mathscr{R}_i f_1 + c_2 \mathscr{R}_i f_2. \tag{3.4}$$

This is easily proved using the definitions of $\mathscr{R}_i$ and $\mathscr{R}$.

The other property is mathematically less rigorous. We would like to say that "if f_1 and f_2 are near each other, then so are $\mathscr{R}_i f_1$ and $\mathscr{R}_i f_2$." Unfortunately, using the distance for functions given in (1.3), a mathematically precise version of this statement would not be always true. Nevertheless, it is reasonable to argue based on the definition of $\mathscr{R}_i$ that if $\hat{f}$ is defined by the previous (i) and (ii), then $\mathscr{R}_i \hat{f}$ will be approximately the same as $\mathscr{R}_i f$. This property is called *continuity*. A basic weakness of the series expansion approach is that this assumption is sometimes badly violated.

Combining these properties we can state that, for $1 \leq i \leq I$,

$$\mathscr{R}_i f \simeq \mathscr{R}_i \hat{f} = \sum_{j=1}^{J} x_j \mathscr{R}_i b_j. \tag{3.5}$$

Since the b_j are user defined functions, usually $\mathscr{R}_i b_j$ can be easily calculated by analytical means. For example, in the case of b_j being defined by (3.1), $\mathscr{R}_i b_j$ is just the length of intersection with the jth pixel of the line of the

ith position of the source–detector pair [more precisely, the line at a distance ℓ_i from the origin making angle θ_i with the positive y axis; see (1.8) and Fig. 2.8]. Unless otherwise stated, we use $r_{i,j}$ to denote our calculated value of $\mathscr{R}_i b_j$. Hence,

$$r_{i,j} \simeq \mathscr{R}_i b_j. \tag{3.6}$$

Recall also that we use y_i to denote the physically obtained estimate of $\mathscr{R}_i f$. Combining this with (3.5) and (3.6), we get that, for $1 \le i \le I$,

$$y_i \simeq \sum_{j=1}^{J} r_{i,j} x_j. \tag{3.7}$$

Let R denote the matrix whose (i, j)th element is $r_{i,j}$. We refer to this matrix as the *projection matrix*. Let e be the I-dimensional column vector whose ith component, e_i, is the difference between the left- and right-hand sides of (3.7). We refer to this as the *error vector*. Then (3.7) can be rewritten as

$$y = Rx + e. \tag{3.8}$$

Thus the series expansion approach leads us to the following *discrete reconstruction problem*: based on (3.8),

given the data y, **estimate** the image vector x.

If the estimate which we find as our solution to the discrete reconstruction problem is the vector x^*, then the estimate f^* to the picture to be reconstructed is given by

$$f^* = \sum_{j=1}^{J} x_j^* b_j. \tag{3.9}$$

We make the following important observation. Our justification for the series expansion approach did *not* need that the functionals $\mathscr{R}_i$ be defined by (1.8). It only needed that $\mathscr{R}_i$ satisfy the property expressed by (3.5). Many different ways of defining the $\mathscr{R}_i$'s will have this property: integration along curved rather than straight lines or even areas (such as strips) rather than lines are potentially relevant to the general reconstruction problem. A major advantage of the series expansion methods over the transform methods is that they are immediately applicable to such more general ways of data collection.

6.4   OPTIMIZATION CRITERIA

In this section we discuss optimization criteria by which the image vector of the series expansion approach is estimated. Although this will not be explicitly indicated, much of what we say is also relevant in estimating the picture using transform methods.

In (3.8) vector e is unknown. The very most we can hope for is that we can specify a random variable of which e is a sample, and in most cases even this is impossible. The simple approach of trying to solve (3.8) by first assuming that e is the zero vector is dangerous: $y = Rx$ may have no solutions, or it may have many solutions possibly none of which is any good for the practical problem at hand. Some criteria have to be developed, indicating what x ought to be chosen as a solution of (3.8).

The criteria that have been used for the reconstruction problem are usually of the form: Choose as the "solution" of (3.8) an image vector x for which the value of some function $\phi_1(x)$ is minimal, and if there is more than one x which minimizes $\phi_1(x)$ choose among these one for which the value of some other function $\phi_2(x)$ is minimal. In this section we survey some of the choices for ϕ_1 and ϕ_2 that have been proposed.

A theoretically attractive approach is the following. Consider both the image vector x and the error vector e to be samples of random variables, denoted by X and E, respectively. Since our discussion in Section 1.2 was restricted to discrete random variables (only a finite number of possible outcomes), while here the outcomes can be column vectors of real numbers, further explanation is needed. [A reader who is not desirous to learn about the foundations of Bayesian estimation may safely skip to (4.8).]

A random variable such as X is defined by a *probability density function* p_X, which is a real number valued function on J-dimensional vectors of real numbers (the possible outcomes of X). This probability density function is defined so that for any J pairs of numbers $\ell_1 < u_1, \ell_2 < u_2, \ldots, \ell_J < u_J$, the following is the case. The probability that a sample x of X will have the property $\ell_j \leq x_j \leq u_j$, for $1 \leq j \leq J$, is

$$\int_{\ell_1}^{u_1} \int_{\ell_2}^{u_2} \cdots \int_{\ell_J}^{u_J} p_X(x)\, dx_J \ldots dx_2\, dx_1. \tag{4.1}$$

For notational convenience we sometimes abbreviate such integrals as

$$\int_{\ell}^{u} p_X(x)\, dx. \tag{4.2}$$

Corresponding to the concepts of mean and variance of a discrete random variable, as defined in (2.4) and (2.5) of Chapter 1, we have the concepts of *mean vector* μ_X and *covariance matrix* V_X, defined as follows.

$$\mu_X = \int_{-\infty}^{\infty} x p_X(x)\, dx, \tag{4.3}$$

$$V_X = \int_{-\infty}^{\infty} (x - \mu_X)(x - \mu_X)^{\mathrm{T}} p_X(x)\, dx, \tag{4.4}$$

where x^T denotes the row vector which is the *transpose* of the column vector x (i.e., a row vector whose ith component is x_i). These integrals are to be interpreted component by component. For example, using $(x - \mu_X)_i$ to denote the ith component of the vector $x - \mu_X$, the (i, j)th component of V_X is given by

$$(V_X)_{i,j} = \int_{-\infty}^{\infty} (x - \mu_X)_i (x - \mu_X)_j p_X(x)\, dx. \tag{4.5}$$

The most commonly used random variable with vector outcomes is the *multivariate Gaussian* random variable, for which the probability density function is uniquely determined by its mean vector and by its covariance matrix as follows:

$$p_X(x) = \frac{1}{(2\pi)^{J/2}(\det V_X)^{1/2}} \exp[-\tfrac{1}{2}(x - \mu_X)^T V_X^{-1}(x - \mu_X)]. \tag{4.6}$$

Note that for $p_X(x)$ to make sense, the determinant of the covariance matrix, $\det V_X$, must be positive. It is not too difficult to check that (4.3), (4.4), and (4.6) are consistent. The probability density function of a multivariate Gaussian distribution peaks at its mean.

The importance of the multivariate Gaussian random variable rests on two facts. One is that many random variables occurring in practice are approximately multivariate Gaussian. The other is that the assumption that an unknown distribution is multivariate Gaussian usually makes the mathematical treatment of the problem much easier than it would be otherwise.

Let us return now to the random variables X and E associated with x and e of (3.8). In this case p_X is referred to as the *a priori* probability density function, since $p_X(x)$ indicates the likelihood of coming across an image vector similar to x. In CT it makes sense to adjust p_X to the area of the body we are imaging; the probabilities of the same picture representing a cross section of the head or of the thorax should be different. Our treating X and E separately is by itself a simplifying assumption, since in practice E is not independent of X, as can be seen from the discussion in Section 3.1. The theory that we are describing can be developed without making this assumption, but it becomes more complicated.

At last we are in position to state an optimization criterion (it assumes that p_X and p_E are known): given the data y, choose the image vector x for which the value of

$$p_E(y - Rx)p_X(x) \tag{4.7}$$

is as large as possible. Note that the second term in the product is large for x's which have large a priori probabilities, while the first term is large for the x's which are consistent with the data (at least if p_E peaks at the zero vector).

The relative importance of the two terms depends on the nature of p_X and p_E. If p_X is flat (many image vectors are equally likely) and p_E is highly peaked near the zero vector, then our criterion will produce an image vector x^* which fits the measured data y in the sense that Rx^* will be nearly the same as y. On the other hand, if p_E is flat (large errors are nearly as likely as small ones) but p_X is highly peaked, our having made our measurements will have only a small effect on our preconceived ideas as to how the image vector should be chosen.

The x^* which maximizes (4.7) is called the *Bayesian estimate*.

A difficulty with using Bayesian estimation is that it presupposes knowledge of p_X and p_E. Precise knowledge of the true a priori distribution of image vectors and of the error vector is usually not available. A second difficulty is that for many p_X and p_E the estimation of x which maximizes (4.7) may be far from trivial.

If we assume that both X and E are multivariate Gaussian, the optimization problem becomes much simpler. In that case it is easy to see from (4.6) that, assuming that μ_E is the zero vector, the x which maximizes (4.7) is the same as the x which minimizes

$$(y - Rx)^T V_E^{-1}(y - Rx) + (x - \mu_X)^T V_X^{-1}(x - \mu_X). \tag{4.8}$$

A less sophisticated approach is to aim at finding a *least squares* solution of (3.8), i.e., an x which minimizes

$$\|e\|^2 = \|y - Rx\|^2 = \sum_{i=1}^{I} \left(y_i - \sum_{j=1}^{J} r_{i,j} x_j \right)^2. \tag{4.9}$$

Such a criterion does not necessarily determine x; there may be more than one vector x which minimizes (4.9). In such a case one has to select an x by a second criterion, choices for which are described in the following.

Another reason why a least squares solution is not necessarily very good is that the criterion expressed in (4.9) does not contain any information regarding the nature of a "desirable" solution x. In the Bayesian approach of (4.8) such information is incorporated into the a priori covariance matrix V_X.

It can be reasonably argued that a desirable property of the solution of (3.8) is that the variance

$$\sum_{j=1}^{J} (x_j - \bar{x})^2, \tag{4.10}$$

where

$$\bar{x} = \sum_{j=1}^{J} x_j / J \tag{4.11}$$

should be small. [If the basis pictures are chosen according to (3.1), $\bar{x}$ is the average density in the digitized picture.] It can be shown that if $\bar{x}$ is considered fixed for all acceptable solutions to (3.8), then the x which minimizes (4.10) is the same x which minimizes the norm $\|x\|$ of x, where

$$\|x\|^2 = \sum_{j=1}^{J} x_j^2. \tag{4.12}$$

In other words, in such a case the *minimum variance* and *minimum norm* solutions are the same.

The critera expressed in (4.10) and (4.12) are not to be used as "primary" criteria in image reconstruction. That is, in terms of the notation introduced at the beginning of this section, it is not reasonable to define $\phi_1(x)$ by (4.10). That would lead to the "solution" in which all components of x are the same, namely $\bar{x}$. The use of (4.10) is either as a secondary criterion, or as a component of the primary criterion, where the other components force the "solution" to be consistent with the measurements, or express other properties of desirable solutions of (3.8).

For example, in the case when the basis pictures are chosen according to (3.1) it may be considered "desirable" that the values x_j assigned to neighboring pixels should be close to one another on the average. Such a criterion can be expressed (see Section 12.3) by saying that we desire to minimize $x^T B x$, where B is an appropriately chosen matrix. This, in conjunction with the desire to minimize (4.9) and (4.12) at the same time, leads us to state that the sought solution x of (3.8) is the one which minimizes

$$a\|y - Rx\|^2 + x^T(bB + U)x, \tag{4.13}$$

where a and b are appropriately chosen positive numbers, indicating the relative importance we attach to minimizing the various expressions previously discussed, and U is the identity matrix.

All these approaches [(4.8), (4.9), (4.10), (4.12), (4.13)] are special cases of a *quadratic optimization* problem which can be stated as follows.

Find an x which minimizes

$$a(y - Rx)^T A(y - Rx) + (x - x_0)^T(bB + cC^{-1})(x - x_0), \tag{4.14}$$

where A is a symmetric $I \times I$ matrix, B and C are $J \times J$ matrices, a, b, and c are nonnegative real numbers, and x_0 is a J-dimensional vector. (Further details on the nature of these matrices, constants, and vectors are given in Section 12.1, which also contains the reasons for writing the matrix in the second term in the cumbersome form $bB + cC^{-1}$.)

There are alternative ways of incorporating a priori information about pictures of interest into the process of selecting a solution to (3.8). One example is to use the knowledge that x_j must lie within a certain range. In many applications all pictures $f(r, \phi)$ which may occur have only nonnegative values. Then it is reasonable to demand that we accept an image vector x based on the digitization process of (3.1) as a solution to (3.8) only if $x_j \geq 0$, for $1 \leq j \leq J$. In fact, one may go further and demand also that for any solution of (3.8), the error should be within a certain bound, i.e., specify positive numbers $\varepsilon_1, \ldots, \varepsilon_I$, and accept as solutions only those x_j's which have the property

$$-\varepsilon_i \leq y_i - \sum_{j=1}^{J} r_{i,j} x_j \leq \varepsilon_i, \qquad (4.15)$$

for $1 \leq i \leq I$. Other inequality constraints may also be introduced.

Using such arguments, we can replace the system of equations (3.8), with the unspecified e and possibly with inequality side conditions, by a system of inequalities of the form

$$\sum_{j=1}^{J} n_{i,j} x_j \leq q_i, \qquad (4.16)$$

which may be written in matrix notation as

$$Nx \leq q, \qquad (4.17)$$

and restate the reconstruction problem as a search for an image vector x which satisfies (4.17). One must bear in mind here that there may be no x which satisfies all inequalities in (4.17), and if there is one such x, then usually there are many others as well. Just as in the case when there is more than one minimizing vector of (4.14), we need a secondary criterion to select one of these vectors as the desired solution.

There have been two different kinds of secondary optimization criteria proposed in the reconstruction literature.

One of these is based on the minimization of the norm $\|x\|$, which we already discussed above. More generally, a unique solution will be ensured, if among all the image vectors which satisfy the primary criterion we require that the one to be chosen minimizes

$$\|D^{-1}x\|, \qquad (4.18)$$

where D is a positive definite symmetric $J \times J$ matrix. (D is *positive definite* if $x^{\mathrm{T}}Dx > 0$ for all nonzero vectors x.) As will be discussed below, some reconstruction techniques minimize (4.18) for different D's.

An alternative secondary criterion is applicable if the average value of the x_j's, $\bar{x}$, is known. In such a case there is at most one vector x for which $x_j \geq 0$, for $1 \leq j \leq J$, whose average value is $\bar{x}$ and which maximizes

$$-\sum_{j=1}^{J} (x_j/J\bar{x}) \ln(x_j/J\bar{x}). \qquad (4.19)$$

This has been referred to as the *maximum entropy* criterion. The use of this criterion is usually justified by arguments (which are too long to be reproduced here) aimed at showing that of all the pictures which satisfy the primary criterion, the maximum entropy solution has the smallest information content, and so it is least likely to mislead the user by the presence of spurious features.

The reason why one may assume that $\bar{x}$ is known is the following. Consider Fig. 2.8. For any source–detector pair, the ray sum divided by the length of intersection of the ray with the picture region (reconstruction region) gives an estimate of the average relative linear attenuation for that ray. If we have many such rays which provide a fairly uniform and dense covering of the reconstruction region, then the sum of all the ray sums divided by the sum of the lengths of intersections is a reasonable estimate of $\bar{x}$. For example, for our standard head phantom $\bar{x} = 0.1468$. The estimate of $\bar{x}$ obtained from the standard projection data (Section 5.6) by the method described above is 0.1461. This in spite of the fact that the standard projection data are contaminated with errors due to photon statistics, beam hardening, scatter, etc. Similarly, the estimate of $\bar{x}$ obtained from the standard parallel projection data is 0.1462. Such experiments justify the use of the method described above for the estimation of $\bar{x}$ in conjunction with optimization criteria, such as maximum entropy or minimum variance.

6.5 COMPUTATIONAL EFFICIENCY

In the succeeding chapters we show reconstructions of our head phantom from the standard projection data (or for the standard parallel data) using many different methods. In each case we also show the plot of the 63rd column and give the picture distance measures defined in Section 5.1.

In addition, we indicate the cost of the reconstruction in terms of computer time. All the algorithms are implemented in the SNARK77 programming system (see Chapter 4), and the times reported are the number of seconds used by the central processor of a Cyber 173 computer.

While these timings are given for the sake of completeness, they are not to be taken too seriously. A general framework of computer programs containing many different algorithms, such as SNARK77, is by necessity not as efficient for any single algorithm as a program specially written for that purpose. Thus the absolute, and even the relative, values of computer times quoted below may be misleading. Implementations of algorithms used in actual CT scanners usually involve machine level programming and even special purpose hardware, making the execution of reconstructions orders of magnitude faster than what is possible using SNARK77. (The reason for using SNARK77 is ease of implementation; it would be quite beyond the capability of an individual to implement all algorithms to be reported on in this book by programming at the machine level of the computer.)

This attitude towards timing reflects the fact that electronic hardware used for calculation is getting cheaper and cheaper at an amazing rate. It is unlikely that an efficacious reconstruction algorithm would for long remain unused solely because of computational considerations.

An illustration of the irrelevance of the timings as far as "honest-to-goodness" CT is concerned is given in Section 10.6.

NOTES AND REFERENCES

Much of the material in this chapter is based on the survey paper on iterative reconstruction algorithms by Herman and Lent (1976a). That paper contains discussions of and references to many earlier publications concerning reconstruction algorithms based on the series expansion approach and optimization criteria.

A good coverage of Lebesgue integrals and square integrable functions, operators, and linear functionals is given by Kolmogorov and Fomin (1957, 1961).

Our treatment of the inverse Radon transform adapted the approach and notation of Rowland (1979). A thorough mathematical discussion of Hilbert transforms can be found in Butzer and Nessel (1971). References to literature on derivations of the Radon inversion formula without assuming properties such as differentiability are given at the end of Chapter 16.

Our treatment of multivariate random variables is based on Sage and Melsa (1971). That book also contains a discussion of Bayes' theorem which provides the mathematical justification for the use of the Bayesian estimate.

The equivalence of the minimum norm and minimum variance criteria is shown, for example, by Herman, Lent, and Lutz (1978).

The maximum entropy formalism is a general scientific approach; there are whole books devoted to the subject; see, e.g., Levine and Tribus (1979). The suggestion that it be used for image reconstruction has first appeared in the open literature in Gordon *et al.* (1970). It has been extensively used in the related field of digital image restoration; see, e.g., Andrews and Hunt (1977). For recent works on the computation of maximum entropy solutions see Elfving (1978) and Minerbo (1979a) and their references.

Additional optimization criteria proposed in the literature include *maximum signal-to-noise power ratio* (Tanaka and Iinuma, 1975), *maximum likelihood* (Rockmore and Macovski, 1977) and *Kalman filter* (Wood *et al.* 1977). Hurwitz and Rumbaugh (1977) defined optimization criteria based on the *point response function* and compare these with the Bayesian criteria. (A discussion of the point response function is given in Section 10.3.).

Evidence regarding the great increase in speed and decrease in cost of electronic computing equipment in recent years can be found in the September 1977 special issue of *Scientific American*, devoted to microelectronics.

7

Backprojection

Backprojection methods of reconstruction do not in general produce as good images as the more sophisticated techniques to be discussed in the succeeding chapters. They are studied mainly because they indicate the nature of parts of the more sophisticated reconstruction procedures (both for transform methods and for some of the series expansion methods), and the need for the other steps in such procedures.

7.1 CONTINUOUS BACKPROJECTION

The simplest algorithm for reconstruction is to estimate the density at a point by adding all the ray sums of the rays through that point. This has been called both the *summation method* and the *backprojection method*.

Note that traditional tomography (see Section 2.2) is essentially a back-projection method. In Fig. 2.4, the linear attenuation at A is estimated by the summing up (integration) of the total density along the path from X_t to A_t as time t varies. Note that A_t is always the same point on the moving photographic plate P, and that A is the only point that two paths from X_t to A_t have in common at different times t. All forms of traditional tomography involving such coordinated movements of x-ray source and film are three-dimensional versions of the backprojection method.

As has been explained in some detail in Section 6.2, given a function p of two variables, the backprojection operator $\mathcal{B}$ produces another function $\mathcal{B}p$ of two polar variables, such that $[\mathcal{B}p](r, \phi)$ is obtained by integrating, as θ varies, the values of $p(\ell, \theta)$ with $\ell = r \cos(\theta - \phi)$. For fixed r, θ, and ϕ, $\ell = r \cos(\theta - \phi)$ denotes the distance from the origin of the line L through (r, ϕ) perpendicular to the line K making angle θ with the x axis (see Fig. 6.1). If $p(\ell, \theta)$ is the ray sum associated with the line L, we see that the mathematical idealization of the summation method described at the beginning of the section is to associate with the projection data p the estimated reconstruction $\mathcal{B}p$.

We first discuss basic objections to such a procedure as a method of reconstruction and then (in Section 7.2) we look at implementations of the procedure from the type of finite data we have to deal with in practice.

We have discussed in Section 6.2 the fact that the inverse of the Radon transform can be obtained by a series of operations: differentiation, Hilbert transform, backprojection, and normalization. Using only backprojection for reconstruction has little justification and is likely to produce blurred pictures. To see how this blurring occurs, consider the following intuitive argument.

Suppose we have taken a number of projections of an object consisting of a single point. The result of the reconstruction from these projections by the summation method would be a star-shaped object whose center is the original point (Fig. 7.1). Let us take equally spaced projections of a point from a full

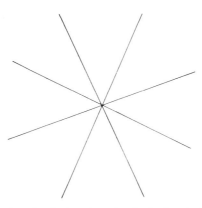

Fig. 7.1. Reconstruction of a single point using the backprojection method. Each line is due to a projection of the point in the corresponding direction.

range of directions. As we increase the number of views, a reconstruction from such projections comes to resemble a density distribution proportional to $1/r$, where r is distance from the point. This is because the limiting case of superposition of a number of equally spaced straight lines through a common point is equivalent to the rotation of a line about the point. The weight of each point of the straight line is distributed during rotation along the length of a circumference $2\pi r$.

This intuitive argument indicates that any implementation of the backprojection method is likely to blur out sharp features in the picture to be reconstructed. There is an even more basic, physical reason why backprojection alone cannot possible serve as a generally acceptable method of reconstruction in CT.

To understand this reason some knowledge of elementary physics is required. Essentially the reason is that the value produced by backprojection is of the wrong *dimensionality*. The relative linear attenuation (reconstruction of which is what we are after in CT) has dimensionality inverse length. That means that the value of relative linear attenuation is inversely proportional to the unit of length used; if it is 0.192 cm^{-1}, then it is 19.2 m^{-1}. As opposed to this, ray sums have no dimensionality, they are just probabilities. The result of summing up ray sums [or even integrating with respect to angle, see (2.6) of Chapter 6] will also be a dimensionless quantity. Hence, the result of the backprojection method does not depend on the unit of length used. If it happens to be a reasonable estimator of the distribution of the relative linear attenuation when the unit of length used is a centimeter, then it will be off by a factor of 100 when the unit of length is a meter. (In the next section we show that correct dimensionality can be reintroduced by certain normalization.)

To see that the same objection cannot be raised to the inverse Radon transform $\mathscr{R}^{-1}$, consider the dimensionality of the output of each step in the sequence of operations shown in (2.8) of the last chapter. If p is dimensionless, $\mathscr{D}_Y p$ has dimensionality inverse length [see (2.3) of Chapter 6]. Neither $\mathscr{H}_Y$, nor $\mathscr{B}$, nor normalization changes the dimensionality [see (2.5) and (2.6) of Chapter 6]. Hence $\mathscr{R}^{-1}p$ has the same dimensionality as $\mathscr{D}_Y p$, which is the correct dimensionality for the relative linear attenuation.

7.2   IMPLEMENTATION OF THE BACKPROJECTION OPERATOR

The summation method can be implemented by various "analog" devices. For example, an oscilloscope screen can be used on which we successively display lines whose positions correspond to rays for which the ray sums have been measured. The oscilloscope pattern is integrated on a photographic film, with the brightness (alternatively length of display) of a line modulated by the ray sum. The resulting picture on the film will be a backprojection reconstruction.

We shall not be concerned with such analog techniques. Our interest is in calculating the value of $[\mathscr{B}p](r, \phi)$ from the data y, where $y_i = p(\ell_i, \theta_i)$ for $1 \le i \le I$ (see Sections 6.1 and 6.2). We restrict our discussion to the parallel mode of data collection, with M equally spaced views and $2N + 1$ equally spaced parallel rays in each view. We use Δ to denote the angles between the views (thus $\Delta = \pi/M$) and d to denote the distance between the

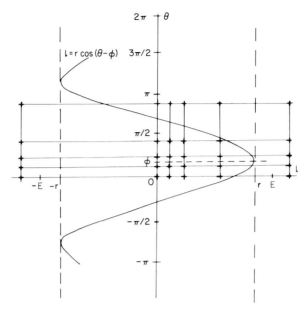

Fig. 7.2. Numerical evaluation of the backprojection operator is done by estimating the line integral along $l = r \cos(\theta - \phi)$ from the known values at the locations marked by a $+$.

parallel rays. We assume that $Nd > E > r$. Figure 7.2 is essentially a super-imposition of Figs 6.2 and 6.1b; it shows both the points at which the value of p is known and the line along which p has to be integrated to obtain

$$[\mathscr{B}p](r, \phi) = \int_0^{\pi} p(r \cos(\theta - \phi), \theta) \, d\theta. \tag{2.1}$$

A commonly used technique for numerically evaluating this integral is the following two-step process.

First we approximate the integral on the right-hand side of (2.1) by the sum

$$\Delta \sum_{m=0}^{M-1} p(r \cos(m\Delta - \phi), m\Delta). \tag{2.2}$$

(This is called a *Riemann sum* for the integral.) Second, we estimate, for each m, the value of $p(r \cos(m\Delta - \phi), m\Delta)$ from the known values $p(nd, m\Delta)$ $(-N \leq n \leq N)$ by *interpolation*.

Two commonly used methods of interpolation in CT are the *nearest neighbor* and the *linear* interpolations. The nearest neighbor interpolation estimates $p(r \cos(m\Delta - \phi), m\Delta)$ by the value of $p(nd, m\Delta)$ where n is chosen so that $|nd - r \cos(m\Delta - \phi)|$ is as small as possible. In linear interpolation, we select n so that $nd \leq r\cos(m\Delta - \phi) < (n + 1)d$ and estimate $p(r\cos(m\Delta - \phi), m\Delta)$ by

$$\frac{(n + 1)d - r\cos(m\Delta - \phi)}{d} p(nd, m\Delta)$$

$$+ \frac{r\cos(m\Delta - \phi) - nd}{d} p((n + 1)d, m\Delta). \quad (2.3)$$

In other words, numerical evaluation of $[\mathscr{B}p](r, \phi)$ using nearest neighbor interpolation is done as follows: add together the ray sums of the rays (one from each view) which are nearest to the point (r, ϕ) and multiply the result by Δ. Linear interpolation is slightly more complicated (and expensive); instead of single ray sums, we add linear interpolates of the ray sums of the two rays which lie on either side of the point (r, ϕ).

In order to produce a digitized picture, this calculation is repeated for the central point of each pixel and the outcome is assigned as the estimated density to the pixel. This digitized picture can be represented as a J-dimensional column vector x^*; see Section 6.3.

In view of the comments at the end of Section 7.1, it should be clear that this method may produce a digitized picture x^* whose average density $\bar{x}^*$ is very different from the average density $\bar{x}$ of the digitization x of the picture to be reconstructed. Since we usually have a good estimate $\bar{\bar{x}}$ of $\bar{x}$ (see the discussion at the end of Section 6.4), we can correct for this by *normalization* which maybe *additive* or *multiplicative*.

Additive normalization produces a digitized picture x^{**}, whose jth component is

$$x_j^{**} = x_j^* + (\bar{\bar{x}} - \bar{x}^*)/J. \quad (2.4)$$

Multiplicative normalization produces a digitized picture x^{**}, whose jth component is

$$x_j^{**} = x_j^*(\bar{\bar{x}}/\bar{x}^*). \quad (2.5)$$

(This is only applicable if $\bar{x}^* \neq 0$.) Note that in either case the average density of x^{**} is $\bar{\bar{x}}$.

An interesting property of multiplicative normalization is that the correct dimensionality is reintroduced. This is because $\bar{x}$ itself has dimensionality inverse length (it is a sum of dimensionless quantities divided by a sum of lengths) and so x_j^{**} has the correct dimensionality. On the other hand, (2.4) makes little physical sense: $\bar{x} - \bar{x}^*$ is the difference between a quantity measured in inverse length ($\bar{x}$) and a dimensionless quantity ($\bar{x}^*$). For this reason, multiplicative rather than additive normalization is recommended.

The methods described above have been applied to the standard parallel projection data using linear interpolation. The results are shown in Fig. 7.3,

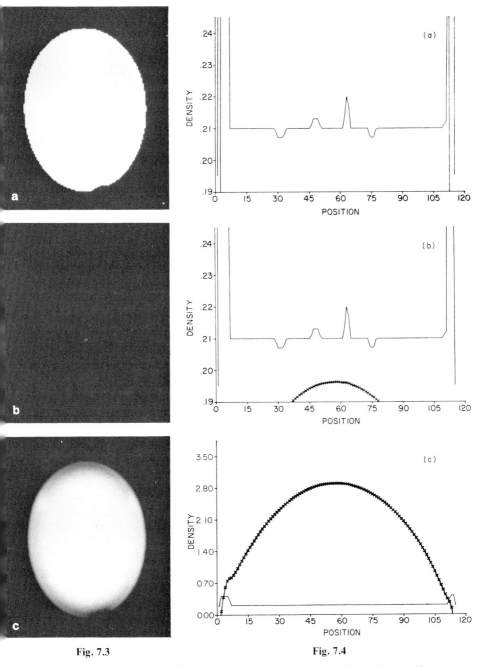

Fig. 7.3   Fig. 7.4

Fig. 7.3. Reconstructions of the standard parallel projection data using continuous backprojection with linear interpolation. (a) Additive normalization. (b) Multiplicative normalization. (c) Using a brightness/contrast setting other than the usual to bring out features in the reconstruction.

Fig. 7.4. Plots of the 63rd column in the reconstructions shown in Fig. 7.3. (a) In additive normalization the values are so large that the reconstruction is only visible as two near vertical lines at the two ends. (b) Multiplicative normalization. (c) Additive normalization plotted on a different scale.

with line plots for the 63rd column in Fig. 7.4. As can be seen, these techniques are not acceptable for examining the contents of the head. The image in Fig. 7.3b appears black, due to our convention of displaying values 0.1945 cm^{-1} or less as black (see Section 4.3). For this reason, we display the same image at a different brightness/contrast setting in Fig. 7.3c. The picture distance measures are given in Table 7.1.

TABLE 7.1

PICTURE DISTANCE MEASURES AND COMPUTER TIMES FOR "CONTINUOUS" BACKPROJECTION RECONSTRUCTIONS FROM STANDARD PARALLEL PROJECTION DATA.

Normalization	d	r	e	t
Additive	14.6040	12.0195	3.9950	125
Multiplicative	0.8111	0.5818	0.2731	125

7.3   DISCRETE BACKPROJECTION

In the last section we have produced a digitized picture by numerically evaluating the integral in (2.1) for the center points of the pixels. An alternative approach is provided by the series expansion method.

Consider the basis pictures which have value 1 within a pixel and 0 outside [defined by (3.1) of Chapter 6]. In this case $r_{i,j}$ is the (calculated) length of intersection of the ith ray with the jth pixel. The following basic criteria describe what we intuitively expect from an implementation of the backprojection method which uses pixels.

(i)   A ray should contribute to those pixels which it intersects and to no others.

(ii)   The contribution of the ith ray to a pixel should be proportional to y_i (the measured ray sum for the ith ray).

(iii)   The contribution of the ith ray to the jth pixel should be proportional to $r_{i,j}$.

All these criteria are satisfied if we estimate the density x_j^* in the jth pixel by

$$x_j^* = \sum_{i=1}^{I} r_{i,j} y_i. \tag{3.1}$$

This can be expressed in matrix notation as

$$x^* = R^{T} y, \tag{3.2}$$

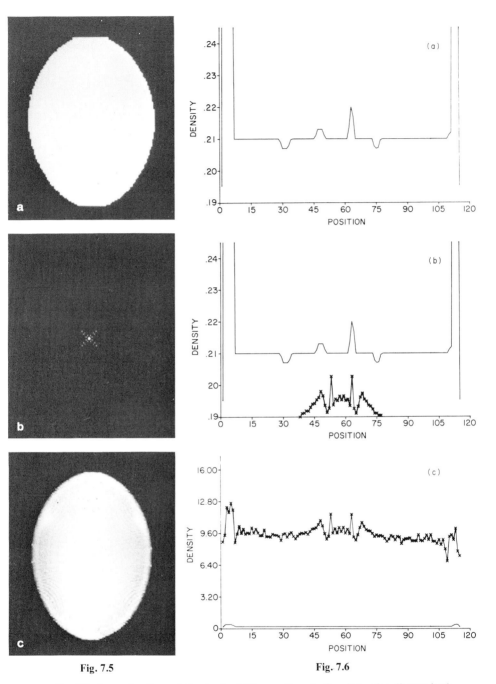

Fig. 7.5   Fig. 7.6

Fig. 7.5. Reconstructions of the standard (divergent) projection data using discrete back-projection. (a) Additive normalization. (b) Multiplicative normalization. (c) Using a brightness/contrast setting other than usual to bring out features in the reconstruction.

Fig. 7.6. Plots of the 63rd column in the reconstructions shown in Fig. 7.5. See comments in legend of Fig. 7.4.

where R^T (the *transpose* of the matrix R) is the matrix whose (i, j)th element is $r_{j,i}$. (Implementational details are deferred until Section 11.1.)

The argument given above does not depend in any essential way on the basis functions being pixels. We consider, in general, (3.2) to be the back-projection solution of the discrete reconstruction problem with projection matrix R. In particular, we refer to multiplication of an (I-dimensional) vector by R^T as *discrete backprojection*.

Just as in the case of continuous backprojection, the average density of x^* may be quite different from that of the picture to be reconstructed. In such a case the additive or multiplicative normalization procedures, see (2.4) and (2.5), can be applied to advantage. This of course only makes sense if the series expansion is a digitization.

Discrete backprojection, as expressed by (3.2), is applicable to any method of data collection. When applied to the standard parallel projection data it gives results very similar in appearance to those shown in Fig. 7.3. When applied to the standard (divergent) projection data it gives slightly different looking results, which are shown in Fig. 7.5, with line plots for the 63rd column in Fig. 7.6. This is further illustrated in Table 7.2.

TABLE 7.2

PICTURE DISTANCE MEASURES AND COMPUTER TIMES FOR
DISCRETE BACKPROJECTION FROM STANDARD (DIVERGENT)
PROJECTION DATA

Normalization	d	r	e	t
Additive	80.5233	66.8735	25.2084	295
Multiplicative	0.8109	0.5818	0.2727	297

NOTES AND REFERENCES

The backprojection method in various analog and digital implementa-tions has been proposed by a number of authors. For a history, see Gordon and Herman (1974). The particular analog technique described in Section 7.2 is taken from Kuhl and Edwards (1963).

Numerical evaluation of integrals, and in particular Riemann sums, are discussed in detail by Davis and Rabinowitz (1967). A discussion of alterna-tive modes of numerical evaluation of the integral in (2.1) is given by Brooks and Weiss (1976).

Interpolation methods other than the ones we have mentioned have been studied by a number of authors in conjunction with the backprojection operator. Rowland (1979) gave an exhaustive evaluation of the Lagrange interpolation methods. Oppenheim (1977) proposed the use of modified cubic splines; this has been further evaluated by Herman, Rowland, and Yau (1979). Weiss and Stein (1978) discuss a "Fourier" interpolation technique.

A backprojection operator for divergent beam geometry [third and fourth scanning modes, see Figs. 3.3c and d] is discussed by Gullberg (1977).

8

Convolution Method for Parallel Beams

The most commonly used methods in CT for parallel beam projection data are the convolution methods. The reason for this is ease of implementation combined with good accuracy. These methods are transform methods, where the taking of the derivative and the Hilbert transform is approximated by the use of a single convolution.

8.1 Convolutions, Hilbert Transforms, Regularization

Given two functions ϕ and ψ over the real numbers, their *convolution* $\phi * \psi$ is another function over the real numbers defined by

$$[\phi * \psi](v) = \int_{-\infty}^{\infty} \phi(u)\psi(v - u) \, du. \tag{1.1}$$

Note that it is possible that, for certain values of v, $[\phi * \psi](v)$ is not defined [because the integral on the right-hand side of (1.1) does not exist]. According to our earlier convention we shall not worry about such mathematical niceties; for now we assume that $[\phi * \psi](v)$ is defined whenever we need it.

Note that convolution is an operator which acting on two functions ϕ and ψ, produces a third function $\phi * \psi$. It is easy to show that $\phi * \psi = \psi * \phi$, in the sense that, for all v,

$$[\phi * \psi](v) = [\psi * \phi](v). \tag{1.2}$$

We have already come across an example of convolution: the *Hilbert transform* $\mathcal{H}\phi$ of a function ϕ can be defined as the convolution of ϕ with the function ρ such that

$$\rho(u) = -(1/\pi u) \tag{1.3}$$

118

In other words, we may write

$$\mathscr{H}\phi = \phi * \rho, \tag{1.4}$$

where ρ is defined by (1.3). Combining (1.1), (1.3), and (1.4) we get

$$[\mathscr{H}\phi](v) = -\frac{1}{\pi}\int_{-\infty}^{\infty}\frac{\phi(u)}{v - u}\,du. \tag{1.5}$$

The right-hand side of (1.5) is what is called an *improper integral* both of the *first kind* and of the *second kind*. It is an improper integral of the first kind because the limits of integration are $-\infty$ and ∞. This does not worry us in image reconstruction, since the values of $\phi(u)$ are zero outside a finite range. This can be seen by comparing (1.5) with (2.4) of Chapter 6. We see that Hilbert transforms arise in image reconstruction with $\phi(u) = q(u, \theta)$, for some fixed θ, where

$$\phi(u) = q(u, \theta) = [\mathscr{D}_Y p](u, \theta) = [\mathscr{D}_Y \mathscr{R}f](u, \theta) = 0 \tag{1.6}$$

if $|u| \geq E$. [See Chapter 6, formulas (2.4), (2.3), and (1.6).]

The right-hand side of (1.5) is also an improper integral of the second kind, since the integrand diverges at $u = v$. We interpret the integral in its Cauchy principal value sense, i.e.,

$$[\mathscr{H}\phi](v) = -\frac{1}{\pi}\lim_{\varepsilon \to 0}\left\{\int_{-\infty}^{v-\varepsilon}\frac{\phi(u)}{v - u}\,du + \int_{v+\varepsilon}^{\infty}\frac{\phi(u)}{v - u}\,du\right\}. \tag{1.7}$$

Even if this integral exists, its numerical evaluation may be far from straightforward. One approach is the method of *regularization*.

This method consists of defining a set $\{\rho_A | A > 0\}$ of functions on the real numbers, where the subscript A is a positive real number. Roughly speaking, the idea is that ρ_A should be so chosen that, for the ϕ's that we are interested in,

$$\lim_{A \to \infty} \phi * \rho_A = \mathscr{H}\phi, \tag{1.8}$$

and for any fixed A the convolution on the left-hand side of (1.8) is easy to evaluate.

To make this more precise we have to define the class of functions ϕ for which (1.8) is true. In Section 16.7 we define precisely the terminology "the function ϕ is *reasonable* at the point v." For now we may simply assume that the functions ϕ we are dealing with are reasonable at all points. We call a set $\{\rho_A | A > 0\}$ of functions a *regularizing family*, if, for any function ϕ over the real numbers and any real number v such that ϕ is reasonable at v,

$$\lim_{A \to \infty} [\phi * \rho_A](v) = [\mathscr{H}\phi](v). \tag{1.9}$$

Numerical evaluation of $[\mathscr{H}\phi](v)$ can now be carried out by numerical evaluation of $[\phi * \rho_A](v)$, with A chosen sufficiently large so that the left-hand side of (1.9) is near enough to its right-hand side for our purpose. If the ρ_A have some nice properties (e.g., boundedness, differentiability, etc.), then $[\phi * \rho_A](v)$ may be quite easy to evaluate numerically. In particular, if ϕ is the derivative of another function, one may use integration by parts to evaluate $[\phi * \rho_A](v)$. This is in fact the case in our application, as can be seen in (1.6).

The preceding discussion hinges on the existence of a regularizing family. In fact, there is a large variety of regularizing families, as can be seen from the following result, which is proved in Section 16.7. We refer to this result as the *regularization theorem*.

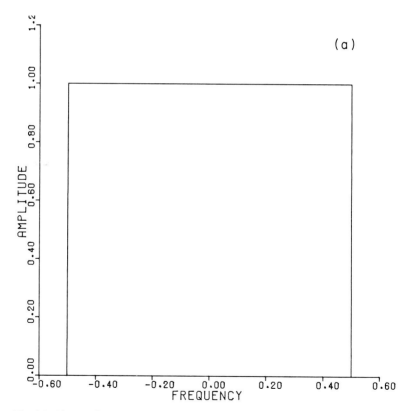

Fig. 8.1. Shapes of the generalized Hamming window for different values of α. (a) $\alpha = 1.0$ (same as bandlimiting). (b) $\alpha = 0.8$. (c) $\alpha = 0.54$. In all cases A is assumed to be 1. The U axis is labeled as "frequency," the $F_A(U)$ axis is labeled as "amplitude," and $F_A(U)$ is defined for negative values of U by assuming that F_A is symmetric.

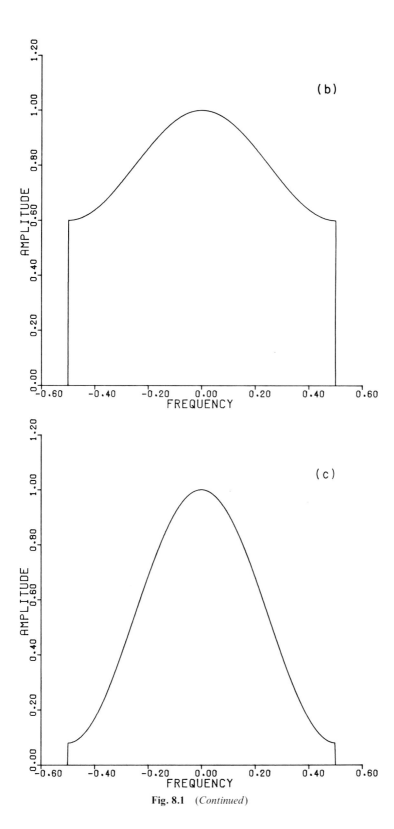

Fig. 8.1 (*Continued*)

For each real number A, let F_A be a real valued integrable function such that for $U \geq 0$

(i) $0 \leq F_A(U) \leq 1$, $F_A(U) = 0$ if $U \geq A/2$,
(ii) $F_A(U)$ is a monotonically nonincreasing function of U,
(iii) $\lim_{A \to \infty} F_A(U) = 1$.

Let

$$\rho_A(u) = -2 \int_0^{A/2} F_A(U)\sin(2\pi U u)\, dU. \tag{1.10}$$

Then $\{\rho_A | A > 0\}$ is a regularizing family of functions.

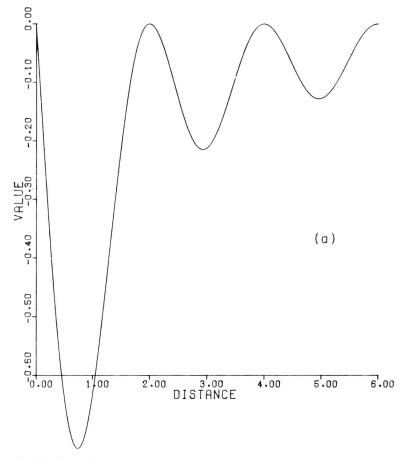

Fig. 8.2. Plots of ρ_A corresponding to the windows in Fig. 8.1. The u axis is labeled as "distance," the $\rho(u)$ axis is labeled as "value." Note that ρ is antisymmetric, i.e., $\rho(-u) = -\rho(u)$ [see (1.10)].

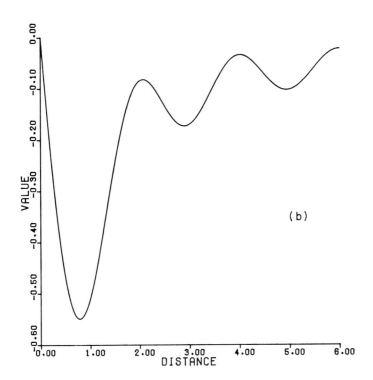

(b)

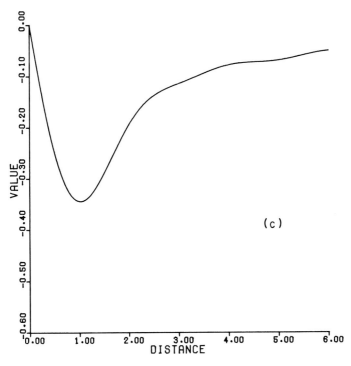

(c)

Fig. 8.2 (*Continued*)

For reasons which become clear later, the F_A in this result is often referred to as a *window with bandwidth A.*

It is easy to produce families of windows satisfying conditions (i)–(iii). In Table 8.1 we give a few examples, together with names commonly used for them. In all cases the definition is valid only for $0 \leq U < A/2$, since for $U \geq A/2$, $F_A(U) = 0$, according to (i). Note that the bandlimiting window is the same as the generalized Hamming window with parameter $\alpha = 1$. The shape of some windows is shown in Fig. 8.1, and the corresponding ρ_A are shown in Fig. 8.2.

TABLE 8.1

Definitions of Some Commonly Used Windows

Name of window	$F_A(U)$
Bandlimiting	1
Cosine	$\cos(\pi U/A)$
Sinc	$\sin(\pi U/A)/(\pi U/A)$
Generalized Hamming[a] with parameter α ($0.5 \leq \alpha \leq 1$)	$\alpha + (1 - \alpha)\cos(2\pi U/A)$

[a] If $\alpha = 0.5$, the generalized Hamming window is called the *hanning* window. If $\alpha = 0.54$, the generalized Hamming window is called the *Hamming* window.

8.2 Derivation of the Convolution Method

We are now going to show that the first two stages of evaluating the inverse Radon transform, namely differentiation of the data and taking the Hilbert transform [see (2.8) of Chapter 6], can be approximated by a simple convolution of the data with a fixed convolving function.

As in Section 6.2, let p be the function of two variables whose inverse Radon transform we wish to find. For the time being, let us consider θ fixed and define

$$p_\theta(\ell) = p(\ell, \theta). \tag{2.1}$$

Then, for any ℓ',

$$[\mathscr{H}_Y \mathscr{D}_Y p](\ell', \theta) = [\mathscr{H} p'_\theta](\ell'), \tag{2.2}$$

where p'_θ is the derivative of p_θ.

In view of (1.9), the right-hand side of (2.2) can be approximated by

$$[p'_\theta * \rho_A](\ell') = \int_{-\infty}^{\infty} p'_\theta(\ell)\rho_A(\ell' - \ell)\, d\ell. \tag{2.3}$$

Now observe that $p'_\theta(\ell) = 0$ if $|\ell| \geq E$. Note also that if ρ_A is defined by (1.10) and F_A satisfies conditions (i)–(iii) in Section 8.1, then the derivative ρ'_A of ρ_A exists and

$$\rho'_A(u) = -4\pi \int_0^{A/2} U F_A(U)\cos(2\pi U u)\, dU. \tag{2.4}$$

(Here we made use of the standard technique which in mathematical analysis is usually referred to as "differentiation under the integral sign.") Using these facts, we can integrate the right-hand side of (2.3) by parts and obtain

$$[p'_\theta * \rho_A](\ell') = \int_{-\infty}^{\infty} p_\theta(\ell)\rho'_A(\ell' - \ell)\, d\ell. \tag{2.5}$$

Let us define p_A by

$$p_A(\ell', 0) = [p_\theta * \rho'_A](\ell'). \tag{2.6}$$

Combining the facts just stated, we can say that $[\mathcal{H}_Y \mathcal{D}_Y p](\ell', 0)$ is approximated by $p_A(\ell', 0)$. This leads us to define the estimate f^* produced by the convolution method as

$$f^* = -(1/2\pi)\mathcal{B}p_A \tag{2.7}$$

[see (2.8) and (2.2) of Chapter 6].

We now introduce notation that allows us to describe concisely the convolution method.

We define a new operator $*_Y$, which we call *convolution with respect to the first variable*. It associates with a function p of two variables and a function q of one variable a new function $p *_Y q$ of two variables, defined by

$$[p *_Y q](\ell, 0) = [p_\theta * q](\ell), \tag{2.8}$$

where p_θ is defined by (2.1).

The mathematical idealization of the convolution method of reconstruction (with *convolving function q*) is the estimate f^* defined by

$$f^* = \mathcal{B}(p *_Y q). \tag{2.9}$$

The functions defined by (2.7) and (2.9) are the same provided that

$$q(u) = -(1/2\pi)\rho'_A(U). \tag{2.10}$$

Substitution into (2.4) gives

$$q(u) = 2 \int_0^{A/2} U F_A(U) \cos(2\pi U u) \, dU. \qquad (2.11)$$

In Fig. 8.3 we show plots of q determined by different choices of F_A.

To summarize, the convolution method of reconstruction approximates the inverse Radon transform in two steps:

(i)   a convolution with respect to the first variable; and
(ii)   a backprojection.

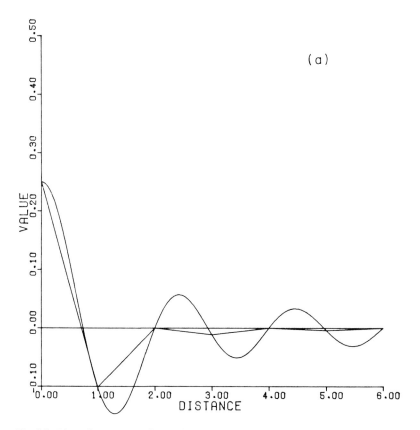

Fig. 8.3. Plots of q corresponding to the windows in Fig. 8.1. The q's are the curves with the continuous derivative. The u axis is labeled as "distance," the $q(u)$ axis is labeled as "value." Note that q is symmetric [see (2.11)]. The piecewise linear curves connect up those values of the q's at which the u's are sampled in the discrete convolution of (3.2), assuming that $d = 1$.

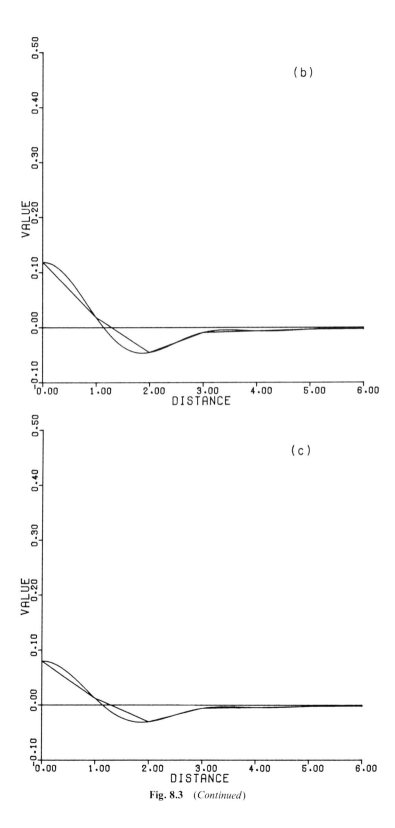

Fig. 8.3 (*Continued*)

The convolving function in the first step is usually chosen by (2.11), where F_A is one of a family of windows satisfying (i)–(iii) of Section 8.1. How this window is to be chosen is discussed in Section 8.6.

8.3   IMPLEMENTATION OF THE CONVOLUTION METHOD

In Section 7.2 we have discussed how the backprojection operator is implemented. That discussion assumed that the function p to be back-projected is known at points $(nd, m\Delta)$, $-N \leq n \leq N, 0 \leq m \leq M - 1$, and $M\Delta = \pi$. In order to apply the techniques developed there we need to calculate the values of $p *_Y q$ at these points from the values of p at the same points.

Combining (2.8) with (1.1) we get

$$[p *_Y q](n'd, m\Delta) = \int_{-\infty}^{\infty} p(\ell, m\Delta)q(n'd - \ell)\,d\ell. \qquad (3.1)$$

Recall that $p(\ell, \theta)$ is projection data [and hence we can assume that $p(\ell, \theta) = 0$ if $|\ell| \geq E$] and our assumption in Section 7.2 that $Nd \geq E$. Then a Riemann sum approximation to the integral on the right-hand side of (3.1) is

$$p_c(n'd, m\Delta) = d \sum_{n=-N}^{N} p(nd, m\Delta)q((n' - n)d). \qquad (3.2)$$

The sum in (3.2) is referred to as a *discrete convolution*.

We now bring together the total process of calculating $f^*(r, \phi)$ for projection data collected along equally spaced parallel rays at equal angular increments. More precisely, we assume that we have estimates $p(nd, m\Delta)$ of $[\mathscr{R}f](nd, m\Delta)$ for integers n and m with $-N \leq n \leq N$ and $0 \leq m \leq M - 1$.

   (i)   For each m, $0 \leq m < M - 1$, we evaluate $p_c(n'd, m\Delta)$ for $-N \leq n' \leq N$ using (3.2). The number of points at which p_c is calculated is $I = (2N + 1)M$, and the associated I-dimensional vector y_c is often referred to as the *convolved projection data*.

   (ii) $f^*(r, \phi)$ is calculated using (2.2) of Chapter 7, but with p_c in place of p. This involves interpolation for estimating $p_c(r \cos(m\Delta - \phi), m\Delta)$ from values of $p_c(n'd, m\Delta)$.

There are a number of computational points which need to be emphasized.

Since $-N \leq n \leq N$ and $-N \leq n' \leq N$, the values of q need to be known for at most $4N + 1$ points. For a fixed geometry of data collection, these values can be precalculated and used with the different sets of measured projection data. [In fact, usually $q(-v) = q(v)$; see (2.11). In such a case q needs to be calculated for only $2N + 1$ points.] See Fig. 8.3, for some of these points for the windows shown in Fig. 8.1.

For any fixed m, the values of $p_c(n'd, m\Delta)$, $-N \leq n' \leq N$, are obtained from the values of $p(nd, m\Delta)$, $-N \leq n \leq N$. Hence the projection data in one view (i.e., in one set of parallel rays) completely determines the convolved projection data in that view. Evaluation of (3.2) for a particular view can begin as soon as all data for that view are collected, and does not need any data from the other views.

Similarly, the contribution to $f^*(r, \phi)$ of the convolved projection data $p_c(nd, m\Delta)$, for any one view (i.e., m fixed, n varies), can be calculated from that view alone, since the interpolations described in Section 7.2 estimate $p_c(r \cos(m\Delta - \phi), m\Delta)$ from values of $p_c(nd, m\Delta)$ with $-N \leq n \leq N$.

Hence, in practice, the process of convolution followed by backprojection need not be repeated for every (r, ϕ) at which $f^*(r, \phi)$ is evaluated. Instead, the computer algorithm operates as follows.

A sequence $f_0, \ldots, f_{M-1}, f_M$ of digitized pictures is produced, by assigning to the jth pixel the value at its center (r_j, ϕ_j). These values are calculated as follows.

$$f_0(r_j, \phi_j) = 0, \tag{3.3}$$

for $1 \leq j \leq J$. For each value of m, $0 \leq m \leq M - 1$, we produce the $(m + 1)$st picture from the mth picture by a two-step process.

(i)   Calculate $p_c(n'd, m\Delta)$ for $-N \leq n' \leq N$, from $p(nd, m\Delta)$ for $-N \leq n \leq N$, using (3.2) and the precalculated values of $q((n' - n)d)$.

(ii)   Let, for $1 \leq j \leq J$,

$$f_{m+1}(r_j, \phi_j) = f_m(r_j, \phi_j) + \Delta p_c(r_j \cos(m\Delta - \phi_j), m\Delta). \tag{3.4}$$

Interpolation may have to be used in evaluating (3.4).

The digitized picture f_M produced by this process is our estimate f^*. Note that once we have calculated $f_{m+1}(r_j, \phi_j)$ we no longer need $f_m(r_j, \phi_j)$, and so the computer can reuse the same memory location for $f_0(r_j, \phi_j)$, $f_1(r_j, \phi_j), \ldots, f^*(r_j, \phi_j)$.

The reader should make careful note of the following. The implementation, as just described, is more efficient than brute force implementation of the convolution/backprojection formulas repeatedly for all points $(r_1, \phi_1), \ldots,$ (r_J, ϕ_J). The efficiency comes from the observation that we do not have to calculate the convolution step described by (3.2) JM times (once for each pixel and each view), but only $(2N + 1)M$ times (once for each ray in each view). Since typically J is of the same order as $(2N + 1)^2$, this is a significant saving.

The only thing we have left vague in our discussion of the implementation of the convolution method is the choice of the convolving function. In order to discuss this choice intelligently, we need to know something about Fourier transforms and sampling.

8.4 FOURIER TRANSFORMS

Fourier transforms are operators which act on functions whose arguments are real, but whose values are *complex numbers*, i.e., numbers of the form $a + ib$, where a and b are real numbers and i denotes $\sqrt{-1}$. In particular, we use the notation $\exp[i\alpha]$ to denote the complex number $\cos \alpha + i(\sin \alpha)$. In fact, any complex number $a + ib$ can be written in the form $r \exp[i\alpha]$, by choosing r to be the positive square root of $a^2 + b^2$ and α so that $a \tan \alpha = b$. In such a case r is called the *modulus* and α is called an *argument* of $a + ib$. The modulus of $a + ib$ is often denoted by $|a + ib|$. Note that this is consistent with the notation $|a|$ for the absolute value of a real number a.

If ϕ is a complex valued function of a real variable, we define

$$\int_s^t \phi(u) \, du = \left(\int_s^t a(u) \, du \right) + i \left(\int_s^t b(u) \, du \right), \tag{4.1}$$

where a and b are the real valued functions such that $a(u) + ib(u) = \phi(u)$.

The *(one-dimensional) Fourier transform* is an operator which associates with a complex valued function ϕ of a real variable another complex valued function $\mathscr{F}\phi$ of a real variable, defined by

$$[\mathscr{F}\phi](U) = \int_{-\infty}^{\infty} \phi(u)\exp[-2\pi iUu] \, du. \tag{4.2}$$

The *(one-dimensional) inverse Fourier transform* is an operator which associates with a complex valued function ϕ of a real variable another complex valued function $\mathscr{F}^{-1}\phi$ of a real variable, defined by

$$[\mathscr{F}^{-1}\phi](u) = \int_{-\infty}^{\infty} \phi(U)\exp[2\pi iUu] \, dU. \tag{4.3}$$

A most important relationship between these operators is that for many functions ϕ (and we assume that the functions we use fall in this category)

$$\mathscr{F}^{-1}\mathscr{F}\phi = \mathscr{F}\mathscr{F}^{-1}\phi = \phi. \tag{4.4}$$

This is why $\mathscr{F}^{-1}$ is called the inverse Fourier transform.

In order to give an intuitive explanation of the relationship between a function and its Fourier transform we need to digress a little.

A *harmonic function* is a function of one of the types $R \cos(2\pi Uu + \alpha)$ or $R \sin(2\pi Uu + \alpha)$, where R, U, and α are constants and u is the variable. The *amplitude* of this function is $|R|$ (i.e., its value lies between $-R$ and $+R$) and the function is *periodic* with *period* $1/|U|$ [i.e., $R \cos(2\pi U(u + 1/|U|) + \alpha) = R \cos(2\pi Uu + \alpha)$, for all u]. The shape of just over a period of a harmonic function can be seen in Fig. 7.2. Since the function has $|U|$ complete periods in a unit interval, U is called the *frequency* of the function. The number α is called the *initial phase* of the function.

To get an intuitive feeling for the relationship between a function ϕ and its Fourier transform Φ consider the following.

$$\phi(u) = \int_{-\infty}^{\infty} |\Phi(U)| \cos(2\pi Uu + \alpha(U)) \, dU$$

$$+ i \int_{-\infty}^{\infty} |\Phi(U)| \sin(2\pi Uu + \alpha(U)) \, dU, \tag{4.5}$$

where $\alpha(U)$ is an argument of $\Phi(U)$. This is easily proved from (4.4), (4.3), and (4.1). Note that, for any fixed value of U, both of the integrands on the right-hand side of (4.5) are harmonic functions of u with frequency U, amplitude the same as the modulus of $\Phi(U)$, and initial phase the same as an argument of $\Phi(U)$. Roughly speaking (4.5) says that both the real and the imaginary part of the function ϕ can be "decomposed" into harmonic functions of different frequencies, and the amplitude and initial phase of the harmonic function with frequency U in this decomposition is determined by the value of the Fourier transform of ϕ at the point U.

It appears reasonable that the smoother the function ϕ is, the less important are the contributions of high frequency harmonic functions, i.e., for a smooth function ϕ we expect $[\mathscr{F}\phi](U)$ to be small for large U. This statement can be made mathematically precise, but this book is not the place for that. We are, however, very interested in functions ϕ which are *bandlimited*; i.e., which are such that $[\mathscr{F}\phi](U) = 0$ if $|U| \geq A/2$. In such a case A is said to be the *bandwidth* of ϕ. A function we are likely to come across in image reconstruction is probably not bandlimited, but usually there exists a bandlimited function which is practically indistinguishable from it.

We have, however, already introduced some bandlimited functions: in fact the convolving functions q as defined by (2.11) are bandlimited. In order to see this, we define

$$\Phi(U) = |U| F_A(|U|). \tag{4.6}$$

Note that $\Phi(U) = 0$ if $|U| \geq A/2$ and $\Phi(-U) = \Phi(U)$. Using these facts, substitution into (4.3) yields that

$$[\mathscr{F}^{-1}\Phi](u) = 2 \int_{0}^{A/2} \Phi(U) \cos(2\pi Uu) \, dU. \tag{4.7}$$

Comparison with (2.11) shows that $q(u) = [\mathscr{F}^{-1}\Phi](u)$, and so $\mathscr{F}q$ is the function Φ defined by (4.6). This shows that a convolving function based on a window of bandwidth A is a bandlimited function of the same bandwidth.

The following argument now appears quite natural. The F_A were introduced in Section 8.1, since they gave rise using (1.10), to a family $\{\rho_A | A > 0\}$ of regularizing functions. The purpose of such a family is to approximate the Hilbert transform; see (1.9). The approximation at any point can be made as accurate as we wish by choosing A large enough. The value of the functions F_A at any fixed point tends to 1 as A increases. So why not use instead of (4.6) its limit as A increases; namely define $\Phi(U) = |U|$? If we did this, it appears reasonable that we would get

$$\mathcal{R}^{-1}p = \mathcal{B}(p *_Y \mathcal{F}^{-1}\Phi); \tag{4.8}$$

i.e., we would have replaced the approximating formula (2.9) by one which gives $\mathcal{R}^{-1}p$ exactly. There is a major flaw in this argument; if Φ is defined by $\Phi(U) = |U|$, then $\mathcal{F}^{-1}\Phi$ is not defined, in the sense that the infinite integral on the right-hand side of the definition of the inverse Fourier transform (4.3) does not exist.

Hence this limiting argument fails, and we are still stuck with the problem of having to choose an F_A. The desire to approximate the Hilbert transform accurately seems to imply that A should be chosen large, but as we shall see, the nature of the data may dictate otherwise.

Let us now recall the notation of Section 8.2. The function of two variables whose inverse Radon transform we wish to estimate is denoted by p. For any angle θ, we define p_θ by (2.1). The convolution step consists of convolving p_θ with q for each θ; see (2.8). One way towards understanding how q should be chosen is to look at what convolving p_θ with q does to the Fourier transform of p_θ.

The important relevant result here is the *convolution theorem*. It states that the Fourier transform of the convolution of two functions is the product of their Fourier transforms, or in symbols

$$[\mathcal{F}[\phi * \psi]](U) = [\mathcal{F}\phi](U) \times [\mathcal{F}\psi](U). \tag{4.9}$$

Applying this theorem to our case we get

$$[\mathcal{F}[p_\theta * q]](U) = |U| F_A(|U|)[\mathcal{F}p_\theta](U). \tag{4.10}$$

What we see is the following. The value of the Fourier transform of $p_\theta * q$ at the point U is $|U| F_A(|U|)$ times the value of the Fourier transform of p_θ at the point U. This has many interesting consequences; for example, $p_\theta * q$ is a bandlimited function with bandwidth A. However, our real interest lies not in the approximate formula to the inverse Radon transform given in (2.9), but in the actual implementation described in Section 8.3. Hence, we need to look at the discrete versions of the convolution and Fourier transform operators.

8.5   SAMPLING AND INTERPOLATION

In (2.9) we have defined the estimate f^* produced by the mathematical idealization of the convolution method as the backprojection of $p *_Y q$, where p is the function of two variables whose inverse Radon transform we wish to find and q is the convolving function. In Section 8.3 we have pointed out that in practice the backprojection is applied not to $p *_Y q$, but to an approximation of it which we have denoted by p_c. In order to apply our approximation of the backprojection operator [see (2.2) of Chapter 7], $p_c(\ell, \theta)$ need to be known for those values of ℓ and θ which are of the form $\ell = r \cos(m\Delta - \phi)$ and $\theta = m\Delta$. Since the point (r, ϕ) at which we wish to estimate the picture can be anywhere in the picture region, p_c need to be defined at all points (ℓ, θ), where $-E \le \ell \le E$ and $\theta = m\Delta$ with m an integer in the range $0 \le m \le M - 1$. Defining p_c at these points has been done in two stages. First in (3.2), we have defined p_c explicitly at points $(n'd, m\Delta)$, where n' is an integer in the range $-N \le n' \le N$, and then we have stated that $p_c(r \cos(m\Delta - \phi), m\Delta)$ is obtained by interpolation from the values of $p_c(n'd, m\Delta)$. In this section we discuss the relationship between $p *_Y q$ and its approximation p_c.

Note, first of all, that the discussion here is concerned with functions which are essentially functions of one variable only. This is because, for any fixed $m\Delta$, $p_c(\ell, m\Delta)$ is defined based on the values of $p(\ell, m\Delta)$, i.e., on the values of $p_{m\Delta}(\ell)$, see (2.1). Hence we can rephrase our problem as follows.

Assume that p_θ is a function of one real variable such that $p_\theta(\ell) = 0$ if $|\ell| \ge E$ (where E is a positive real number) and that q is another function of one variable. Let d be a real number and N be an integer such that $Nd > E$. Define a new function t as follows. For integer values of n',

$$t(n'd) = d \sum_{n=-N}^{N} p_\theta(nd)q((n' - n)d). \tag{5.1}$$

For all values of the real variable ℓ, $t(\ell)$ is defined by interpolation from the values of $t(n'd)$.

Problem: Investigate how the choices of q and the method of interpolation influence the relationship between p_θ and t.

We have stated the problem in this particular form, since p_θ represents our projection data, which is given to us by our physical device. On the other hand, the choices of convolving function and of interpolation method are ours; it is the effect of these choices which is our current interest.

In order to be able to solve our problem, we have to discuss the nature of interpolation more precisely than we had to do until now. For every positive real number d (called the *sampling interval*) and every function on the real numbers ψ (called the *interpolating function*) we define an operator $\mathscr{I}_d^\psi$ (called the *interpolation operator* with sampling interval d and interpolating function ψ), which associates with any function ϕ of one real variable another function $\mathscr{I}_d^\psi \phi$ of one real variable defined by

$$[\mathscr{I}_d^\psi \phi](v) = \sum_{n=-\infty}^{\infty} \phi(nd)\psi(v - nd). \tag{5.2}$$

In practice the sum in (5.2) is usually finite, since in most applications the interpolating function assumes zero value outside a small interval. For example, for the nearest neighbor interpolation we can use the function ψ_n, defined by

$$\psi_n(u) = \begin{cases} 1 & \text{if} \quad -d/2 < u < d/2, \\ 0.5 & \text{if} \quad |u| = d/2, \\ 0 & \text{if} \quad |u| > d/2 \end{cases} \tag{5.3}$$

(we assume that the average is desired at a point exactly half-way between two sample points), and for linear interpolation we can use the function ψ_ℓ, defined by

$$\psi_\ell(u) = \begin{cases} 1 - |u/d| & \text{if} \quad |u| < d, \\ 0 & \text{if} \quad |u| \geq d. \end{cases} \tag{5.4}$$

Note that for both these interpolating functions

$$[\mathscr{I}_d^\psi \phi](nd) = \phi(nd), \tag{5.5}$$

for any function ϕ and any integer n. We call interpolating functions satisfying this property *proper interpolating functions*.

Let us assume that the function t of our problem is to be defined using a proper interpolating function ψ. The precise method of definition is the following. Define t at points $n'd$ (for all integers n') using (5.1). Then, using (5.2) with t in place of ϕ, we define $t \, (= \mathscr{I}_d^\psi t)$ at all real numbers u. Under these circumstances, we can characterize the Fourier transform of t as follows.

Let

$$F_1(U) = \sum_{k=-\infty}^{\infty} [\mathscr{F} p_\theta](U + k/d), \tag{5.6}$$

$$F_2(U) = \sum_{k=-\infty}^{\infty} [\mathscr{F} q](U + k/d), \tag{5.7}$$

and

$$F_3(U) = [\mathscr{F} \psi](U)/d. \tag{5.8}$$

Then

$$[\mathscr{F}t](U) = F_1(U) \times F_2(U) \times F_3(U). \tag{5.9}$$

The proof of this claim requires a more thorough mathematical background than what we have assumed in writing this book. This is unfortunate, since the claim has important implications for the convolution method. Our discussion in the next section of the choice of convolving and interpolating functions is based entirely on (5.6)–(5.9).

8.6   THE CHOICE OF CONVOLVING
AND INTERPOLATING FUNCTIONS

Equations (5.6)–(5.9) provide us with a handle on how to choose the convolving function q and the interpolating function ψ. The function t is supposed to be an approximation to $p_\theta * q$. By the convolution theorem (Section 8.4), the Fourier transform of $p_\theta * q$ is the product of the Fourier transforms of p_θ and of q. On the other hand the Fourier transform of t is expressed as the product of three terms in (5.9): $F_1(U)$, which depends on the projection data p_θ; $F_2(U)$, which depends on the convolving function q; and $F_3(U)$, which depends on the interpolating function ψ. Roughly speaking, we aim to identify F_1 with $\mathscr{F}p_\theta$, F_2 with $\mathscr{F}q$, and F_3 with a function whose value is always 1. However, the interrelations between the three functions are also important, especially since our aim previously stated turns out to be unachievable in practice. We deal with the functions F_1, F_2 and F_3 one by one.

The function F_1 in (5.6) is a periodic function with period $1/d$. (Recall that d is the sampling interval in the ℓ variable; in other words, d is the spacing between the parallel rays along which ray sums are collected.) If the projection data are reasonably smooth compared with the sampling distance, one finds that the value of $|[\mathscr{F}p_\theta](U)|$ is very small for $|U| > 1/2d$. (In other words, the amplitudes of high frequency harmonic functions in the Fourier decomposition of p_θ are small.) In such a case, for $|U| < 1/2d$,

$$F_1(U) \simeq [\mathscr{F}p_\theta](U), \tag{6.1}$$

which is desirable, since we wish to identify F_1 with $\mathscr{F}p_\theta$. However, (6.1) is clearly violated for $U > 1/2d$, since the values of F_1 outside the range $-1/2d \le U \le 1/2d$ are just periodic repeats of the values inside that range, while the values of $\mathscr{F}p_\theta$ for projection functions p_θ do not have this property. It follows that while we may use $F_1(U)$ to be an approximation to $[\mathscr{F}p_\theta](U)$ in the range $-1/2d < U < 1/2d$, we must not do this outside this range. If we can assume that the function p_θ is smooth relative to the sampling distance, a reasonable approximation to $[\mathscr{F}p_\theta](U)$ for $|U| \ge 1/2d$ is zero.

A very important point to consider is the following. If the values of $[\mathscr{F}p_\theta](U)$ are not insignificant for $|U| \geq 1/2d$, then we are in a serious difficulty. In such a case we have no idea how to approximate $\mathscr{F}p_\theta$ for large values of $|U|$. Even worse, (6.1) is no longer valid even in the range $-1/2d < U < 1/2d$ as can be seen by comparing (5.6), which defines $F_1(U)$, with (6.1), since the values $[\mathscr{F}p_\theta](U + k/d)$ cannot be ignored for $k \neq 0$. Thus, the amplitudes of high frequency components of p_θ influence the values of $F_1(U)$ for small values of $|U|$. This phenomenon is called *aliasing*; it is demonstrated in Fig. 8.4.

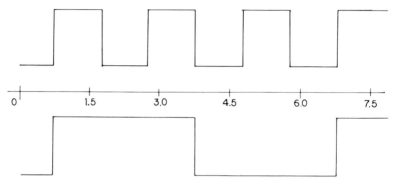

Fig. 8.4. Illustration of aliasing. The periodic function (shown on the top) with period 2 (frequency $\frac{1}{2}$) is sampled at the sampling interval 1.5. Nearest neighbor interpolation gives a function (shown on the bottom) with period 6 (frequency $\frac{1}{6}$).

What is happening here is the following. If we do not sample p_θ finely enough, not only do we lose information about the high frequency components of our data, but we also contaminate the low frequency components. A priori knowledge (see Section 6.4) may help us to recover from such a situation, but the convolution method does not make use of such knowledge. If we cannot sample finer (and machine design usually limits our sampling rate), we just have to accept that in those cases where the projection data have significant high frequency components we obtain low quality reconstructions.

Of course, the change in amplitude is unlikely to be abrupt at the frequency $1/2d$. It is to be expected that the amplitudes slightly over $1/2d$ are small but not totally insignificant. In this case aliasing does not affect the amplitudes at significantly smaller frequencies than $1/2d$ see Fig. 8.5. We thus have a fairly typical intermediate situation between the ideal (but unobtainable) case of bandlimited projection data (with bandwidth $1/d$) and the totally hopeless case where frequencies up to $3/2d$ have large amplitudes. In this intermediate situation $F_1(U)$ approximates $[\mathscr{F}p_\theta](U)$ well for small

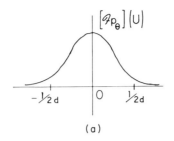

(a)

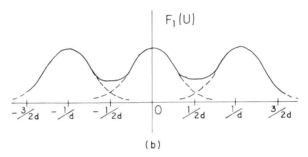

(b)

Fig. 8.5. The amplitudes at frequencies near $\pm 1/2d$ in $\mathscr{F}p_\theta$ affect the values of $F_1(U)$ only near $\pm 1/2d$. In the illustration both (a) $\mathscr{F}p_\theta$ and (b) F_1 are shown as if they were real valued. In practice they will be complex valued, but the moduli of their values have the behavior indicated in the figure.

values of $|U|$, but the approximation deteriorates as U approaches $\pm 1/2d$, becoming useless past those points.

One other point needs to be mentioned in our consideration of F_1 as an approximation to $\mathscr{F}p_\theta$. Since we are discussing data obtained from physical experiments, the values of p_θ only approximate the values of the Radon transform of the picture f we wish to reconstruct. We may write p_θ as

$$p_\theta = \mathscr{R}_\theta f + n_\theta, \tag{6.2}$$

where

$$[\mathscr{R}_\theta f](\ell) = [\mathscr{R}f](\ell, \theta). \tag{6.3}$$

From the definition of Fourier transform (4.2) we see that, for all U,

$$[\mathscr{F}p_\theta](U) = [\mathscr{F}\mathscr{R}_\theta f](U) + [\mathscr{F}n_\theta](U). \tag{6.4}$$

Since n_θ represents the noise in our data, $|[\mathscr{F}n_\theta](U)|$ (amplitude in the noise at frequency U) can be considered as a sample from a random variable. (Recall the discussion in Chapter 3, especially Section 3.1). The expected value of this random variable is about the same for all values of U. On the other hand, for sufficiently smooth $\mathscr{R}_\theta f$, $|[\mathscr{F}\mathscr{R}_\theta f](U)|$ gets to be small as $|U|$ approaches $1/2d$. Hence the values $[\mathscr{F}p_\theta](U)$ when $|U|$ is near $1/2d$ are often determined more by the noise in the data than by the Radon transform of the function we wish to reconstruct. This observation also influences our selection of the convolving and interpolating functions.

We illustrate the nature of the function F_1 by plotting, in Fig. 8.6, $|F_1(U)|$ for the standard parallel projection data for the angle $\theta = 0$.

The function F_2 defined by (5.7) appears to have the same relationship

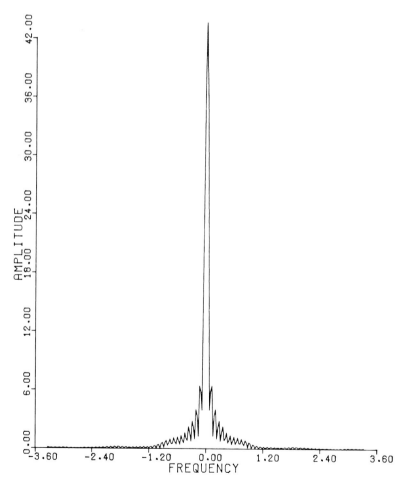

Fig. 8.6. The function $|F_1(U)|$ for the standard projection data for angle $\theta = 0$. Since the sampling interval is $d = 0.1504$, the value of $1/2d$ is slightly smaller than 3.33. Past $\pm 1/2d$ the values of the function are periodic repeats of the values between $-1/2d$ and $+1/2d$.

to q as F_1 has to p_θ. However, the situation here is much simpler, since the choice of q is under our control.

In the first place, we can select q so that it is bandlimited with bandwidth no greater than $1/d$. If we do that, then, for $|U| < 1/2d$,

$$F_2(U) = [\mathscr{F}q](U), \tag{6.5}$$

where we now have a precise equality, rather than an approximation as in (6.1).

The discussion in Section 8.4 shows that the convolving functions which arise out of the regularization arguments of Sections 8.1 and 8.2 are indeed bandlimited. In fact, $\mathscr{F}q$ is the function Φ defined by (4.6). If we choose A to be no greater than $1/d$, then (6.5) is satisfied.

We now have to resolve a dilemma: the regularization argument suggested that A should be as large as possible, but now we are talking about restricting it to $1/d$. The resolution of the dilemma comes from the recognition that we are working in two different contexts. In the mathematical idealization a high value of A appears desirable. In the practical implementation there appears to be just about no point in having A higher than $1/d$. $F_2(U)$ is used as one term in a product where another term is $F_1(U)$. This term is already known to be totally unreliable for $|U| > 1/2d$; we may as well give up making $F_2(U)$ reliable for such values of U. On the other hand, by making $F_2(U)$ equal to $[\mathscr{F}q](U)$ within the range $-1/2d < U < 1/2d$, we make our second approximation as precise as possible in the range where it matters.

It also appears that there is no reason to choose A anything but $1/d$. This is the highest possible value within the constraints just discussed, hence it is desirable based on the regularization argument. Often the values of q at multiples of d become easy to calculate when q is defined as $[\mathscr{F}^{-1}\Phi]$, with $\Phi(U) = |U|F_{1/d}(|U|)$ [see (4.6), and Fig. 8.3, especially the bandlimiting window]. Finally, if for some family of windows $\{F_A\}$ a choice of A which is $A_0 < 1/d$ appears ideal, then there is very likely to be another family of windows $\{G_A\}$, such that $G_{1/d} = F_{A_0}$. From now on, therefore, we assume that $A = 1/d$, i.e., that the bandwidth of our window is the inverse of our sampling interval.

Assuming that we remain with the formulation that q is $\mathscr{F}^{-1}\Phi$, where Φ is defined by (4.6), the question still remains: How do we choose the window $F_A(U)$? The regularization argument in Section 8.4 indicates, that for the families of windows under discussion the ideal limiting value of Φ is given by $\Phi(U) = |U|$. One may therefore argue that the bandlimiting window, which sets Φ to this ideal value in the range up to $A/2$, may be the best. However, the regularization argument is based on the assumption of perfect data. As we have seen in our discussion on the nature of F_1, the values of $F_1(U)$ for U

near $1/2d$ may be far from the ideal assumed in the regularization argument. Furthermore, since in this case we would have $F_2(U) = |U|$, F_2 would multiply F_1 by the largest values where F_1 is least reliable.

From all this we may conclude the following. If the data collection is very reliable and if $\mathscr{F}p_\theta$ is very nearly bandlimited with bandwidth $1/d$, then it is appropriate to choose q so that $[\mathscr{F}_2 q](U) = F_2(U) = |U|$ for $-1/2d \leq U \leq 1/2d$. However, if there is considerable noise in the data or if there are aliasing errors near $1/2d$, then a choice of an $F_A(U)$ which is small for U near $1/2d$ is more likely to produce good results, since it avoids multiplication of the erroneous amplitudes at frequencies near $1/2d$ by the relatively large value of $|U|$. The exact choice of the filter must be dependent on the data collection method and the type of object which is to be reconstructed.

Finally, we come to the discussion of F_3. Under ideal circumstances $F_3(U)$ should have the value 1 everywhere. In real life a very different objective occurs. We have assumed that $[\mathscr{F}p_\theta](U)$; and hence the product $[\mathscr{F}p_\theta](U) \times [\mathscr{F}q](U)$, is nearly zero if $|U| > 1/2d$. However, both F_1 and F_2 are periodic with period $1/d$. Thus, for $|U| > 1/2d$, the product $F_1(U) \times F_2(U)$ is unlikely to be near zero. We can use $F_3(U)$ to remedy this situation. Thus, it is desirable to have $|F_3(U)|$ small if $|U| > 1/2d$. Even for $|U| < 1/2d$, we may not wish $F_3(U)$ to have the value 1. This is because $F_3(U)$ can be used, in conjunction with $F_2(U)$, to suppress the erroneous values in $F_1(U)$ when $|U|$ is near $1/2d$. Hence, a desirable F_3 is one which has value 1 at the origin, but dies away as it nears $1/2d$ and remains near zero past $1/2d$.

In Fig. 8.7 we plot the values of $F_3(U)$ for the nearest neighbor and the linear interpolation. In view of the comments just made, it is not surprising that linear interpolation usually leads to better reconstructions than the nearest neighbor interpolation.

We illustrate this discussion using a number of experiments all involving the standard parallel projection data. (Further discussion of the choice of the convolving function is given in Section 10.2.)

In Fig. 8.8 we show reconstructions using linear interpolation and the generalized Hamming window with three different values of the parameter α. The case $\alpha = 1$ is the same as the bandlimiting window; there is no suppression of frequencies near $U = 1/2d$. The case $\alpha = 0.54$ is near the other extreme; it is the Hamming window. The case $\alpha = 0.8$ is in between these extremes. Note that smaller values of α give smoother looking pictures (suppression of high frequency harmonics), but this may eliminate tumors as well as noise. Figure 8.9 plots values along the 63rd column and Table 8.2 reports on the picture distance measures and the computer times.

In Figs. 8.10 and 8.11 and Table 8.3, we compare the linear and nearest neighbor methods of interpolation, when the filter is the Hamming filter with $\alpha = 0.8$. Both the figures indicate that linear interpolation is clearly

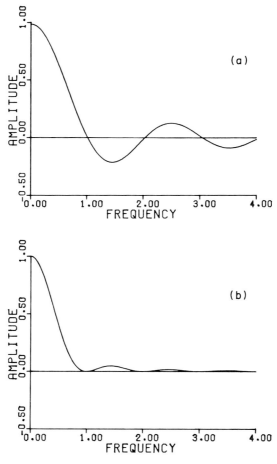

Fig. 8.7. Plots of F_3 for (a) nearest neighbor interpolation, and (b) linear interpolation; assuming $d = 1$.

TABLE 8.2

PICTURE DISTANCE MEASURES FOR THE
RECONSTRUCTIONS IN FIG. 8.8

α	d	r	e	t
1.0	0.0944	0.0427	0.0471	157
0.8	0.1178	0.0484	0.0657	160
0.54	0.1556	0.0574	0.0899	161

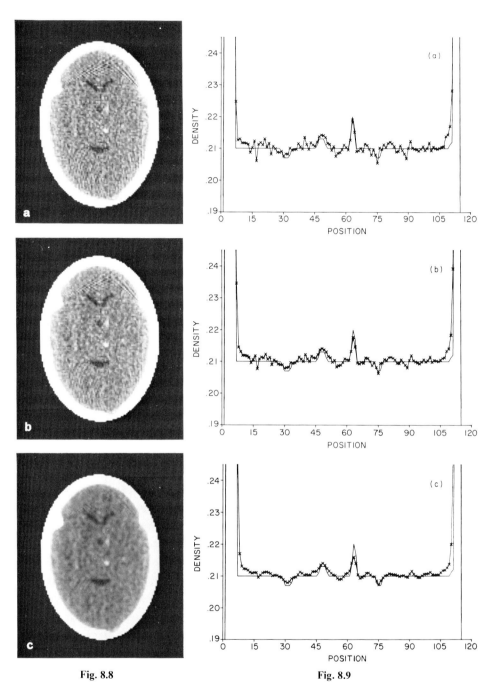

Fig. 8.8 **Fig. 8.9**

Fig. 8.8. Reconstructions from the standard parallel projection data using parallel beam convolution method with the generalized Hamming window and linear interpolation. (a) $\alpha = 1.0$. (b) $\alpha = 0.8$. (c) $\alpha = 0.54$.

Fig. 8.9. Plots of the 63rd columns of the reconstructions shown in Fig. 8.8.

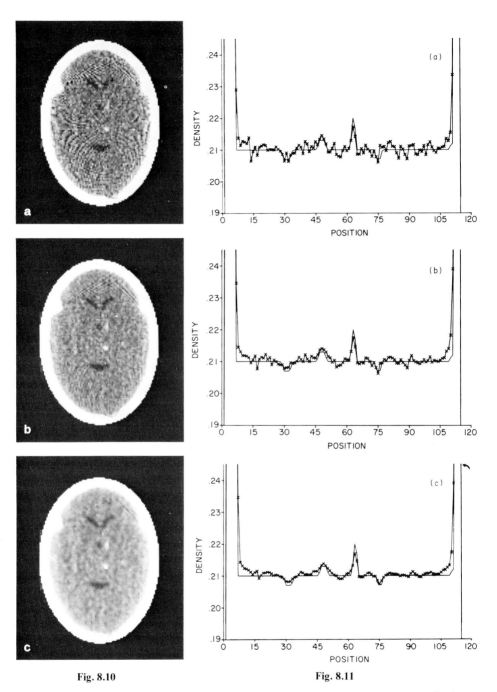

Fig. 8.10   Fig. 8.11

Fig. 8.10. Reconstructions using the parallel beam convolution method with generalized Hamming window $\alpha = 0.8$. (a) Nearest neighbor interpolation. (b) Linear interpolation. (c) Linear interpolation and nonlinear smoothing.

Fig. 8.11. Plots of the 63rd columns in the reconstructions shown in Fig. 8.10.

TABLE 8.3

PICTURE DISTANCE MEASURES FOR THE RECONSTRUCTIONS IN
FIG. 8.10

	d	r	e	t
Nearest neighbor	0.1168	0.0589	0.0652	144
Linear interpolation	0.1178	0.0484	0.0657	160
Nonlinear smoothing	0.1175	0.0470	0.0657	166

superior to nearest neighbor interpolation. Nevertheless, the picture distance measures d and e indicate that nearest neighbor is superior to linear interpolation. The reason for this is that both of these measures are highly influenced by the accuracy of the reconstruction of the skull. Linear interpolation is less accurate than nearest neighbor interpolation for the region of the picture occupied by the skull, but is more accurate than nearest neighbor interpolation for the region in the interior of the skull. This is a prime example of a general principle in CT: the appropriate choices of the free parameters in a reconstruction algorithm are dependent on the information we wish to obtain about the picture to be reconstructed. The third reconstruction of this set is a reproduction of our standard reconstruction method in Chapter 5. It is obtained from the reconstruction with linear interpolation by the process of nonlinear smoothing. This is an image processing procedure which is discussed in Section 11.4.

8.7 WHY SO POPULAR?

The convolution method is the most widely used method for reconstruction from data obtained by the parallel modes of data collection. There are many reasons for this.

The major reason is its computational simplicity. As we have discussed in Section 8.3, the demands of the convolution method on computer time and core are surprisingly small, even when implemented on a traditional computer. Examination of the method reveals that it is relatively easy to build special purpose computing hardware which implements the convolution method very efficiently. The data from each view can be convolved and backprojected independently of the other views; the final outcome is simply a sum of such convolved and backprojected views. In state of the art scanners, large digitized pictures (e.g., 512×512) are reconstructed from many views (over 500) in times under a minute.

The quality of the reconstructions produced by the convolution method is generally as good as by any other procedure, and often better than those produced by other methods. That is not to say that there are no situations where other reconstruction techniques would not produce more reliable images than the convolution method; but when accurate data is available in abundance (x-ray reconstruction appears to fall in this category), the convolution method seems to be as efficacious as any other.

The electrical engineering and physics background of many people involved in scanner design also makes the convolution method popular. The type of analysis we have carried out in the last section, using the Fourier transforms of the functions involved to explain the effects of our choices, is very familiar to scientists and engineers. In fact, this familiarity leads to statements of the type "the convolution method is preferable to series expansion techniques, because the underlying mathematics is well understood." This particular reason for the popularity of the convolution method appears weak; the theory that we develop for the series expansion methods is every bit as rigorous as the theory underlying the convolution and other transform methods. Different aspects of the problem are more easily explained in the different theories: while it is difficult to explain the behavior of some of the series expansion techniques using Fourier analysis, it is easier to incorporate a priori knowledge into the series expansion techniques than into a transform method. We shall return to this point later.

In conclusion, the convolution method produces efficacious reconstructions at a small cost. Unless evidence is available to the contrary in a particular application area, it is more likely to be an appropriate method to use than any other method designed for the parallel mode of data collection.

NOTES AND REFERENCES

The mathematical form of the convolution method was first proposed for image reconstruction from data collected along parallel rays by Bracewell and Riddle (1967). Ramachandran and Lakshminarayanan (1971) described an implementation which took care of the discrete nature of the data. Both these approaches used the bandlimiting window, as it has been made explicit in the derivation provided by Herman and Rowland (1973). Shepp and Logan (1974) introduced the idea of using windows other than the bandlimiting window: they have suggested the use of the sinc window, combined with linear interpolation. The use of Hamming window was proposed by Chesler and Riederer (1975). As it was shown, e.g., by Rowland (1979), the use of the generalized Hamming window is equivalent to applying the bandlimiting window to the data which have been smoothed by a three-point averaging process of the type discussed, e.g., by Shepp and Logan (1974). An exhaustive study of these windows was carried out by Rowland (1979), who was the first to carefully separate the convolving function and the interpolating function. Our presentation is highly influenced by Rowland's work.

The notion of a regularizing family was introduced into the image reconstruction literature by Herman and Naparstek (1978). We have followed the approach of Chang and Herman (1978).

A precise statement of the theorem used to differentiate under the integral sign can be found in most standard books on mathematical analysis; see, e.g., Apostol (1957, Theorem 9-37).

The general context of our approach to Fourier transforms, sampling and interpolation can be easily obtained from a basic text on these topics, such as Bracewell (1978). Discussion of different windows can be found in standard texts on signal processing, such as Rabiner and Gold (1975).

Examples of difficulties with the convolution method when the data have high frequency components have been given by Herman, Lakshminarayanan, and Rowland (1975).

There have been a number of publications comparing the performance of the convolution method with series expansion techniques, examples are Herman and Rowland (1973) and Shepp and Logan (1974).

9

Other Transform Methods
for Parallel Beams

In this chapter we discuss two alternative transform methods for image reconstruction from data collected along parallel rays: the Fourier method and the method of rho-filtered layergrams. Both these methods make use of the concept of the two-dimensional Fourier transform.

9.1 Two-Dimensional Fourier Transform

The *two-dimensional Fourier transform* is an operator which associates with a complex valued function f of two polar variables another complex valued function $\mathscr{F}_2 f$ of two polar variables defined by

$$[\mathscr{F}_2 f](R, \Phi) = \int_0^\pi \int_{-\infty}^\infty |r| f(r, \phi) \exp[-2\pi i r R \cos(\Phi - \phi)] \, dr \, d\phi. \quad (1.1)$$

The *inverse two-dimensional Fourier transform* is an operator which associates with a complex valued function F of two polar variables another complex valued function $\mathscr{F}_2^{-1} F$ of two polar variables defined by

$$[\mathscr{F}_2^{-1} F](r, \phi) = \int_0^\pi \int_{-\infty}^\infty |R| F(R, \Phi) \exp[2\pi i R r \cos(\phi - \Phi)] \, dR \, d\Phi. \quad (1.2)$$

For many functions f (including all in this book, except where otherwise stated)

$$\mathscr{F}_2^{-1} \mathscr{F}_2 f = \mathscr{F}_2 \mathscr{F}_2^{-1} f = f. \quad (1.3)$$

Similarly to the one-dimensional case [see (4.5) of Chapter 8] a function f of two polar variables can be "decomposed" into harmonic functions of two variables, and the two-dimensional Fourier transform indicates the nature of these harmonic components. We now explain the details.

Let f be a function of two polar variables and F be its two-dimensional Fourier transform. Let $\alpha(R, \Phi)$ denote an argument of $F(R, \Phi)$. Then it follows from (1.3) and (1.2) that

$$f(r, \phi) = \int_0^\pi \int_{-\infty}^\infty |R||F(R, \Phi)|\cos[2\pi Rr \cos(\phi - \Phi) + \alpha(R, \Phi)]\, dR\, d\Phi$$

$$+ i \int_0^\pi \int_{-\infty}^\infty |R||F(R, \Phi)|\sin[2\pi Rr\, \cos(\phi - \Phi) + \alpha(R, \Phi)]\, dR\, d\Phi.$$

$$(1.4)$$

For any fixed R and Φ, the functions

$$|F(R, \Phi)|\cos[2\pi Rr \cos(\phi - \Phi) + \alpha(R, \Phi)]$$

and

$$|F(R, \Phi)|\sin[2\pi Rr \cos(\phi - \Phi) + \alpha(R, \Phi)]$$

are *harmonic functions of two polar variables* (r, ϕ) with *frequency* $|R|$, *direction* Φ, *amplitude* $|F(R, \Phi)|$, and *initial phase* $\alpha(R, \Phi)$.

What do harmonic functions of two polar variables look like? Note first of all that if we fix ϕ, then the resulting function of r is a harmonic function with amplitude $|F(R, \Phi)|$, initial phase $\alpha(R, \Phi)$, and frequency $|R \cos(\phi - \Phi)|$. In particular, on the line L through the origin which makes an angle Φ with the x axis (the line $\phi = \Phi$), the resulting harmonic function has frequency

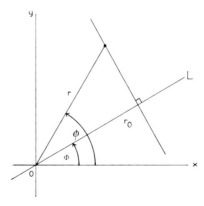

Fig. 9.1. A harmonic function of two polar variables (r, ϕ) with frequency R and direction Φ, restricted to the line L ($\phi = \Phi$), is a harmonic function of the variable r with frequency R. On any line perpendicular to L [$r \cos(\phi - \Phi) = r_0$], the value of the harmonic function of two polar variables is constant.

$|R|$. On any line perpendicular to L [i.e., on any line with equation $r \cos(\phi - \Phi) = r_0$, where r_0 is constant], the harmonic function of two polar variables is constant (see Fig. 9.1).

If a function f is smooth, we expect a small amplitude $|F(R, \Phi)|$ for components with large frequency $|R|$ in the decomposition (1.4). A function f is said to be *bandlimited* if $[\mathscr{F}_2 f](R, \Phi) = 0$ if $|R| \geq A/2$, where A is a positive real number, called the *bandwidth* of f. (See similar definitions for functions of one variable in Section 8.4.)

Of the many interesting and useful properties of the two-dimensional Fourier transform the most important for image reconstruction is the so-called *projection theorem*. It gives a basic relationship between the Radon transform, the two-dimensional Fourier transform, and an operator $\mathscr{F}_Y$, which is a two-dimensional version of the one-dimensional Fourier transform, defined as follows.

Let p be a function of two variables, and let p_θ be defined, as in (2.1) of Chapter 8, by $p_\theta(\ell) = p(\ell, \theta)$. Then $\mathscr{F}_Y p$ is another function of two variables defined by

$$[\mathscr{F}_Y p](L, \theta) = [\mathscr{F} p_\theta](L). \tag{1.5}$$

In other words, $\mathscr{F}_Y$ is a *Fourier transform with respect to the first variable*.

The projection theorem can now be stated as the operator equation:

$$\mathscr{F}_2 = \mathscr{F}_Y \mathscr{R}. \tag{1.6}$$

In words, taking the two-dimensional Fourier transform is the same as taking the Radon transform and then applying the Fourier transform with respect to the first variable. The projection theorem follows easily from the definitions of the Radon and Fourier transform; we omit the details.

9.2   THE FOURIER METHOD OF RECONSTRUCTION

From (1.3) and (1.6) we see that for a function f of two polar variables

$$f = \mathscr{F}_2^{-1} \mathscr{F}_Y \mathscr{R} f. \tag{2.1}$$

This leads to the mathematical idealization of the Fourier method of reconstruction. For any function p, representing projection data of a picture, we estimate the picture by

$$\mathscr{R}^{-1} p = \mathscr{F}_2^{-1} \mathscr{F}_Y p. \tag{2.2}$$

The major difficulty with the Fourier method lies in its implementation on real data. We look at what is involved step by step.

Let us recall our assumption that in the parallel mode of data collection p is known at points $(nd, m\Delta)$, where $-N \leq n \leq N$ and $0 \leq m \leq M - 1$.

For any value of R, we may calculate $[\mathscr{F}_Y p](R, m\Delta)$ using (1.5) in conjunction with (2.1) and (4.2) of Chapter 8 as

$$[\mathscr{F}_Y p](R, m\Delta) = \int_{-E}^{E} p(\ell, m\Delta)\exp[-2\pi iR\ell]\, d\ell. \tag{2.3}$$

We have made use of the fact that $p_\theta(\ell) = 0$ if $|\ell| \geq E$.

The right-hand side of (2.3) has to be numerically evaluated for some selected values of R. A Riemann sum approximation using the sample points gives:

$$[\mathscr{F}_Y p](R, m\Delta) \simeq d \sum_{n=-N}^{N} p(nd, m\Delta)\exp[-2\pi iRnd]. \tag{2.4}$$

In fact, this approximation is accurate for at most a limited range of values of R. In fact, the right-hand side of (2.4) is equal to

$$F_1(R) = \sum_{k=-\infty}^{\infty} [\mathscr{F}_Y p](R + k/d, m\Delta). \tag{2.5}$$

The use of the same function name, F_1, that has been defined in (5.6) of Chapter 8 and discussed in detail in Section 8.6 is not accidental; as simple observation will show, the function defined in (2.5) is the same function that was called F_1 in Chapter 8. As it has been discussed in Section 8.6, $F_1(R)$ can only be an accurate approximation of $[\mathscr{F}_Y p](R, m\Delta)$ $(=[\mathscr{F} p_{m\Delta}](R))$ if $|R| < 1/2d$, and it may be inaccurate even within that interval, especially near the edges. For $|R| > 1/2d$, it is probably better to approximate $[\mathscr{F}_Y p](R, m\Delta)$ by zero, than by the use of (2.4).

Also, we have to make a decision as to the points R in the interval $-1/2d \leq R \leq 1/2d$, at which we wish to evaluate $[\mathscr{F}_Y p](R, m\Delta)$. It is computationally desirable, for reasons that are now given, to select values of R which are multiples of $1/(2N + 1)d$. Note that this is not a real restriction on how finely these sample points are spaced, since the evaluation in (2.4) would not change if we decide to use a larger value for N. [Recall that $p(nd, m\Delta) = 0$ if $nd \geq E$.]

Combining these statements we see that the first stage of the Fourier method is to estimate, for $0 \leq m \leq M - 1$, $-N \leq n' \leq N$, $[\mathscr{F}_Y p](n'/(2N + 1)d, m\Delta)$ by

$$[\mathscr{F}_Y p](n'/(2N + 1)d, m\Delta) \simeq d \sum_{n=-N}^{N} p(nd, m\Delta)\exp[-2\pi inn'/(2N + 1)]. \tag{2.6}$$

The right-hand side of (2.6) is d multiplied by what is called the *discrete Fourier transform* in the first variable of the sampled version of p. We introduce the abbreviation

$$[\mathscr{D}\mathscr{F}_Y p](n', m) = \sum_{n=-N}^{N} p(nd, m\Delta)\exp[-2\pi inn'/(2N + 1)]. \tag{2.7}$$

The evaluation of $\overline{\mathscr{D}\mathscr{F}}_Y p$ at the $M(2N + 1)$ points ($0 \leq m \leq M - 1$, $-N \leq n' \leq N$) is much less expensive than it would appear at first sight. Note first of all that, just as in the convolution method, we deal with each view separately. The $2N + 1$ different values of $[\mathscr{D}\mathscr{F}_Y p](n', m)$ for a fixed m but varying n', are evaluated from the $2N + 1$ values of $p(nd, m\Delta)$, for the same fixed m and varying n. Since the values of $\exp[-2\pi i n n'/(2N + 1)]$ can be precalculated and stored (they do not depend on the data), it appears that the evaluation of (2.7), for a fixed m but varying n', requires $2(2N + 1)^2$ multiplications. (The factor 2 in the front comes from the fact that in each term of the sum a real number is multiplied by a complex number, which requires two real multiplications.) However, there is a much more efficient way of evaluating (2.7) for $-N \leq n' \leq N$ than the method which evaluates the expression for each value of n' separately. This method is called the *fast Fourier transform* (FFT). Its description is beyond the scope of this book, but we must comment on its performance, since this is essential in appreciating the computational efficiency of the Fourier reconstruction method.

Using FFT, the calculation of (2.7), for a fixed m but for all the $2N + 1$ values of n' between $-N$ and N, requires approximately $N(3 + \lceil \log_2 N \rceil)$ multiplications, where $\lceil \log_2 N \rceil$ is the smallest integer not smaller than the base 2 logarithm of N.

Consider the case of the standard parallel projection data. In this case $M = 144$ and $N = 82$. Hence, the straightforward evaluation of (2.7) requires $2M(2N + 1)^2 = 7,840,800 \simeq 8 \times 10^6$ multiplications. Using the FFT, we need $MN(3 + \lceil \log_2 N \rceil) = 118,080 \simeq 10^5$. This is a reduction by two orders of magnitude, a very considerable saving. In commercial scanners, where N may be several times larger than in our example, the saving is even more substantial.

Thus, using the FFT, the first stage of the Fourier method [evaluation of (2.7) for $0 \leq m \leq M - 1$, $-N \leq n' \leq N$] can be done at a relatively low cost.

We are now faced with the problem of numerically evaluating $\mathscr{F}_2^{-1}\mathscr{F}_Y p$ based on the estimated values of $\mathscr{F}_Y p$ at the points $(n/(2N + 1)d, m\Delta)$. One possible way of doing this is to combine our claim that $[\mathscr{F}_Y p](R, m\Delta)$ is best approximated by zero for $|R| \geq E$ with Riemann sum approximation of (1.2) and obtain the estimated picture

$$f^*(r, \phi) = \frac{\Delta}{2N + 1} \sum_{m=0}^{M-1} \sum_{n=-N}^{N} \left| \frac{n}{(2N + 1)d} \right| [\mathscr{D}\mathscr{F}_Y p](n, m)$$

$$\times \exp\left[2\pi i \frac{n}{(2N + 1)d} r \cos(\phi - m\Delta)\right]. \quad (2.8)$$

In fact, the Fourier reconstruction method is usually not implemented in this way. The reason for this is computational. Getting back to our example of the head phantom and the standard parallel projection data, we see that f^*

is to be evaluated at $J = 115 \times 115 = 13{,}225$ points. If (2.8) is used separately for each point, then the total number of multiplications required is

$$2JM(2N + 1) > 6 \times 10^8,$$

even if we assume that the values

$$\frac{\Delta}{2N + 1} \left| \frac{n}{(2N + 1)d} \right| \exp\left[2\pi i \frac{n}{(2N + 1)d} r \cos(\phi - m\Delta) \right]$$

are precalculated and stored. This is quite a sizable computational require-ment, especially when we consider that our example is actually small as compared to a commercial scanner, for which the number of calculations would be at least an order of magnitude larger. Another way of indicating the unreasonableness of implementing the Fourier method using (2.8) is to consider the total number of multiplications needed for the convolution method for the head phantom and standard parallel projection data. As the reader can easily work out, it is between 10^6 and 10^7 (depending on the method of interpolation used). In any case, it is about two orders of magnitude less than what was calculated for evaluating (2.8).

Clearly, an alternative method has to be found of numerically evaluating $\mathscr{F}_2^{-1}\mathscr{F}_Y p$ based on the estimated values of $\mathscr{F}_Y p$ at the points $(n/(2N + 1)d, m\Delta)$.

One way is to break up the evaluation of (2.8) into a two-stage process:

(i)   For each m, $0 \leq m \leq M - 1$, we evaluate $p_c(n' d, m\Delta)$ for $-N \leq n' \leq N$, using

$$p_c(n'd, m\Delta) = \frac{1}{(2N + 1)^2 d} \sum_{n = -N}^{N} |n| [\overline{\mathscr{D}\mathscr{F}}_Y p](n, m) \exp\left[2\pi i \frac{nn'}{2N + 1} \right]. \quad (2.9)$$

(ii) $f^*(r, \phi)$ is estimated by

$$f^*(r, \phi) = \Delta \sum_{m = 0}^{M - 1} p_c(r \cos(\phi - m\Delta), m\Delta). \quad (2.10)$$

This involves interpolation for estimating $p_c(r \cos(\phi - m\Delta), m\Delta)$ from values of $p_c(n'd, m\Delta)$.

This approach is just about identical to the convolution method, except that p_c is defined by (2.9) rather than by (3.2) of Chapter 8. In fact, (2.9) can be rewritten as a discrete convolution of p with a convolving function q, and so the approach just described is essentially identical to the convolution method. We therefore say no more about it in this chapter.

An alternative efficient implementation, and this is the alternative which we refer to as the Fourier method, makes use of the availability of a two-dimensional fast Fourier transform. There is a version of the FFT which can be used to estimate the values of the two-dimensional inverse Fourier transform $\mathscr{F}_2^{-1}F$ at J points from the values of F at J points, and the number of multiplications required for this process is of the order $J \log_2 J$. (The point-by-point Riemann sum evaluation discussed previously requires J^2 multiplications.)

The difficulty with this process is that the points at which $\mathscr{F}_2^{-1}F$ are to be calculated and the points at which the values of F have to be given must lie in a regular rectangular arrangement (such as the centers of pixels provided by an n-element grid, see Section 4.1). For our application this is not a restriction as far as the output is concerned, since we desire to estimate $f^* = \mathscr{F}_2^{-1}\mathscr{F}_Y p$ at points which are centers of pixels. The input is a different matter. The first stage of the Fourier method provides us with values at points with polar coordinates $(n/(2N + 1)d, m\Delta)$. These points lie in a radial arrangement, rather than in a rectangular one (see Fig. 9.2).

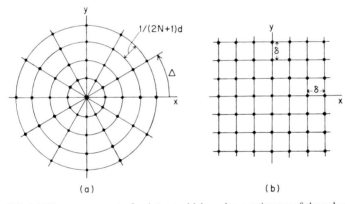

Fig. 9.2. (a) The arrangement of points at which we have estimates of the values of $\mathscr{F}_Y p$. (b) The arrangement of points at which we need to know the values of a function before the inverse two-dimensional fast Fourier transform can be applied.

Hence, the Fourier method of reconstruction has two stages beyond the already described first stage. The second stage is the estimation of the values of $\mathscr{F}_Y p$ at points on a rectangular grid from the values of $\mathscr{F}_Y p$ produced by the first stage (on a radial grid). The third stage is the use of the fast Fourier transform to obtain f^* at the centers of pixels. It is beyond the scope of this book to give a detailed description of both these stages, but we mention some considerations which go into the design of a Fourier method to ensure that it provides acceptable reconstructions.

The major difficulty comes from the fact that the FFT algorithm only provides an estimate of the two-dimensional inverse Fourier transform.

The relationship between the output of the FFT and the true inverse Fourier transform is similar to the one between the function F_1 of (2.5) and $\mathscr{F}p_{m\Delta}$. In particular, if the spacing between the points at which values of $\mathscr{F}_Y p$ are interpolated is δ (see Fig. 9.2), then the output of the FFT can only be accurate in the rectangular region defined by $|r \cos \phi| < 1/2\delta$ and $|r \sin \phi| < 1/2\delta$. Furthermore, near the edges of this region it is likely to be contaminated with aliasing errors (see Section 8.6). Hence, to get an accurate reconstruction, we have to select δ small enough so that $1/\delta$ is considerably larger than E. This has two computationally undesirable consequences.

First, the FFT has to be calculated for a number of points much larger than J (the number of pixels in the final display), corresponding to additional pixels which are introduced to make the picture region $1/\delta \times 1/\delta$ instead of $E \times E$. The desirable increase maybe as large as a factor of 9 (if $1/\delta = 3E$), removing much of the computational advantage of FFT. This can also put excessive demands on the available computer memory.

Second, in order to have accurate estimates of $\mathscr{F}_Y p$ at the rectangular grid with spacing δ, we may have to evaluate during the first stage of the process $\mathscr{F}_Y p$ at points $(n'/(2N' + 1)d, m\Delta)$ with an N' which is larger than N, where $2N + 1$ is the number of rays in a view. This would have to be done for all points n' such that $-N' \le n' \le N'$, resulting in a further increase in computational cost.

In practice, we should bear in mind that the calculated values of $[\mathscr{F}_Y p](n'/(2N' + 1)d, m\Delta)$ for $|n'|$ near N' may be inaccurate [see (2.5) and the discussion in Section 8.6]. It sometimes improves the result if, prior to interpolation, $\mathscr{F}_Y p$ is multiplied pointwise by a window function $F_{1/d}$ of the type defined in Table 8.1. That is, instead of $[\mathscr{F}_Y p](n/(2N + 1)d, m\Delta)$, use $[\mathscr{F}_Y p](n/(2N + 1)d, m\Delta) \times F_{1/d}(|n|/(2N + 1)d)$.

Finally, we have to say something about the method of interpolation from the polar to the rectangular grid. There are a number of ways of doing this. A relatively inexpensive method is *bilinear interpolation*.

Observe Fig. 9.3. Let P be the point in the rectangular grid at which we wish to evaluate $\mathscr{F}_Y p$, and let A, B, C, and D be four points on the radial grid at which estimates of $\mathscr{F}_Y p$ are already known. These are chosen so that the region between the line AB and CD and the arcs AC and BD contains P and that this region is the smallest possible such region containing P. Let $\mathscr{F}(Q)$ denote the estimate of $\mathscr{F}_Y p$ at a point Q and let $\overline{Q_1 Q_2}$ denote the distance between points Q_1 and Q_2. We first estimate

$$\mathscr{F}(E) = \frac{\overline{BE} \times \mathscr{F}(A) + \overline{AE} \times \mathscr{F}(B)}{\overline{AB}},$$

$$\mathscr{F}(F) = \frac{\overline{DF} \times \mathscr{F}(C) + \overline{CF} \times \mathscr{F}(D)}{\overline{CD}}. \tag{2.11}$$

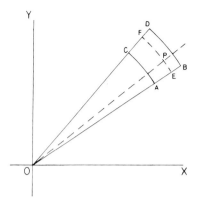

Fig. 9.3. Bilinear interpolation at point P.

Let $\overline{PE}$ (respectively, $\overline{PF}$) be the distance along the arc connecting P and E (respectively, P and F). Then

$$\mathscr{F}(P) = \frac{\overline{PE} \times \mathscr{F}(F) + \overline{PF} \times \mathscr{F}(E)}{\overline{PE} + \overline{PF}}. \tag{2.12}$$

The performance of the Fourier reconstruction method on the standard parallel projection data is reported in Figs. 9.4 and 9.5 and Table 9.1. Two reconstructions have been carried out. In one of them the two-dimensional inverse FFT was calculated using $J \, (= 115 \times 115)$ points and the N' in the first stage of the process was N, where $2N + 1 \, (= 165)$ is the number of rays in one view in the data set. In the second reconstruction we have attempted to reduce aliasing errors by choosing 345×345 points for the two-dimensional inverse FFT. The size of the extended reconstruction region is therefore 51.888 cm (recall that each pixel is 0.1504×0.1504 cm), and so $\delta = 1/51.888 = 0.0193$. We want to choose N' so that $1/(2N' + 1)d$ is

TABLE 9.1

PICTURE DISTANCE MEASURES FOR THE RECONSTRUCTIONS IN
FIG. 9.4[a]

J	d	r	e	t
115×115	0.2780	0.1747	0.1417	Not available
345×345	0.1100	0.0524	0.0592	Not available

[a] Value of t is not available, since due to the limited size of the core memory on the Cyber 173, these two reconstructions were done on a different computer.

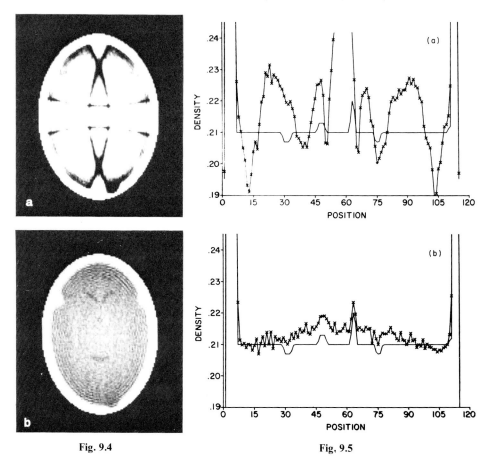

Fig. 9.4   **Fig, 9.5**

Fig. 9.4. Reconstructions using the Fourier reconstruction method with (a) 115 × 115 grid and $N' = 82$, and (b) 345 × 345 grid with $N' = 244$.

Fig. 9.5. Plots of the 63rd columns in the reconstructions shown in Fig. 9.4.

significantly smaller than δ, to ensure the accuracy of the interpolation during the second stage. We used $N' = 244$. In both these reconstructions, we have multiplied pointwise the calculated values of $\mathscr{F}_Y p$ with the value of the generalized Hamming window with $\alpha = 0.8$ prior to interpolation. This should make the output comparable to that of the convolution method using the same window. Clearly a better numerical procedure is necessary for the Fourier method to achieve the quality of the convolution method, see Figs. 8.8b and 8.9b.

9.3   RHO-FILTERED LAYERGRAM

In our discussion of the continuous backprojection method we have
pointed out that the method produces a blurred version of the original
picture, where the contribution of the original density at a point A to the
reconstructed density at a point B is inversely proportional to the distance
between the two points. The rho-filtered layergram is a method which
attempts to deblur the picture which is obtained by backprojection alone.

The method of deblurring is based on a relationship between the two-
dimensional Fourier transform of a picture and the two-dimensional Fourier
transform of the backprojected Radon transform of the picture. This relationship is given by

$$[\mathscr{F}_2 f](R, \Phi) = |R| \times [\mathscr{F}_2 \mathscr{B}\mathscr{R}f](R, \Phi), \tag{3.1}$$

for any point (R, Φ) with $R \neq 0$.

Equation (3.1) gives rise to a four-stage process for estimating a picture
f from projection data p:

   (i)   Backproject p, to obtain $\mathscr{B}p$.
   (ii)   Calculate the two-dimensional Fourier transform $\mathscr{F}_2 \mathscr{B}p$.
   (iii)   Obtain a new function F of two polar variables by

$$F(R, \Phi) = |R| \times [\mathscr{F}_2 \mathscr{B}p](R, \Phi). \tag{3.2}$$

   (iv)   Estimate the picture by

$$f^* = \mathscr{F}_2^{-1} F. \tag{3.3}$$

The reason for the name of the method is the following. The result of the
process of backprojection has sometimes been called in the literature a
layergram. In the articles which introduced the concept of the rho-filtered
layergram, the first polar variable of the two-dimensional Fourier transform
was denoted by the greek letter ρ (rho), and hence the operations described
in (ii)–(iv) were given the name rho filtering.

The difficulty with the rho-filtered layergram is its implementation. We
discuss the implementation of the four steps just described one by one.

It is easy to estimate the value of $\mathscr{B}p$ at any point (r, ϕ) using a Riemann
sum approximation combined with an interpolation (see Section 7.2). How-
ever, note that even though $p(\ell, \theta) = 0$ for $|\ell| \geq E$, there is no value of E'
such that $[\mathscr{B}p](r, \phi) = 0$ for $r \geq E'$. In other words, the set of points at
which $\mathscr{B}p$ is not zero is unbounded. On the other hand, as the reader can easily
prove it for himself, it is the case that

$$\lim_{r \to \infty} \sup_{0 \leq \phi \leq 2\pi} [\mathscr{B}p](r, \phi) = 0, \tag{3.4}$$

i.e., $[\mathscr{B}p](r, \phi)$ is guaranteed to be arbitrarily small provided r is large enough.

In practice, we can evaluate $\mathscr{B}p$ only at finitely many points. In view of the fact that the next thing to be done is to apply the two-dimensional Fourier transform to $\mathscr{B}p$, it makes sense to evaluate $\mathscr{B}p$ on equally spaced points on a rectangular grid. (Recall our discussion on the FTT for two-dimensional Fourier transforms.) The central part of this grid should form the picture region, with the pixel centers being points on the rectangular grid. The rest of the grid should form a frame around the picture region. The frame should be big enough so that the values of $\mathscr{B}p$ outside it can be ignored with relative safety.

For the second stage of the rho-filtered layergram, we apply the FFT to estimate $\mathscr{F}_2\mathscr{B}p$ from values of $\mathscr{B}p$. As discussed before, the number of points at which the FFT provides us with estimates of $\mathscr{F}_2\mathscr{B}p$ is the same as the number of points at which we had estimates for $\mathscr{B}p$. The spacing (parallel to the rectangular axis) between the points at which we have estimates of $\mathscr{F}_2\mathscr{B}p$ is the inverse of the size of the backprojection region (i.e, the picture region plus the border around it that we discussed previously). Estimates of $\mathscr{F}_2\mathscr{B}p$ at points near the edge of the rectangular grid on which it is estimated are usually unreliable, because of aliasing and noise in the data. (This statement is not supported by anything we said in this section. However, the reader should be able to argue this out, based on similar arguments given for the convolution and the Fourier methods.)

Implementation of the third stage is a trivial matter. However, for reasons which are similar to those given in previous sections, rather than multiplying by $|R|$, we multiply by $|R| \times F_{1/d}(|R|)$, where $F_{1/d}$ is a window function whose bandwidth is the inverse of the sampling distance.

Note an important fact: $F(0, \Phi) = 0$. Looking at (3.3), (1.3), and (1.1), we see that this means that

$$\int_0^\pi \int_{-\infty}^\infty |r|\, f^*(r, \phi)\, dr\, d\phi = 0, \tag{3.5}$$

i.e, that the total density of f^* is zero. This seems to be very undesirable. It implies that whatever picture we are estimating, the total density of the estimate is the same. Two comments are in order.

First, (3.3) is somewhat misleading. The function f^* defined by it may (and usually does) have nonzero values everywhere in the plane. Knowing that we are estimating a picture, we can set all values outside the picture region to zero. The resulting picture function may very well have a total density which is nearly the same as that of the picture we are attempting to reconstruct.

Second, the problem is not new, but it has never been so obvious before. In the convolution method, the convolved projection data $p_{m\Delta} * \mathscr{F}^{-1}\Phi$

has zero total density [see (4.6) of Chapter 8]. In the implementation of the Fourier method which is indicated by (2.8), $[\mathscr{D}\mathscr{F}_Y p](0, m)$ is always multiplied by zero, and the value of the total density of $p_{m\Delta}$ is irrelevant. Nevertheless, by both these techniques we have obtained reconstructions whose total density (inside the picture region) is quite accurate.

However, in the case of the rho-filtered layergram this problem often does not resolve itself as nicely as with the other methods. Since the fourth stage is to be implemented by the use of the FFT, we end up with values of f^* on a rectangular grid which is identical in size and location with the grid onto which we backprojected in the first stage. The sums of the values of f^* on this grid is zero. Unless this grid is very much bigger than the grid associated with the digitized picture region, the total density even in the picture region will be noticeably inaccurate. Fortunately, this can be easily corrected by additive normalization (see Section 7.2). Note that, in this case, multiplicative normalization is not appropriate.

We do not report in this book on reconstructions using the rho-filtered layergram method.

NOTES AND REFERENCES

The relationship between the Radon transform and the Fourier transforms has been studied in a number of mathematical texts; see, for example, Ludwig (1966) and its references. The first mention (and proof) of the projection theorem in application oriented image reconstruction is in Bracewell (1956).

The equivalence of (2.9) to (3.2) of Chapter 8 follows from the convolution theorem for the discrete Fourier transform; see, e.g., Bracewell (1978).

Some researchers, e.g., Shepp and Logan (1974), refer to all transform methods, in particular the convolution method, as "Fourier reconstruction." Since neither the derivation nor the implementation of the convolution method requires the use of Fourier transforms (although both can be done that way), this name seems inappropriate; especially in view of the fact that the implementational differences between what we called the convolution method and what we called the Fourier method are sufficiently significant· to require separate names to distinguish them. A good overview of what is known about the Fourier method can be obtained by reading Mersereau (1976) and its references, especially the paper by Crowther, *et al.* (1970). A report by Lutz (1975) on some experimental results concludes that in practical implementation the convolution method is superior to the Fourier method, confirming the claim of Ramachandran and Lakshminarayanan (1971). Wee and Prakash (1978) discuss the possibility of using the Fourier method when the number of views is small.

The FFT, very important for the implementation of both methods in this chapter, is of sufficient general importance that there have been whole books essentially devoted to the topic, e.g., Brigham (1974).

The phrase rho-filtered layergram has been introduced by Smith *et al.* (1973). Our development is based on the more detailed study of Rowland (1979), which also contains reports on experiments with this technique using different windows and interpolating functions. The reader should consult these works for other relevant literature. The method has been extended to the divergent beam data collection techniques by Gullberg (1979); see also Budinger and Gullberg (1975).

For exact implementational details of the two reconstruction methods in this chapter the reader should consult Herman and Rowland (1978), which was used for producing Figs. 9.4 and 9.5, or Huesman *et al.* (1977).

10

Convolution Methods for Divergent Beams

An alternative to the parallel mode of data collection is when data are collected so that they naturally divide into subsets with each subset containing estimated ray sums for rays diverging from a single point. Our standard projection data are of this type.

There are two basic approaches to designing a convolution-type algorithm for this type of data. The first is to find a convolution-type implementation of the Radon inversion formula that is appropriate for the divergent mode of data collection. The second is to use interpolation in the (ℓ, θ) space to estimate ray sums for sets of parallel rays from the measured ray sums for sets of divergent rays (this process is called *rebinning*) and then apply the parallel beam convolution method.

In this chapter both these methods are discussed. We also return to the topic of window selection; this time in the context of the divergent beam convolution method.

10.1 The Divergent Beam Convolution Algorithm

The data collection geometry we deal with is described in Fig. 10.1. The x-ray source is always on a circle of radius D around the origin. The detector strip is an arc centered at the source. Each ray can be considered as one of a set of divergent rays (σ, β), where β determines the source position and σ determines which of the rays divergent from this source position we are considering. This is an alternative way of specifying lines to the (ℓ, θ) notation used previously (in particular in Fig. 2.8). Of course, each (σ, β) ray is also an (ℓ, θ) ray, for some values of ℓ and θ which depend on σ and β. In fact, as it is easily seen from Fig. 10.1, the ray (σ, β) corresponds to the point $(D \sin \sigma, \beta + \sigma)$ in (ℓ, θ) space.

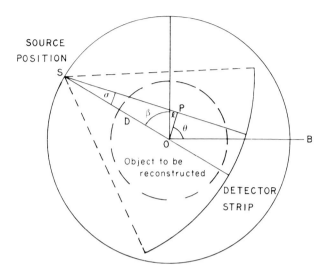

Fig. 10.1. Geometry of divergent data collection. Every ray is determined by two para-meters β and σ. Let O be the origin and S be the position of the source, which always lies on a circle of radius D around O. Then $\beta + \pi/2$ is the angle the line OS makes with the baseline B, and σ is the angle the ray makes with SO. The same ray is also one of a set of parallel rays. As such it is determined by the parameters θ and ℓ. Let P be the point at which the ray meets the line through the origin which is perpendicular to the ray. Then θ is the angle OP makes with the baseline and ℓ is the distance from O to P. [Reproduced from Herman (1980), with permission.]

As usual in this book, we use f to denote the function of two polar variables r and ϕ which we wish to reconstruct. Recall that $f(r, \phi) = 0$ if $r \geq E$. We assume that $D > E$ and use δ to denote the inverse sine of E/D, Note that

$$0 < \delta = \sin^{-1}(E/D) < \pi/2. \tag{1.1}$$

We use $g(\sigma, \beta)$ to denote the line integral of f along the ray (σ, β). That is,

$$g(\sigma, \beta) = [\mathscr{R}f](D \sin \sigma, \beta + \sigma). \tag{1.2}$$

It follows from (1.1) that $g(\sigma, \beta) = 0$ if $|\sigma| > \delta$.

Suppose we have all possible projection data $g(\sigma, \beta)$ for $0 \leq \beta < 2\pi$ and $|\sigma| \leq \delta$. It can be shown that the Radon inversion formula gives rise to the following. If the derivatives of $g(\sigma, \beta)$ with respect to σ and β both exist and are denoted by $g_1(\sigma, \beta)$ and $g_2(\sigma, \beta)$, then

$$f(r, \phi) = \frac{1}{4\pi^2} \int_0^{2\pi} \int_{-\infty}^{\infty} \frac{1}{\sigma' - \sigma} G(\sigma, \beta, \sigma') \, d\sigma \, d\beta, \tag{1.3}$$

with

$$G(\sigma, \beta, \sigma') = \begin{cases} \dfrac{\sigma' - \sigma}{\sin(\sigma' - \sigma)} \left[\dfrac{1}{W} g_1(\sigma, \beta) - \dfrac{1}{W} g_2(\sigma, \beta) \right] & \text{if } |\sigma| \le \delta, \\ 0 & \text{if } |\sigma| > \delta, \end{cases}$$

(1.4)

where

$$\sigma' = \tan^{-1} \frac{r \cos(\beta - \phi)}{D + r \sin(\beta - \phi)}, \qquad -\frac{\pi}{2} < \sigma' < \frac{\pi}{2}, \qquad (1.5)$$

and

$$W = \{[r \cos(\beta - \phi)]^2 + [D + r \sin(\beta - \phi)]^2\}^{1/2}, \qquad W > 0. \qquad (1.6)$$

Note that σ' and W depend on β, r, and ϕ, but not on σ. The geometrical meanings of σ' and W are that when the source is at angle β, the ray that goes through (r, ϕ) is (σ', β) and the distance between the source and (r, ϕ) is W.

Note that (1.3), called the *Radon inversion formula for divergent rays*, is in the form of a singular integral. The inner integral is essentially a Hilbert transform of the function $G(\sigma, \beta, \sigma')$ considered as a function of σ alone. Hence our discussion of regularization in Section 8.1 is applicable here as well.

Let us assume that the function $G(\sigma, \beta, \sigma')$, as a function of σ, is reasonable at the point σ'. Then, for any choice of $\{F_A | A > 0\}$ which satisfies the conditions stated prior to (1.10) of Chapter 8, we get a family of regularizing functions $\{\rho_A | A > 0\}$ such that (1.3) can be written in the following form:

$$f(r, \phi) = \lim_{A \to \infty} \frac{1}{4\pi^2} \int_0^{2\pi} \int_{-\infty}^{\infty} \rho_A(\sigma' - \sigma) G(\sigma, \beta, \sigma') \, d\sigma \, d\beta \qquad (1.7)$$

[see (1.9) and (1.10) of Chapter 8]. The advantage of rewriting (1.3) as (1.7) is that for any fixed A the inner integral in (1.7) is easy to handle, since one can evaluate it using integration by parts. We denote the approximation to f provided by a fixed A by $\tilde{f}$, i.e.,

$$\tilde{f}(r, \phi) = \frac{1}{4\pi^2} \int_0^{2\pi} \int_{-\infty}^{\infty} \rho_A(\sigma' - \sigma) G(\sigma, \beta, \sigma') \, d\sigma \, d\beta. \qquad (1.8)$$

Having chosen a particular function ρ_A as the regularizing function, substitution of the value of $G(\sigma, \beta, \sigma')$ into (1.8) and integration by parts [note that ρ_A is differentiable, see (2.4) of Chapter 8] leads to

$$\tilde{f}(r, \phi) = \frac{D}{4\pi^2} \int_0^{2\pi} \frac{1}{W^2} \int_{-\delta}^{\delta} [q^{(1)}(\sigma' - \sigma)\cos \sigma$$

$$+ q^{(2)}(\sigma' - \sigma)\cos \sigma']g(\sigma, \beta) \, d\sigma \, d\beta, \qquad (1.9)$$

where

$$q^{(1)}(u) = -u\rho_A(u)/\sin^2 u, \tag{1.10}$$

and

$$q^{(2)}(u) = (\rho_A(u) + u\rho'_A(u))/\sin u, \tag{1.11}$$

for $u \neq 0$, and (1.10) and (1.11) are assigned their limit values for $u = 0$. (We omit the somewhat cumbersome details.) Equation (1.9) gives the convolution reconstruction formula for the fan beam geometry.

We have thus far presented an easy way to generate convolution-type reconstruction formulas for fan beam x-ray data. There are two choices to be made. First, a family of windows F_A has to be selected. Second, a value has to be assigned to A. Once these choices are made, we find the *convolving functions* $q^{(1)}$ and $q^{(2)}$ from (1.10) and (1.11) and get the formula for approximating $f(r, \phi)$ from (1.9).

Up to this point, we have assumed for the simplicity of mathematical analysis that the projection data are available for all possible σ and β. In practice, we can have only finitely many source positions, and for each source position we can have only finitely many detector readings. As shown in Fig. 5.2, we assume that projections are taken for M equally spaced values of β with angular spacing Δ, and that for each projection the projected values are sampled at $2N + 1$ equally spaced angles with angular spacing λ. Thus g is known at points $(n\lambda, m\Delta)$, $-N \leq n \leq N, 0 \leq m \leq M - 1$, and $M\Delta = 2\pi$. Our standard projection data are collected this way (see Section 5.2). Even though the projection data consist of estimates (based on measurements) of $g(n\lambda, m\Delta)$, we use the same notation $g(n\lambda, m\Delta)$ for these estimates for the rest of this chapter.

Similarly to the parallel beam convolution method, the numerical implementation of (1.9) is carried out in two stages.

First, the inner integral in (1.9) is evaluated using a Riemann sum approximation for values of σ' which are multiples of λ. We obtain

$$g_c(n'\lambda, m\Delta) = \lambda \sum_{n=-N}^{N} \cos(n\lambda)g(n\lambda, m\Delta)q^{(1)}((n' - n)\lambda)$$

$$+ \lambda \cos(n'\lambda) \sum_{n=-N}^{N} g(n\lambda, m\Delta)q^{(2)}((n' - n)\lambda). \tag{1.12}$$

[This corresponds to (3.2) of Chapter 8.] Note that the first sum is a discrete convolution of $q^{(1)}$ and the projection data weighted by a cosine function, and the second sum is a discrete convolution of $q^{(2)}$ and the projection data.

Second, the outer integral in (1.9) is evaluated using a Riemann sum approximation. We obtain

$$f^*(r, \phi) = \frac{D\Delta}{4\pi^2} \sum_{m=0}^{M-1} \frac{1}{W^2} g_c(\sigma', m\Delta), \tag{1.13}$$

where σ' and W are defined by (1.5) and (1.6), but with $m\Delta$ in place of β. Implementation of (1.13) involves interpolation for estimating $g_c(\sigma', m\Delta)$ from values of $g_c(n'\lambda, m\Delta)$. The nature of such an interpolation has been discussed in some detail in Section 8.5. Note that (1.13) can be described as a "weighted backprojection." Given a point (r, ϕ) and a source position $m\Delta$ the ray $(\sigma', m\Delta)$ is exactly the ray from the source position $m\Delta$ through the point (r, ϕ). The contribution of the convolved ray sum $g_c(\sigma', m\Delta)$ to the value of f^* at points (r, ϕ) which the ray goes through is inversely proportional to the square of the distance of the point (r, ϕ) from the source position $m\Delta$.

The actual computer implementation of this process is nearly identical to the computer implementation of the parallel convolution method, as described by (3.3) and (3.4) in Chapter 8. We do not repeat this discussion for the divergent case; we turn our attention instead to the choice of the window F_A.

10.2   CHOICE OF THE CONVOLVING FUNCTION

In Section 8.6 we have given a general discussion of some of the principles involved in choosing the convolving and interpolating functions for the parallel beam convolution method. Linear interpolation was found to be clearly superior to nearest neighbor interpolation; for the divergent method we adopt linear interpolation without further discussion in this book.

The purpose of this section is to answer the question: How does the selection of the window F_A influence the quality of the reconstruction? Two approaches which may be taken to answer this question are the following.

(i)   Specify some criteria for measuring the quality of reconstructions and find windows which are "optimal" by these criteria.

(ii)   Take a representative selection of window functions and investigate these according to some basic criteria (such as reconstruction of signal and resistance to noise) and also according to their behavior on test cases typical of the intended application area.

While the former approach is mathematically more attractive, it may not lead to efficacious windows for the following reasons. It is hard to translate the desirable properties of a window for a particular application into mathematical terms. (How does one translate into mathematics: "I want a window which produces diagnostically informative head cross sections from x-ray projections"?) More easily expressed general properties are likely to have some arbitrary parameters in them, and the "optimal" window may be strongly dependent on the values assigned to these parameters. (We see an example of this in the following.) Once the criterion according to which the optimality of the window is determined is fixed, it may still be very difficult to find the optimal window. Usually, simplifying assumptions are made in its derivation (such as the availability of projections from all directions, or that the noise in the measurement is independent of the signal) making it doubtful that the derived window is really optimal for the actual method of data collection. Even with simplifying assumptions, it is often hard to find a closed form solution for the optimal window.

For the reasons just listed, we use the second approach in investigating the influence of the window on reconstruction quality. In choosing our windows we take the following considerations into account.

Under ideal circumstances, we should use a window whose value is 1 within its bandwidth and whose bandwidth is as large as possible. The purpose of using any other window is to reduce the effect of errors introduced by using finite numbers of views, by discretizing the projection data, and by various kinds of noise. Generally, the Fourier transform of the projection data dies away rapidly at higher frequencies, and so the effects of aliasing due to sampling of the projection data and the effects of noise are usually more significant at high frequencies than at low frequencies. A "good" window tends to de-emphasize these effects.

According to the conditions for F_A together with the consideration of de-emphasizing the errors without too much loss of information, windows of interest should be nonincreasing functions of U with $(1 - 2U/A) \leq F_A(U) \leq 1$ over the interval $[0, A/2]$. In order to investigate a range of possibilities, we look at the generalized Hamming window with three different values of the parameter α, namely 1.0, 0.8, and 0.54 (see Table 8.1 and Section 8.6). In all cases the bandwidth A was chosen to be $1/\lambda$, for reasons which should be clear in view of the discussion in Section 8.6.

For each of the three windows mentioned in the last paragraph we have carried out three experiments: one to test the ability of the method to reconstruct signal in the absence of noise, the other to evaluate the noise resistance of the method, and the last one to test the efficacy of the method for reconstructing from x-ray data cross sections of the human head.

In all experiments we have used the standard geometry of data collection (see Section 5.2), and the function to be reconstructed has been estimated at the center of a 115-element grid (see Section 4.1). The spacing between these points is 0.1504 cm.

The three experiments are discussed in separate sections.

10.3   POINT RESPONSE FUNCTION

Since the projection process and the divergent beam convolution reconstruction process are both linear (see Section 6.3), a reasonable choice of
the reconstruction algorithm is the one which gives the most desirable
reconstruction when the original picture to be reconstructed is a single point.
Unfortunately, looking at the reconstruction formula one finds that the
reconstruction of a point is not *stationary*; i.e., the dependence of reconstruction on the point location is not simply translational. Although the shape of
the point reconstruction depends on the point location, we are using the
reconstruction of a point situated at the origin as an example for the analysis
below. Therefore the ray sum is 1 for the center ray in each projection and
zero elsewhere.

We use $P^*(r, \phi)$ to denote the value of reconstructed point response
function at the point (r, ϕ). This value is provided by substitution of the
discrete projection data into (1.12) and (1.13).

Figure 10.2 shows a three-dimensional display of the reconstructed point
response function associated with the generalized Hamming window with

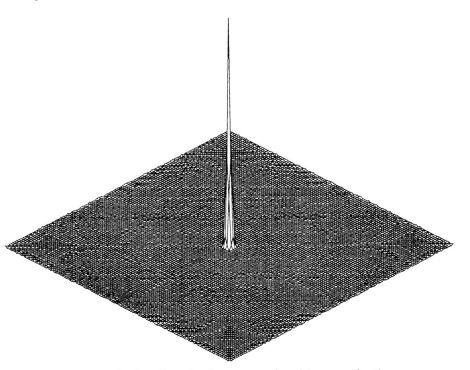

Fig. 10.2. The three-dimensional appearance of a point response function.

$\alpha = 0.54$. The oscillations away from the peak are too small to be visible in this mode of display. A better indication of these oscillations is given in Fig. 10.3.

Ideally, $P^*(r, \phi)$ should have value zero at all $r \neq 0$. In practice this is not the case. The danger is that oscillations in the reconstruction due to a point at which the original has a large value (see Fig. 10.2) will hide the reconstructed value at another point where the original has a smaller value. This motivates us to look at the normalized reconstructed point response function, defined by

$$P_N^*(r, \phi) = P^*(r, \phi)/P^*(0, 0). \tag{3.1}$$

A discrete one-dimensional representation of this function is given by

$$B(\ell) = 10 \log_{10} |P_N^*(\ell d, 0)|, \tag{3.2}$$

where d is the sampling distance in the display; in our case 0.1504 cm. Clearly, $B(0) = 0$. For $\ell \neq 0$, we would like the value of $B(\ell)$ to be as small as possible, with $-\infty$ being the ideal. Figure 10.3 shows plots of $B(\ell)$ for our three windows.

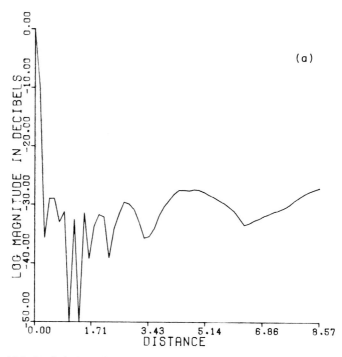

Fig. 10.3. Decibel plots of the normalized point response functions for the generalized Hamming window with (a) $\alpha = 1.0$, (b) $\alpha = 0.8$, (c) $\alpha = 0.54$.

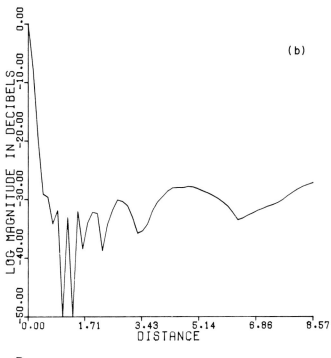

(b)

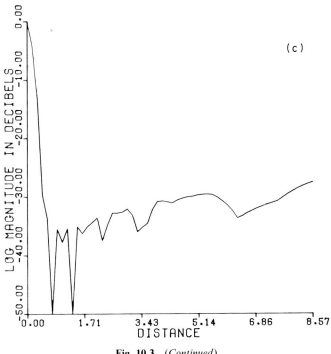

(c)

Fig. 10.3 (*Continued*)

TABLE 10.1

MEASURES OF DESIRABILITY OF THE GENERALIZED HAMMING WINDOW FOR DIFFERENT VALUES OF α[a]

α	HWHM	First overshoot	Distant tail	$10^5 \times \mathscr{D}_{3.0} P_N^*$	$10^4 \times \mathscr{D}_{6.0} P_N^*$	$10^2 \times \mathscr{D}_{12.0} P_N^*$	S
1.0	0.5586	−29.945	−27.098	5.6777	9.6478	2.5619	0.2494
0.8	0.5984	−31.820	−27.186	8.6949	8.5270	2.1138	0.1783
0.54	0.8106	−35.505	−27.506	52.0823	9.1819	1.0325	0.1012

[a] The first six measures relate to the point response function (ability to reconstruct the signal) and the seventh measure refers to the ability to suppress noise. For all seven measures it is desirable to have the values as small as possible.

In Table 10.1 we report on some measures of desirability of $B(\ell)$. These are defined as follows. (The smaller these values are the more desirable is the point response function.)

(i) *Half-width at half-maximum* (HWHM) is the smallest positive ℓ such that $B(\ell) = 10 \log_{10} 0.5$.

(ii) Size of the *first overshoot* is the value of $B(\ell)$ at the smallest positive integer ℓ such that $B(\ell) > B(\ell - 1)$ and $B(\ell) > B(\ell + 1)$.

(iii) Size of the *distant tail* is $B(57)$. (This corresponds to the last pixel on the x axis.)

Looking at the reconstructed point response functions, we immediately observe the difficulty with our measures of desirability: they are not consistent. As far as HWHM is concerned $\alpha = 1.0$ is the best and $\alpha = 0.54$ is the worst, but the first overshoot and distant tail give exactly the opposite result. So the "optimality" of a window is dependent on the chosen criterion.

To emphasize this point further, consider the following way of evaluating the goodness of a normalized point response function. Large values very near the point are "acceptable" since they indicate only a slight blurring. As we go further away from the point large values become less desirable, since they now indicate much blurring (or overshoot). However, a large value very far from the point may well be irrelevant, since the artifact caused is possibly outside the cross section in which we are interested and so would not disturb the medical diagnosis. We can define a family of *desirability functionals* $\mathscr{D}_R$ for normalized point response functions as follows

$$\mathscr{D}_R P_N^* = \int_0^{2\pi} \int_0^R |rP_N^*(r, \phi)|^2 r \, dr \, d\phi. \tag{3.3}$$

Similar to our previously defined measures, small values of $\mathscr{D}_R P_N^*$ indicate desirability.

In Table 10.1 we give the desirability measures of the point response functions associated with $\alpha = 1$, $\alpha = 0.80$, and $\alpha = 0.54$ for three different values of R. As can be seen, each window has a claim of being the best, depending on how R is chosen.

One can approach the problem of window selection quite differently. Given a normalized point response function, it is possible to produce a window that would give rise to that normalized point response function, or something very similar to it. However, our previous discussion on the difficulty of measuring the desirability of a point response function indicates that such an approach to window design is not guaranteed to produce reconstructions of amazing quality; the question has only been shifted from "which window produces a good reconstruction?" to "which point response function is associated with good reconstructions?". Since the harmonic decomposition of a function may well be the most appropriate framework in which such a question should be discussed (see Section 8.6), it is not clear that much can be gained by such a shift.

10.4   NOISE RECONSTRUCTION

In addition to the point response, the efficacy of a reconstruction algorithm is affected by its immunity to noise in the data. Let us assume that the projection data are corrupted with additive noise. Due to the linearity of the convolution method, the reconstruction is the sum of the reconstruction provided by the true signal and the reconstruction of the noise. Hence we concentrate on the behavior of the algorithm on pure noise.

In order to get a rough feeling for the relationship between the noise in the reconstruction and the noise in the data, we investigate the nature of the reconstruction of a very simple (and for our application, unrealistic) type of noise. We assume that each measurement of $g(n\lambda, m\Delta)$ is an independent sample of the same random variable R such that $\mu_R = 0$ (see Section 1.2). Then the reconstructed value at the point (r, ϕ), as determined by (1.13), is also a random variable, which we denote by $F^*(r, \phi)$. It is easy to show that $\mu_{F^*(r, \phi)} = 0$. In words, if the data are zero mean noise, then the reconstructed value at a point has also zero mean. The variance $V_{F^*(r, \phi)}$ depends on a number of things: the variance of the data V_R, the convolving functions $q^{(1)}$ and $q^{(2)}$ used in the reconstruction, the interpolating function ψ for the interpolation used in (1.13), the number of views M, the sampling angle λ, and the location of the point (r, ϕ). The precise formula is

$$V_{F^*(r, \phi)} = [C(r, \phi)]^2 V_R, \tag{4.1}$$

where

$$[C(r, \phi)]^2 = \frac{\lambda^2 D^2}{4M^2\pi^2} \sum_{m=0}^{M-1} \frac{1}{W^2} \sum_{n=-N}^{N} \left[\sum_{n'=-N}^{N} \psi(\sigma' - n'\lambda)q_{n',n} \right]^2, \quad (4.2)$$

with

$$q_{n',n} = q^{(1)}((n' - n)\lambda)\cos n\lambda + q^{(2)}((n' - n)\lambda)\cos n'\lambda. \quad (4.3)$$

In order to determine the sensitivity to noise of a reconstruction algorithm, a global measure of noise effect, rather than a measure at an individual point, is needed. One way of obtaining such a measure is to average the value of $C(r, \phi)$ for a number of points (r, ϕ). We had done this for our noise reconstructions, based on (4.1)–(4.3), using the values at 49 points of a 7×7 grid with spacing 2.8576 cm. The results are incorporated into Table 10.1 under heading S. The averaged standard deviation of the reconstruction is $S\sqrt{V_R}$; see (4.1).

In view of the discussion in Section 8.6 it is not surprising that the window which most suppresses higher frequency components ($\alpha = 0.54$) is the one which is most resistant to noise.

Note that while the value of S indicates how different windows suppress the influence of noise in the data at individual points in the reconstruction, it says nothing about the way noise in the reconstruction is correlated. It may be the case that a window with low value of S is nevertheless considered undesirable in case of noisy data, because it produces structured noise, i.e., noise which influences reconstructed values at neighboring points in a sufficiently similar way as to introduce a false feature spreading over a relatively large area.

10.5   REBINNING

As has been pointed out in Section 10.1, a ray (σ, β) in the divergent geometry corresponds to a point in (ℓ, θ) space. In Chapter 6 we have already given a convolution method for estimating the inverse Radon transform of a function p of two real variables from its (estimated) values at points $(ud, v\Gamma)$, where $-U \leq u \leq U$ and $0 \leq v \leq V - 1$, with $Ud \geq E$ and $V\Gamma = \pi$. The data collected in the divergent mode of data collection, $g(n\lambda, m\Delta)$, where $-N \leq n \leq N$, $0 \leq m \leq M - 1$, with $N\lambda \geq \delta$ and $M\Delta = 2\pi$, can be considered, in view of (1.2), to provide us with values of p according to the rule

$$p(D \sin n\lambda, m\Delta + n\lambda) = g(n\lambda, m\Delta). \quad (5.1)$$

Figure 10.4 shows the points in (ℓ, θ) space at which p is determined according to (5.1). This should be compared to Fig. 6.2.

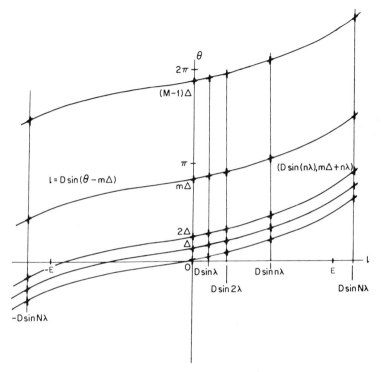

Fig. 10.4. The locations in (ℓ, θ) space of the points for which measurements have been collected in the divergent mode of data collection shown in Fig. 5.2. A typical point is $(D \sin(n\lambda), m\Delta + n\lambda)$, which lies at the intersection of the straight line $\ell = D \sin(n\lambda)$ and the sinusoidal $\ell = D \sin(\theta - m\Delta)$. [Reproduced from Herman (1980), with permission.]

Rewriting (1.5) of Chapter 6 we get

$$p(D \sin n\lambda, m\Delta + n\lambda) = p(D \sin(-n)\lambda, m\Delta + n\lambda + \pi)$$
$$= p(D \sin(-n)\lambda, m\Delta + n\lambda - \pi). \qquad (5.2)$$

Thus, values of $p(D \sin n\lambda, m\Delta + n\lambda)$ in (5.1), with $m\Delta + n\lambda$ outside the range 0 to π, provide us with values of $p(\ell, \theta)$ with $\ell = D \sin n\lambda$ for some n, $-N \leq n \leq N$, and $0 \leq \theta < \pi$.

In summary, the divergent ray projection data provides us with values of $p(\ell_n, \theta_{n,k})$, where $\ell_n = D \sin n\lambda$, for $-N \leq n \leq N$, and $0 \leq \theta_{n,k} < \pi$. From these values we wish to estimate $p(ud, v\Gamma)$ for $-U \leq u \leq U$ and $0 \leq v \leq V - 1$.

One way of doing this is the following two-stage process called *rebinning*.

During the first stage, we do the following for each n, $-N \leq n \leq N$. We consider n fixed, and we estimate, for $0 \leq v \leq V - 1$, the value of $p(\ell_n, v\Gamma)$ from the values of $p(\ell_n, \theta_{n,k})$. This is done by interpolation (for example, linear interpolation) in the second variable. Thus, the first stage gives us ray sums for sets of parallel, but unequally spaced rays.

During the second stage, we do the following for each $v, 0 \leq v \leq V - 1$. We consider v fixed, and we estimate for $-U \leq u \leq U$, the value of $p(ud, v\Gamma)$ from the values of $p(\ell_n, v\Gamma)$. This is done by interpolation (for example, linear interpolation) in the first variable. Thus, the second stage gives us ray sums for sets of parallel and equally spaced rays, as desired. The parallel beam convolution method can now be applied to this data set.

10.6 COMPARISON OF RECONSTRUCTIONS
FROM THE STANDARD PROJECTION DATA

We applied both the reconstruction methods discussed in this chapter to the standard projection data. In the case of rebinning, the parallel geometry into which the data were rebinned is the standard parallel geometry, see Section 5.6. For both methods we used linear interpolation and the generalized Hamming window with three settings of α: 1.0, 0.8, and 0.54. The reconstructions are reported in Figs. 10.5 and 10.6, as well as Table 10.2. The process of nonlinear smoothing with threshold 0.04 and weights 9, 4, and 1 (for the meaning of these terms see Section 11.4) has been applied to the output of the divergent beam convolution method; the resulting processed reconstructions are also reported. The method used in Chapter 5 to show the effects of the different physical sources of error is the divergent beam convolution method with generalized Hamming window, $\alpha = 0.8$, and nonlinear smoothing with parameters just described.

We can draw the following conclusions from these results.

First, there is very little difference between the reconstructions obtained using the divergent beam convolution method and the reconstructions obtained using rebinning and the parallel beam convolution method with the same window and interpolating function. Hence the choice of method is not determined by the quality of the reconstructions.

It does appear from our timings that rebinning and then parallel convolution is faster than divergent convolution. This is not surprising, since the divergent convolution method uses twice as many views and requires multiplication by a weighting factor during its backprojection stage. However, one should not pay too much attention to the exact values of these timings. As it has been explained in Section 6.5, the timings depend on many things which are not necessarily essential to the nature of the method. To illustrate this point, we have applied to the standard projection data the divergent beam reconstruction algorithm as implemented on a minicomputer (the Eclipse S/200) which had a "special tomographic processor" (a device

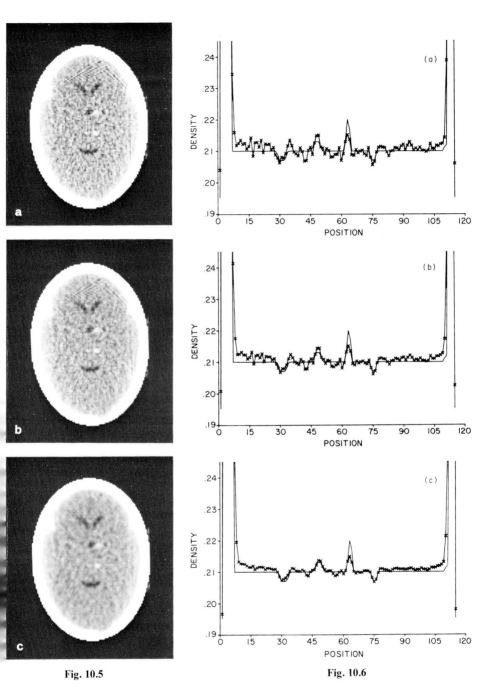

Fig. 10.5   **Fig. 10.6**

Fig. 10.5. Reconstructions from the standard projection data using convolution methods. (a), (b), and (c) are the results of rebinning to the standard parallel geometry and then applying the convolution method for parallel beams, linear interpolation, and Hamming window with $\alpha = 1.0$, 0.8, and 0.54, respectively. (d), (e), and (f) are reconstructions with the convolution method with divergent beams, linear interpolation, and Hamming window with $\alpha = 1.0$, 0.8, and 0.54, respectively. (g), (h), and (i) are the results of applying nonlinear smoothing to (d), (e), and (f), respectively, with threshold and weights given in the text (in Section 11.4).

Fig. 10.6. Plots of the 63rd columns in the reconstructions of Fig. 10.5.

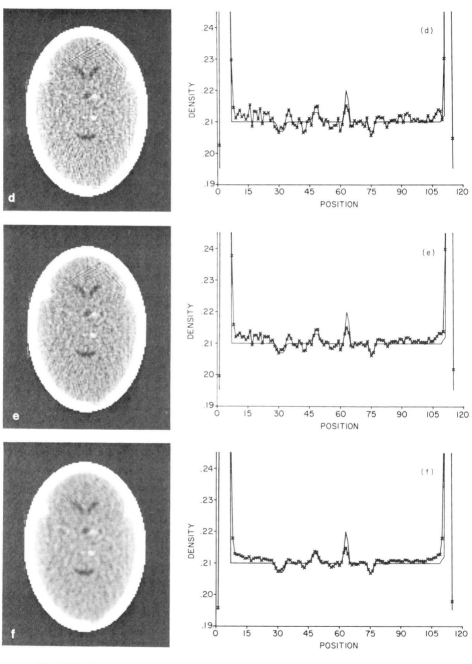

Fig. 10.5   (*Continued*)   Fig. 10.6   (*Continued*)

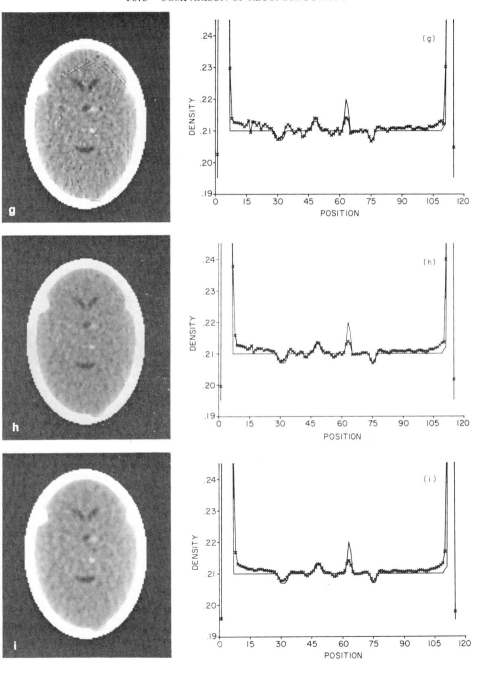

Fig. 10.5 (*Continued*)   Fig. 10.6 (*Continued*)

TABLE 10.2

PICTURE DISTANCE MEASUREMENTS FOR THE RECONSTRUCTIONS IN
FIG. 10.5

		d	r	e	t
Parallel	$\alpha = 1.0$	0.1038	0.0447	0.0597	158
convolution on	$\alpha = 0.8$	0.1278	0.0510	0.0756	164
rebinned data:	$\alpha = 0.54$	0.1629	0.0602	0.0962	162
Divergent	$\alpha = 1.0$	0.0918	0.0422	0.0500	835
convolution	$\alpha = 0.8$	0.1162	0.0480	0.0674	847
unsmoothed:	$\alpha = 0.54$	0.1545	0.0570	0.0900	863
Divergent	$\alpha = 1.0$	0.0913	0.0406	0.0497	841
convolution	$\alpha = 0.8$	0.1159	0.0465	0.0674	853
smoothed:	$\alpha = 0.54$	0.1544	0.0558	0.0900	868

built by Data General for the General Electric Company to be used with their early CT scanners). The reconstruction took only 90 sec, which is much less than the time of 847 sec reported in Table 10.2. (That time is for a large computer, Cyber 173, using SNARK77.) Since processors much faster than the special tomographic processor can be inexpensively built, timing is also unlikely to be the deciding factor between the two methods discussed in this section.

A situation where reconstruction without rebinning may be advantageous is when data are collected so fast (and possibly in such large quantities) that the storing of the data, necessary for rebinning, becomes difficult to manage. Such a situation can arise with the fifth scanning mode shown in Fig. 3.3e (see Section 3.4). In such a case the divergent beam convolution method, which processes each view separately, is probably simpler to implement in a sufficiently fast hardware device.

The choice of window makes a definite difference to the quality of reconstruction. However, it is not easy to decide which reconstruction is the "best." The value $\alpha = 1.0$ is the best according to the picture distance measures, but certainly not visually. The reason for this (and for most other occurrences of the same phenomenon in this book) is that the accuracy of the reconstruction of the skull has a large influence on the picture distance measures, but no influence on the displays (at least at the settings of black and white that we have chosen). In the interior of the skull both $\alpha = 0.8$ and $\alpha = 0.54$ seem to perform better than $\alpha = 1.0$, with no overall advantage to either of those two. We used the same threshold for nonlinear smoothing for all three windows. This resulted in actually emphasizing some of the artifacts in case $\alpha = 1.0$ and, to a lesser extent, when $\alpha = 0.8$. We may conclude from all this that the choice of window and nonlinear smoothing is dependent on the information which we wish to obtain about the picture we are reconstructing.

NOTES AND REFERENCES

The earliest development, as far as this author knows, of a convolution reconstruction method for divergent beams without rebinning is due to Pavkovich (1979). His results did not become publicly available until some time after the appearance of an independent development by Lakshmina-rayanan (1975).

Detailed derivations of the Radon inversion formula for divergent rays (1.3) as well as of (1.9) are given by Herman and Naparstek (1977).

Our presentation of the convolution method for divergent beams without rebinning and our discussion of the choice of the convolving function is based on Chang and Herman (1978). That paper references earlier literature on related approaches. (A noteworthy, missing reference is Tretiak (1975) on the point response function.) It also contains some details, for example on finding an "optimal" window, which were not included in this book. The mathematical theory underlying the inversion of the transform which corresponds to the divergent beam method of data collection has been studied by Smith *et al.* (1978).

The superiority of linear interpolation to nearest neighbor in conjunction with the divergent beam convolution algorithm has been illustrated, for example, by Herman and Naparstek (1977).

Our discussion of rebinning is based on Herman and Lung (1979), which gives references to earlier work on which it is based. See, in particular, Dreike and Boyd (1976).

Devices capable of implementing the divergent beam reconstruction algorithm so that each reconstruction takes less than one hundredth of a second (1/100 sec) are presently being built; see Gilbert *et al.* (1979).

11

The Algebraic Reconstruction Techniques

In this and the next two chapters we discuss series expansion methods for image reconstruction.

The *algebraic reconstruction techniques* (ART) form a large family of reconstruction algorithms. The name is a historical accident; there is nothing more "algebraic" about these techniques than about the techniques which are to be discussed in the next chapter. The distinguishing feature of ART needs careful discussion, which is given in the next section.

11.1   WHAT IS ART?

All series expansion methods are procedures for the solution of the discrete reconstruction problem. As it has been discussed in Section 6.3, this is the problem of estimating an image vector x such that $y = Rx + e$, given a measurement vector y. The estimation is done by requiring x, and the error vector e, to satisfy some specified optimization criterion of the type discussed in Section 6.4. We use x^* to denote the required estimate.

All ART methods of image reconstruction are *iterative procedures*. That is, they produce a sequence of vectors $x^{(0)}$, $x^{(1)}$, $x^{(2)}$, ... such that the sequence *converges* to x^*. This means that, for $1 \leq j \leq J$, $x_j^{(k)}$ (the jth component of the kth iterate) is guaranteed to be arbitrarily near to x_j^*, provided that k is chosen large enough. The process of producing $x^{(k+1)}$ from $x^{(k)}$ is referred to as an *iterative step*.

In ART, $x^{(k+1)}$ is obtained from $x^{(k)}$ by considering a single one of the I approximate equations [see (3.7) of Chapter 6]. In fact, the equations are used in a cyclic order. We use i_k to denote $[k \pmod{I} + 1]$; i.e., $i_0 = 1$, $i_1 = 2, \ldots, i_{I-1} = I, i_I = 1, i_{I+1} = 2, \ldots$. For $1 \leq i \leq I$, we use r_i to denote the J-dimensional column vector whose jth component is $r_{i,j}$. In other words, r_i is the transpose of the ith row of R.

The kth iterative step in ART can be described by a function α_k whose arguments are two J-dimensional vectors and one real number and whose value is a J-dimensional vector. (In mathematical jargon, $\alpha_k : R^J \times R^J \times R \rightarrow R^J$, where R denotes the set of real numbers.) Then,

$$x^{(k+1)} = \alpha_k(x^{(k)}, r_{i_k}, y_{i_k}). \tag{1.1}$$

In words, a particular algebraic reconstruction technique is defined by a sequence of functions $\alpha_0, \alpha_1, \alpha_2 \ldots$. In order to get the $(k + 1)$st iterate we apply α_k to the kth iterate, the i_kth row of the projection matrix R, and the i_kth component of the measurement vector y. Such algorithms have been referred to as *storage efficient*, because the J-dimensional vector $x^{(k+1)}$ can be stored in the same part of computer memory where $x^{(k)}$ has been kept, since $x^{(k)}$ is not needed by the algorithm after the kth step. (Note that the implementation of the convolution method described near the end of Section 8.3 is also storage efficient. The same can not be said for the iterative procedures which are discussed in the next chapter.)

Various ART methods differ from each other in the way the sequence of α_k's is chosen. We now illustrate the previous discussion on a particularly simple example.

One way of choosing the α_k's is the following. For any J-dimensional vectors x and t and for any real number z,

$$\alpha_k(x, t, z) = \begin{cases} x + \dfrac{z - \langle t, x \rangle}{\langle t, t \rangle} t & \text{if } \langle t, t \rangle \neq 0, \\ x & \text{if } \langle t, t \rangle = 0. \end{cases} \tag{1.2}$$

where $\langle \ , \ \rangle$ denotes the *inner product* of two J-dimensional vectors; i.e.,

$$\langle t, x \rangle = \sum_{j=1}^{J} t_j x_j, \tag{1.3}$$

Note that, in this case, the α_k's are the same for all k.

Defining α_k in this way has a number of attractive properties. One is that, if $\langle r_{i_k}, r_{i_k} \rangle \neq 0$, then

$$y_{i_k} = \sum_{j=1}^{J} r_{i_k, j} x_j^{(k+1)}; \tag{1.4}$$

i.e., the i_kth approximate equality is exactly satisfied after the kth step. To see this, combine (1.1) and (1.2), and make use of the notation of (1.3).

The right-hand side of (1.4) can be written as

$$\langle r_{i_k}, x^{(k+1)} \rangle = \langle r_{i_k}, \alpha_k(x^{(k)}, r_{i_k}, y_{i_k}) \rangle$$

$$= \langle r_{i_k}, x^{(k)} \rangle + \frac{y_{i_k} - \langle r_{i_k}, x^{(k)} \rangle}{\langle r_{i_k}, r_{i_k} \rangle} \langle r_{i_k}, r_{i_k} \rangle$$

$$= y_{i_k},$$

as claimed in (1.4).

Another attractive property of defining α_k by (1.2) is that the updating of $x^{(k)}$ becomes very simple: we just add to $x^{(k)}$ a multiple of the vector r_{i_k}. In practice, this updating of $x^{(k)}$ can be computationally very inexpensive.

Consider, for example, the case when the basis pictures are the ones associated with digitization [see (3.1) of Chapter 6]. Then $r_{i,j}$ is just the length of intersection of the ith ray with the jth pixel. This has two consequences. First, most of the components of the vector r_{i_k} are zero. At most $2\ell - 1$ pixels can be intersected by a straight line in an $\ell \times \ell$ digitization of a picture. Thus, of the ℓ^2 components of r_{i_k} at most $2\ell - 1$ (and typically only about ℓ) are nonzero. Second, the location and size of the nonzero components of r_{i_k} can be easily calculated from the geometrical location of the i_kth ray relative to the $\ell \times \ell$ grid. Thus, the projection matrix R need never be stored in the computer. Only one row of the matrix is needed at a time, and all essential information about this row is easily calculable.

We investigate this point further, since it is basic to the understanding of the computational efficacy of ART.

Suppose that we have a list $j_1, \ldots, j_U$ of numbers such that $t_j = 0$ unless j is one of the $j_1, \ldots, j_U$. Then evaluation of (1.3) requires only U multiplications, which in our application is much smaller than J, as discussed previously. Similarly $\langle t, t \rangle$ can be evaluated using U multiplications. Having evaluated $[(z - \langle t, x \rangle)/\langle t, t \rangle]$ using $2U$ multiplications (and one division), the updating of x can be achieved by a further U multiplications. This is because only those x_j need be altered for which $j = j_u$ for some u, $1 \le u \le U$, and the alteration requires adding to x_j a fixed multiple of t_j.

We see that a single step of the algorithm, as described by (1.2), is very simple to implement in a computationally efficient way.

Apart from its computational efficiency, (1.2) is an intuitively reasonable way of producing $x^{(k+1)}$ from $x^{(k)}$. Suppose that, in addition to requiring the satisfaction of (1.4) after the kth iterative step, we impose the following conditions on the way the kth step should be carried out.

(i)   Only those pixels which are intersected by the i_kth ray should have their densities changed.

(ii)   The change in the density of a pixel should be proportional to $y_{i_k} - \langle r_{i_k}, x^{(k)} \rangle$ (the "error" in the i_kth approximate equality prior to the kth step).

(iii)   The change in the jth pixel should be proportional to $r_{i_k, j}$.

These conditions, nearly identical to the conditions for discrete back-projection stated in Section 7.3, uniquely determine how the α_k's are to be defined; and they lead to (1.2). The early literature on ART relied on justifying the algorithms by showing that they are derived from such intuitively reasonable conditions.

Before we get into the details of specific ART methods, two comments are in order.

First, for (1.1) to specify the sequence $x^{(0)}, x^{(1)}, x^{(2)}, \ldots$ precisely, we need to specify the *initial vector* $x^{(0)}$. The choice of $x^{(0)}$ is quite important in the practical behavior of these algorithms. More is said about this in the following.

Second, if the version of the discrete reconstruction problem which is represented by the system of inequalities $Nx \leq q$ (see Section 6.4) is used, then the general description of ART given by (1.1) is not always adequate. In such a case, a slightly more complicated general framework may be required, but one which has essentially similar computational requirements. We discuss a similar situation in Section 11.3 in some detail.

11.2   RELAXATION METHODS FOR SOLVING SYSTEMS OF INEQUALITIES AND EQUALITIES

In this section we give the mathematical background to ART. We do this in the framework of the mathematical problem "find a vector, which satisfies all of a given set of linear inequalities." In other words, we are interested in finding a J-dimensional vector x such that

$$\langle n_i, x \rangle \leq q_i, \qquad 1 \leq i \leq P, \tag{2.1}$$

where the n_i are given J-dimensional vectors and the q_i are given real numbers. [Equation (2.1) is a rewrite of (4.17) of Chapter 6.]

In all that follows we assume that n_i has at least one nonzero component. A physical interpretation of this assumption is that we do not make use of a measurement if none of the pixels contributed to it. The reason for making the assumption is that we wish to avoid having to make special cases all the time when $\langle n_i, n_i \rangle = 0$, like we had to do in (1.2).

We introduce some sets of vectors N_i $(1 \leq i \leq P)$ and N. For $1 \leq i \leq P$,

$$N_i = \{x \mid \langle n_i, x \rangle \leq q_i\} \tag{2.2}$$

and

$$N = \bigcap_{i=1}^{P} N_i. \qquad (2.3)$$

In words, N_i is the set of vectors which satisfies the ith of the P inequalities in (2.1), and N is the set of vectors which satisfies all the P inequalities. Our aim, for now, is to find an element of N.

More precisely, we need an algorithm, which, given $n_1, \ldots, n_P, q_1, \ldots, q_P$ finds an x in N. We propose an ART-type method. It is defined by the sequence of functions

$$\alpha_k(x, t, z) = \begin{cases} x & \text{if } \langle t, x \rangle \leq z, \\ x + \lambda^{(k)}[(z - \langle t, x \rangle)/\langle t, t \rangle]t & \text{otherwise,} \end{cases} \qquad (2.4)$$

where $\lambda^{(k)}$ is a real number, which is referred to in this context as the *relaxation parameter*.

Consider the following procedure, which we refer to as the *relaxation method for inequalities*.

$$\begin{aligned} & x^{(0)} \text{ is arbitrary,} \\ & x^{(k+1)} = \alpha_k(x^{(k)}, n_{i_k}, q_{i_k}), \end{aligned} \qquad (2.5)$$

where α_k is defined by (2.4) and $i_k = [k(\text{mod } P) + 1]$. If the relaxation parameters satisfy the weak condition that for all k,

$$0 < \varepsilon_1 \leq \lambda^{(k)} \leq \varepsilon_2 < 2, \qquad (2.6)$$

then the relaxation method for inequalities produces a sequence, $x^{(0)}, x^{(1)}, x^{(2)}, \ldots$, which converges to a vector in N, provided only that N is not empty. Proof of this result appears in Section 16.8.

For now we wish to discuss the geometrical nature of the relaxation method for inequalities and, in particular, the role of the relaxation parameters. Let

$$H_i = \{x \mid \langle n_i, x \rangle = q_i\}. \qquad (2.7)$$

In words, H_i is the set of vectors x for which the ith inequality is satisfied by the two sides of the inequality being actually equal. Note that H_i is a subset of N_i. Each of the H_i is what mathematicians call a *hyperplane*. If the dimension J of x is three, a hyperplane is a plane in three-dimensional space. If the dimension J of x is two, a hyperplane is a straight line in two-dimensional space (i.e., in a plane).

The two-dimensional situation is illustrated in Fig. 11.1. There are two

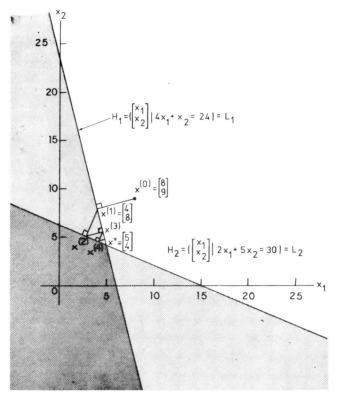

Fig. 11.1. Demonstration of the relaxation method (with $\lambda^{(k)} = 1$ for all k) for the simple case when $I = J = 2$. In the demonstration n_1 and n_2 are given by (2.8) and q_1 and q_2 by (2.9). [Illustration based on Herman and Lent (1976a) with permission. Copyright 1976, Pergamon Press, Ltd.]

hyperplanes H_1 and H_2. For these hyperplanes

$$n_1 = \begin{bmatrix} 4 \\ 1 \end{bmatrix}, \qquad n_2 = \begin{bmatrix} 2 \\ 5 \end{bmatrix}, \tag{2.8}$$

and

$$q_1 = 24, \qquad q_2 = 30. \tag{2.9}$$

Observe the following simple geometrical fact: The vector n_i (think of its as the line drawn from the origin to the point n_i in the plane) is perpendicular to the line H_i. This statement generalizes to any dimensions, as a reader acquainted with analytic geometry can easily see from (2.7).

Since in the relaxation method for inequalities, (2.5), the role of t in (2.4) is taken by n_{i_k}, we see that if $x^{(k+1)}$ differs from $x^{(k)}$ at all, then $x^{(k+1)} - x^{(k)}$ (which is a multiple of n_{i_k}) is perpendicular to H_{i_k}.

Let us look now at the geometrical interpretation of the N_i's. In the two-dimensional case, N_i is clearly a set of points lying on one side of the line H_i (including the line H_i). For example, in Fig. 11.1, both N_1 and N_2 are those half-planes which include the origin. Their intersection N, is shown dark-dotted in Fig. 11.1. This notion also generalizes, and we say that N_i is a *half-space* which is the set of points lying on one side of the hyperplane H_i (including the hyperplane H_i). N, as defined by (2.3), is an intersection of such half-spaces.

In the relaxation method for inequalities, as described by (2.4) and (2.5), if $x^{(k)}$ is in the half-space N_{i_k}, then we do not change our estimate during the kth iterative step [i.e., $x^{(k+1)} = x^{(k)}$]. If $x^{(k)}$ is not in the half-space N_{i_k}, then we move our estimate perpendicular to the bounding hyperplane H_{i_k} of N_{i_k} [i.e., $x^{(k+1)} - x^{(k)}$ is perpendicular to H_{i_k}]. The amount of movement depends on the size of $\lambda^{(k)}$.

If $\lambda^{(k)} = 1$, then by an argument identical to (1.3), we can prove that $\langle n_{i_k}, x^{(k+1)} \rangle = q_{i_k}$, i.e., that $x^{(k+1)}$ is in the hyperplane H_{i_k}. The following statement can be shown in a similarly easy fashion. During the kth step of the relaxation method for inequalities with $x^{(k)}$ not in N_{i_k}, the move from $x^{(k)}$ to $x^{(k+1)}$ is perpendicular to H_{i_k} and has the following geometrical property:

if $\lambda^{(k)} < 0$, move is away from H_{i_k};
if $\lambda^{(k)} = 0$, there is no movement;
if $0 < \lambda^{(k)} < 1$, move is toward H_{i_k}, but does not quite reach it;
if $\lambda^{(k)} = 1$, move is to H_{i_k} exactly;
if $1 < \lambda^{(k)} < 2$, move is past H_{i_k}, but $x^{(k+1)}$ is nearer to H_{i_k} than $x^{(k)}$ was;
if $\lambda^{(k)} = 2$, $x^{(k+1)}$ is the mirror image of $x^{(k)}$ in H_{i_k};
if $\lambda^{(k)} > 2$, $x^{(k+1)}$ is on the other side of H_{i_k}, further from H_{i_k} than $x^{(k)}$ was.

To illustrate the relaxation method for inequalities, consider again Fig. 11.1. Two inequalities are involved (i.e., $P = 2$), and the vectors n_1, n_2 and the scalars q_1, q_2 are defined by (2.8) and (2.9), respectively. Suppose we choose $\lambda^{(k)} = 1$, for all k. We also have to choose the initial vector. If we let

$$x^{(0)} = \begin{bmatrix} 8 \\ 9 \end{bmatrix}, \tag{2.10}$$

then, as it is easily checked,

$$x^{(1)} = \begin{bmatrix} 4 \\ 8 \end{bmatrix} \quad \text{and} \quad x^{(2)} = \begin{bmatrix} \frac{80}{29} \\ \frac{142}{29} \end{bmatrix}. \tag{2.11}$$

Since $x^{(2)}$ is both in N_1 and N_2, all values of $x^{(k)}$, for $k \geq 2$, are the same as $x^{(2)}$. Hence the method converges to $x^* = x^{(2)}$, which is in N.

The convergence that takes place in the previous example is called *finite convergence* since the $x^{(k)}$ remain constant after the first few iterative steps.

It is *not* the case that the relaxation method for inequalities always provides us with finite convergence if the $\lambda^{(k)}$ are chosen according to (2.6).

Now we turn to study systems of equations. Suppose we are given J-dimensional vectors a_i and real numbers b_i, for $1 \le i \le I$. Let,

$$L_i = \{x \,|\, \langle a_i, x \rangle = b_i\}, \tag{2.12}$$

and

$$L = \bigcap_{i=1}^{I} L_i. \tag{2.13}$$

We observe the following fact: L can also be expressed as the intersection of a set of half-spaces. In fact, if we let $P = 2I$ and define, for $1 \le i \le I$,

$$N_{2i-1} = \{x \,|\, \langle -a_i, x \rangle \le -b_i\}, \tag{2.14}$$
$$N_{2i} = \{x \,|\, \langle a_i, x \rangle \le b_i\}, \tag{2.15}$$

then

$$L_i = N_{2i-1} \cap N_{2i} \tag{2.16}$$

and, consequently, L defined by (2.13) is the same as N defined by (2.3), provided that the N_i are defined by (2.14) and (2.15). Hence we can apply the relaxation method for a system of inequalities to find an element of L. Here we assume that, for $1 \le i \le I$, $\langle a_i, a_i \rangle > 0$.

However, note that

$$L_i = H_{2i-1} = H_{2i}, \tag{2.17}$$

where H_i is the bounding hyperplane of the half-space N_i, as defined by (2.7). Hence the combined effect of the $(2k - 1)$st and $(2k)$th iterative steps is to move (if at all) perpendicular to the hyperplane L_{i_k}. We can combine these two steps into one and obtain the following *relaxation method for systems of equalities*:

$$\begin{aligned} &x^{(0)} \text{ is arbitrary,} \\ &x^{(k+1)} = x^{(k)} + c^{(k)} a_{i_k}. \end{aligned} \tag{2.18}$$

It easily follows from the result stated for the convergence of the relaxation method for inequalities that if, for all k,

$$c^{(k)} = \lambda^{(k)} \frac{b_{i_k} - \langle a_{i_k}, x^{(k)} \rangle}{\langle a_{i_k}, a_{i_k} \rangle}, \tag{2.19}$$

with $\lambda^{(k)}$ satisfying (2.6), then the relaxation method for equalities produces a sequence $x^{(0)}, x^{(1)}, x^{(2)}, \ldots$, which converges to a vector in L, provided only that L is not empty.

The algorithm described by (1.1) and (1.2) is a special case of the relaxation method for equalities, with $\lambda^{(k)} = 1$, for all k. We illustrate this special case in Fig. 11.1. Letting $a_1 = n_1$, $a_2 = n_2$, $b_1 = q_1$, and $b_2 = q_2$ be defined by (2.8) and (2.9), we see that if we start with $x^{(0)}$ defined by (2.10), then we get $x^{(1)}$ and $x^{(2)}$ as defined by (2.11). From this point on, the sequence produced by the relaxation method for equalities differs from the relaxation method for inequalities which we discussed before. This is because $x^{(2)}$ does not lie in L_2 and so further steps are necessary to get nearer and nearer to an element of L, which, in this case, is the unique intersection x^* of the two lines L_1 and L_2. Due to the geometrical interpretation given before, we see that the sequence of vectors is produced by dropping perpendiculars alternatively onto L_1 and L_2, see Fig. 11.1.

In general, L has more than one element. With a little extra care in choosing $x^{(0)}$, we can ensure that the relaxation method for equalities converges to an element of L which satisfies an optimization criterion, namely, the minimum norm criterion; see Section 6.4. To do this, we introduce a set S of vectors, which is the set of all linear combinations of the a_i; i.e.,

$$S = \left\{ x \,\middle|\, x = \sum_{i=1}^{I} \beta_i a_i \text{ for some real numbers } \beta_i \right\}. \qquad (2.20)$$

The following result is sometimes referred to as the *minimum norm theorem*. If L is not empty, then there exists one and only one element x^* in $L \cap S$; furthermore, for all x in L other than x^*,

$$\|x^*\| < \|x\|. \qquad (2.21)$$

$[\|x\|^2 = \langle x, x \rangle$; see (4.12) in Chapter 6.]

We refer to x^* as the minimum norm element of L. We have already discussed in Section 6.4 why choosing a minimum norm element may be considered useful in picture reconstruction.

It is clear from (2.18) that if we choose $x^{(0)}$ to be an element of S, then $x^{(k)}$ is an element of S, for all k. It follows, using basic linear algebra, that the limit x^* of the sequence $x^{(0)}, x^{(1)}, x^{(2)}, \ldots,$ is also in S. Since the limit x^* is also in L (by the convergence of the relaxation method for equalities), x^* is in $L \cap S$. Hence, by the minimum norm theorem, x^* is the minimum norm element of L.

In the example for Fig. 11.1, S is the set of all two-dimensional vectors. Hence $x^{(0)}$ is in S, however it is chosen. Since in that simple example there is only one solution, it is by necessity the minimum norm solution. This is, however, not typical. If there are more unknowns than equations, there will invariably be many solutions, and care has to be taken in choosing $x^{(0)}$, if the minimum norm solution is desired.

There are versions of the relaxation method which provide us with the minimum norm solution for a system of inequalities. These are more complex in their nature than the methods previously discussed and are beyond the scope of this book. In the next section we discuss a method whose implementation is similar to the implementation of relaxation methods for finding the minimum norm solution for a system of inequalities.

11.3   Additive ART

In this section we discuss the application of the relaxation methods of the last section to image reconstruction. Such methods are referred to as *additive* ART, since in a single iterative step the estimate is altered by adding to it a scalar multiple of the transpose of a row of the projection matrix; see, e.g., (1.1) and (1.2).

The simplest approach is to use the relaxation method for equalities, described by (2.18) and (2.19), with $a_i = r_i$ and $b_i = y_i$. By the result stated in the previous section this provides us with a sequence of vectors $x^{(0)}$, $x^{(1)}$, $x^{(2)}$, ..., which converges to an x^* such that $Rx^* = y$, provided there is such an x^*. The problem is that the relationship between the image vector x and the measurement vector y [see (3.8) of Chapter 6] is such that there may not exist such an x^*, or that if such an x^* exists, it is not a desirable solution to the discrete reconstruction problem. In view of this, it is pleasantly surprising that even this simple approach leads to acceptable reconstructions, especially if the relaxation parameters are chosen to be rather small (e.g., 0.05). This is illustrated in Section 11.5.

One way of making the theory of the last section applicable to the image reconstruction problem is by using the formulation which involves a system of inequalities [see (4.17) of Chapter 6]. Much work has been done in that direction. In particular, ART-type procedures exist which find the minimum norm solution of a system of inequalities. Such procedures require a formulation more complicated than what is provided by the framework of (1.1). In addition to the sequence of J-dimensional vectors $x^{(0)}$, $x^{(1)}$, $x^{(2)}$, ..., they produce and make use of a sequence of I-dimensional vectors $u^{(0)}$, $u^{(1)}$, $u^{(2)}$, ...

In this book we discuss an alternative approach, but one which has a similar implementation. We give an additive ART method for finding the Bayesian estimate (see Section 6.4) under certain restrictive assumptions.

In the terminology of Section 6.4 the assumptions we make are the following. Both X and E are multivariate Gaussian random variables, with μ_E the zero vector, and V_X and V_E both multiples of identity matrices of appropriate sizes. In other words, we assume that components of a sample of $X - \mu_X$ are uncorrelated, and that each component is a sample from the same Gaussian random variable; and we also assume that components of a sample of E are uncorrelated and that each component is a sample from the same zero mean Gaussian random variable.

We use t^2 to denote the diagonal entries of V_X and s^2 to denote the diagonal entries of V_E and let $r = t/s$. According to (4.8) of Chapter 6, the Bayesian estimate is the vector x which minimizes

$$r^2 \|y - Rx\|^2 + \|x - \mu_X\|^2. \tag{3.1}$$

Note that a small value of r indicates that a priori knowledge of the expected value of the image vector is important relative to the measured data, while a large value of r indicates that the opposite is true.

What we are going to do now is essentially the following. We look at the equation $Rx + e = y$ as an equation in $I + J$ unknowns, namely all the components of x and all the components of e. This is a consistent system of equations; for any x, $e = y - Rx$ provides a solution. Methods for solving consistent systems can therefore be applied. However, in order to find the x which minimizes (3.1) a slightly more complicated approach is needed.

We denote column vectors of dimension $I + J$ by

$$\begin{bmatrix} u \\ z \end{bmatrix},$$

where u has I components and z has J components. We also use the notation

$$[E \quad rR]$$

for the $I \times (I + J)$ matrix, whose first I columns form the $I \times I$ identity matrix E and whose last J columns form the matrix R with every component multiplied by r.

The system of equations

$$[E \quad rR]\begin{bmatrix} u \\ z \end{bmatrix} = r(y - R\mu_X), \tag{3.2}$$

is a consistent system of equations. This is because, if we let $\hat{z}$ be an arbitrary J-dimensional vector and we let

$$\hat{u} = r(y - R\mu_X - R\hat{z}), \tag{3.3}$$

then $\begin{bmatrix} \hat{u} \\ \hat{z} \end{bmatrix}$ satisfies (3.2).

The reason for introducing (3.2) is the following. If u^* and z^* are vectors such that $\begin{bmatrix} u^* \\ z^* \end{bmatrix}$ is the minimum norm solution of (3.2), and if

$$x^* = z^* + \mu_X, \tag{3.4}$$

then x^* minimizes (3.1).

In order to verify this claim consider any J-dimensional vector $\hat{x}$. Let

$$\hat{z} = \hat{x} - \mu_X \tag{3.5}$$

and $\hat{u}$ be defined by (3.3). Then

$$\hat{u} = r(y - R\hat{x}). \tag{3.6}$$

It follows that

$$r^2 \|y - R\hat{x}\|^2 + \|\hat{x} - \mu_X\|^2 = \|\hat{u}\|^2 + \|\hat{z}\|^2 \geq \|u^*\|^2 + \|z^*\|^2, \tag{3.7}$$

since $\begin{bmatrix} u^* \\ z^* \end{bmatrix}$ is the minimum norm solution of (3.2) and $\begin{bmatrix} \hat{u} \\ \hat{z} \end{bmatrix}$ is also a solution of (3.2).

From the fact that u^*, z^*, and x^* satisfy (3.2) and (3.4) we get that

$$u^* = r(y - Rx^*). \tag{3.8}$$

This combined with (3.4) and (3.7) gives that

$$r^2 \|y - R\hat{x}\|^2 + \|\hat{x} - \mu_X\|^2 \geq r^2 \|y - Rx^*\|^2 + \|x^* - \mu_X\|^2. \tag{3.9}$$

Since $\hat{x}$ is an arbitrary J-dimensional vector, this shows that x^* minimizes (3.1).

It follows therefore that any method which provides us with the minimum norm solution of (3.2) automatically gives us the vector which minimizes (3.1). One way of finding the minimum norm solution of a consistent system of equalities is the relaxation method for equalities. Note that the iterative step of (2.18) applied to (3.2) is

$$\begin{bmatrix} u^{(k+1)} \\ z^{(k+1)} \end{bmatrix} = \begin{bmatrix} u^{(k)} \\ z^{(k)} \end{bmatrix} + c^{(k)} \begin{bmatrix} e_{i_k} \\ r \times r_{i_k} \end{bmatrix}, \tag{3.10}$$

where e_i denotes the transpose of the ith row of E (which happens to be the same as the ith column of E, since E is an identity matrix), and

$$c^{(k)} = \lambda^{(k)} \frac{r(y_{i_k} - \langle r_{i_k}, \mu_X \rangle) - (u_{ik}^{(k)} + r\langle r_{i_k}, z^{(k)} \rangle)}{1 + r^2 \|r_{i_k}\|^2}. \tag{3.11}$$

Note that, if S is defined by (2.20), then the zero vector is in S. Hence, one way of ensuring that the relaxation method for equalities, with iterative steps as in (3.10), converges to the minimum norm solution of (3.2) is to choose both $u^{(0)}$ and $z^{(0)}$ to be the zero vector of appropriate dimension.

We define, for all k,

$$x^{(k)} = z^{(k)} + \mu_X. \tag{3.12}$$

If the sequence $z^{(0)}, z^{(1)}, z^{(2)}, \ldots$, converges to z^*, then the sequence $x^{(0)}, x^{(1)}, x^{(2)}, \ldots$, converges to x^*, defined by (3.4). This x^* minimizes (3.1).

There is in fact no need to explicitly introduce the $z^{(k)}$ into the algorithm. Combining (3.10), (3.11), and (3.12) with the fact that both $u^{(0)}$ and $z^{(0)}$ are chosen to be zero vectors, we get the following algorithm. The sequence $x^{(0)}, x^{(1)}, x^{(2)}, \ldots$ produced by it converges to the Bayesian estimate x^*, provided that the relaxation parameters $\lambda^{(k)}$ satisfy (2.6).

$$u^{(0)} \text{ is the } I\text{-dimensional zero vector,}$$
$$x^{(0)} = \mu_X,$$
$$u^{(k+1)} = u^{(k)} + c^{(k)} e_{i_k}, \tag{3.13}$$
$$x^{(k+1)} = x^{(k)} + r c^{(k)} r_{i_k},$$

where

$$c^{(k)} = \lambda^{(k)} \frac{r(y_{i_k} - \langle r_{i_k}, x^{(k)} \rangle) - u_{i_k}^{(k)}}{1 + r^2 \|r_{i_k}\|^2}. \tag{3.14}$$

Note that this algorithm cannot be brought into the framework of (1.1). However, its implementation is hardly more complicated than the implementation of the method described by (1.2). We need an additional sequence of I-dimensional vectors $u^{(k)}$, but in the kth iterative step, only one component of $u^{(k)}$ (namely the i_kth component) is needed or altered. Since the i_k's are defined by a cyclic order ($i_0 = 1$, $i_1 = 2$, etc.), the components of the vector $u^{(k)}$ can be stored in a sequentially accessed auxiliary memory of the computer and can be brought into its main memory one by one (or a few at a time) as needed. A similar comment applies to the elements of the measurement vector y. As it is pointed out in Section 11.1, in our application area the r_{i_k} are usually not stored at all, but the location and size of their nonzero elements are calculated as and when needed. Hence the algorithm described by (3.13) and (3.14) shares the storage efficient nature of the simple ART method described in Section 11.1. It is easy to see that the computational requirements are also essentially the same.

The algorithm described by (3.13) and (3.14) is a typical additive ART algorithm. To illustrate this further, we now state, without proof, an additive ART algorithm which produces a sequence $x^{(0)}, x^{(1)}, x^{(2)}, \ldots$, which converges to the minimum norm solution of

$$\gamma_i \leq \langle r_i, x \rangle \leq \delta_i, \tag{3.15}$$

$1 \leq i \leq I$ [cf. (4.15) of Chapter 6].

$$u^{(0)} \text{ is the } I\text{-dimensional zero vector,}$$
$$x^{(0)} \text{ is the } J\text{-dimensional zero vector,}$$
$$u^{(k+1)} = u^{(k)} - c^{(k)} e_{i_k}, \tag{3.16}$$
$$x^{(k+1)} = x^{(k)} + c^{(k)} r_{i_k},$$

where

$$c^{(k)} = \text{mid}\{u_{i_k}^{(k)}, (\delta_{i_k} - \langle r_{i_k}, x^{(k)}\rangle)/\|r_{i_k}\|^2, (\gamma_{i_k} - \langle r_{i_k}, x^{(k)}\rangle)/\|r_{i_k}\|^2\},$$

(3.17)

where mid(u, v, w) denotes the median of the three real numbers u, v, and w.

The algorithm described by (3.16) and (3.17) has been referred to as ART4 in the literature, in order to distinguish it from other versions of ART, which have different convergence properties.

11.4 TRICKS

It has been found in practice that the efficiency of iterative procedures for image reconstruction can often be improved by applying between iterative steps certain processes to the image vectors. These processes have been referred to as *tricks* in the literature.

More precisely, consider the iterative step in ART as described by (1.1). Let τ_k be functions mapping J-dimensional vectors into J-dimensional vectors. Then the iterative method of (1.1) combined with the sequence of tricks τ_k produces a sequence $x^{(0)}, x^{(1)}, x^{(2)}, \ldots$, defined by

$$\hat{x}^{(k+1)} = \alpha_k(x^{(k)}, r_{i_k}, y_{i_k}),$$

(4.1)

$$x^{(k+1)} = \tau_{k+1}(\hat{x}^{(k+1)}).$$

(4.2)

Tricks are useful if they incorporate a priori knowledge about the space of desirable image vectors. Sometimes they can be used to accelerate convergence towards the image vector which satisfies the specified optimization criterion. Other times, they actually cause the process to move towards an image vector other than the one optimizing the specified function, but which is nevertheless a better approximation of the picture to be reconstructed according to the picture distance measures of Section 5.1. The latter happens, for instance, if the desirable digitized pictures have a common property which cannot be expressed by a simple function, but which may be obtained by the application of an appropriate trick.

In the discussions that follow, the intuitive justifications for all the tricks are based on the assumption that the basis pictures are those associated with an $n \times n$ digitization. They are defined by (3.1) of Chapter 6.

A trick which has been already referred to repeatedly is *selective smoothing*. In many applications, pictures are made up from regions within which the values are largely uniform and distinguishable from those in other regions. Selective smoothing produces pictures of this type in the following way.

Let $v_1, v_2, \ldots, v_9$ denote the densities in a pixel p and its neighbors as indicated by the following diagram.

$$
\begin{array}{ccc}
v_6 & v_2 & v_7 \\
v_3 & v_1 & v_4 \\
v_8 & v_5 & v_9
\end{array}
$$

Let t, w_1, w_2, and w_3 be real nonnegative numbers, called the *threshold* and *smoothing weights*, respectively. After the selective smoothing, the density in p is

$$
\frac{w_1 v_1 + w_2 \sum_{i=2}^{5} f_i v_i + w_3 \sum_{i=6}^{9} f_i v_i}{w_1 + w_2 \sum_{i=2}^{5} f_i + w_3 \sum_{i=6}^{9} f_i}, \tag{4.3}
$$

where

$$
f_i = \begin{cases} 1 & \text{if } |v_i - v_1| \le t, \\ 0 & \text{otherwise.} \end{cases} \tag{4.4}
$$

If p is a border pixel, and so v_i is undefined for some of the i's, then we set $f_i = 0$ for the corresponding i's.

Figures 8.10 and 10.5 illustrate the effect of a single application of the trick of selective smoothing (also referred to as nonlinear smoothing in previous sections) to the output of the parallel and divergent beam convolution methods, respectively. Tables 8.3 and 10.2 show the improvements of the picture distance measures which are achieved using this trick. In all cases we used $t = 0.004$ and $w_1 = 9, w_2 = 4; w_3 = 1$.

When such a trick is used in conjunction with ART, typically we choose τ_k in (4.2) to represent selective smoothing only infrequently, for example, only when k is a multiple of I (the number of measurements). For other values of k, we choose τ_k to be the identity function which does not change the image vector.

In contrast, the trick of *constraining* is usually applied at every iterative step of ART. Constraining is justified in case we have a priori information about the range within which the values of the components of acceptable image vectors must lie. For example, the linear attenuation coefficient (at any energy) is always nonnegative, and in medical applications we may usually assume that it is always bounded above by the linear attenuation coefficient of compact bone.

Such constraints may be introduced into series expansion methods in various ways. They may simply be made part of the set of inequalities (2.1). Or they may be introduced into the iterative algorithm as tricks.

For example, if we know that, for $1 \le j \le J$,

$$
\lambda \le x_j \le \mu, \tag{4.5}
$$

then the following trick is appropriate.

$$\tau_k(\hat{x}) = x, \tag{4.6}$$

where, for $1 \le j \le J$,

$$x_j = \begin{cases} \lambda & \text{if } \hat{x}_j < \lambda, \\ \hat{x}_j & \text{if } \lambda \le \hat{x}_j \le \mu, \\ \mu & \text{if } \mu < \hat{x}_j. \end{cases} \tag{4.7}$$

Such a trick can be easily incorporated into ART. To demonstrate this, consider the relaxation method for inequalities. The following is claimed to be true.

If N, as defined by (2.3), contains at least one vector x whose components satisfy (4.5), then the algorithm specified below produces a sequence $x^{(0)}, x^{(1)}$, $x^{(2)}, \ldots$, which converges to an element of N whose components satisfy (4.5).

$$\begin{aligned} x^{(0)} &\text{ is arbitrary,} \\ \hat{x}^{(k+1)} &= \alpha_k(x^{(k)}, n_{i_k}, q_{i_k}), \\ x^{(k+1)} &= \tau_{k+1}(\hat{x}^{(k+1)}), \end{aligned} \tag{4.8}$$

where α_k is defined by (2.4) with the $\lambda^{(k)}$ satisfying (2.6), and τ_k is defined by (4.6).

The verification of this claim follows easily from the convergence of the relaxation method for inequalities. This is because the set of vectors M which satisfy (4.5) can be characterized as follows. Let, for $1 \le j \le J$,

$$M_{2j-1} = \{x \mid x_j \le \mu\} \tag{4.9}$$

and

$$M_{2j} = \{x \mid -x_j \le -\lambda\}. \tag{4.10}$$

Then

$$M = \bigcap_{i=1}^{2J} M_j. \tag{4.11}$$

Thus M, the set of vectors satisfying (4.5), can be described in a way strictly analogous to the way N is described in Section 11.2. The reader can easily check that applying the relaxation method for inequalities based on M instead of N, with relaxation parameter 1 and initial vector $\hat{x}$, produces in $2J$ iterative steps the vector $\tau_k(\hat{x})$, where τ_k is defined by (4.6). Thus, the trick of constraining in this case is equivalent to applying the relaxation method to a larger set of inequalities. This completes the verification of the claim on the convergence of (4.8).

There are other versions of constraining in use besides the one specified by (4.6) and (4.7). For example, there is a way of defining the constraining τ_k's so that, when used in conjunction with the algorithm described in (3.16), the method converges to the minimum norm solution of the combined system (3.15) and (4.5). Another method, which is useful when it is known a priori that there are only two different densities in the picture (as is the case in certain nondestructive testing applications), is to use τ_k's which set the values of $\hat{x}_j$ to either one or the other of the two densities.

Another trick which we have already come across is *normalization*. This is discussed in conjunction with the backprojection method in Section 7.2. Repeated normalization during the iterative procedure has sometimes been found to improve the speed of convergence of ART to a desirable result.

Although there are other tricks whose use has been reported in the literature, we now complete this section by a discussion of four topics related to, but somewhat different from, tricks.

An essential tool available to us with ART is the relaxation parameter. We have already mentioned that choosing a low value for the relaxation parameter has been found to result in good reconstructions using ART-type algorithms, even on experimentally obtained data. A low relaxation parameter, *underrelaxation*, seems to reduce the effect of inaccuracies in the equations, and prevents the production of the "salt and pepper" often seen in ART-type reconstructions using a high relaxation parameter.

In certain situations a limited use of a high relaxation parameter is advisable. When solving a system of inequalities, the process can be markedly shortened if whenever an inequality is only slightly violated a relaxation parameter with value 2 is used, resulting in a mirror *reflection* of the estimate before the iteration in the hyperplane associated with the inequality. Selective use of reflections can, under certain circumstances, ensure finite convergence.

The choice of *initialization* (i.e., of $x^{(0)}$) has a large effect on the outcome of the iterative procedure, especially since due to time and cost constraints the number of iterative steps may be rather limited. For example, in the algorithm (3.13) $x^{(0)}$ is supposed to be μ_X. In practice, it may be very difficult to find the mean of the multivariate random variable which reflects the actual situation. Instead outputs of other methods (such as convolution or back-projection) have often been used as $x^{(0)}$ for ART. Even more frequent in practice is the use of a uniformly gray picture, possibly with the estimated average density (or even blank) in every pixel.

Rearrangement of the order of inequalities (or equalities) in the system can also have a significant effect on the practical performance of the algorithm. With data collection such as our standard geometry, it has been found advantageous to deal consecutively with the equations arising from all the rays in one view, but then move on to the rays from a view in which the source position makes a large angle (such as 60°) with the previous source position.

11.5   EFFICACY OF ART

In this section we illustrate some of the algebraic reconstruction techniques proposed previously. All illustrations are done on the standard projection data.

In all illustrations, the output at the end of the Ith, $2I$th, $3I$th, and $4I$th iteration are shown. In I iterations, the measurements for all source–detector positions have been made use of exactly once. For one source position all rays are dealt with consecutively, but the source positions are selected so that two source positions which are successively dealt with subtend an angle of approximately 60° at the center of rotation (see Fig. 5.2).

Figures 11.2 and 11.3 show what happens if the relaxation method for equalities, (2.18) and (2.19), is applied to the inconsistent system of equations $Rx = y$, with relaxation parameter $\lambda^{(k)}$ equal to 1 for all k. [This is the same as the algorithm of (1.1) and (1.2).] We have chosen $x^{(0)}$ to be the output of the discrete backprojection method with multiplicative normalization, see Fig. 7.5b. The results are quite unacceptable, and they do not significantly improve by further iterations. See Table 11.1 for the picture distance measures and timings.

Underrelaxation significantly improves the results. Figures 11.4 and 11.5 report on a computer run identical in every respect to that which produced Figs. 11.2 and 11.3, except that $\lambda^{(k)}$ was set equal to 0.05 for all k. We see that there is an amazing improvement due to a simple change of relaxation parameter.

Using further tricks described in Section 11.4 (namely, selective smoothing, constraining, and normalization) we obtain Figs. 11.6 and 11.7. A disturbing aspect of these results is that selective smoothing has actually emphasized some of the nondesirable features of the previous output. This could have been avoided by using a variable threshold for the selective smoothing (initially large and then reducing), but for the sake of uniformity we have decided to use at the end of each I iterations the same parameters for selective smoothing as we have used everywhere else in this book, namely $t = 0.004$, $w_1 = 9$, $w_2 = 4$, and $w_3 = 1$ [see (4.3) and (4.4)].

If exactly the same tricks are applied to the additive ART algorithm described in (3.13) and (3.14), we get much better results, provided that μ_X and r are chosen appropriately. This algorithm converges to the Bayesian estimate x which minimizes (3.1). By choosing μ_X to be the selectively smoothed output of the convolution method based on the generalized

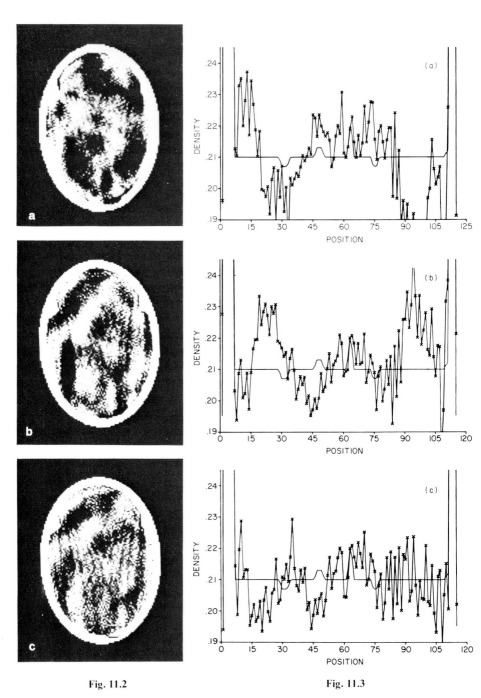

Fig. 11.2   Fig. 11.3

Fig. 11.2. Reconstructions using (2.18) and (2.19), with $x^{(0)}$ same as Fig. 7.5b and $\lambda^{(k)} = 1$ for all k. (a) $x^{(1)}$, (b) $x^{(21)}$, (c) $x^{(31)}$ (d) $x^{(41)}$.

Fig. 11.3. Plots of the 63rd columns of the reconstructions in Fig. 11.2.

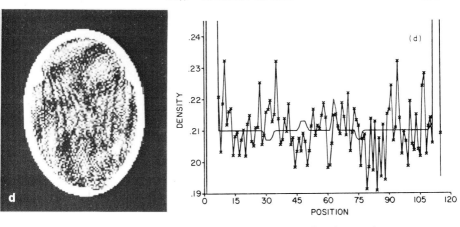

Fig. 11.2 (*Continued*)   **Fig. 11.3** (*Continued*)

Hamming window with $\alpha = 0.8$ (see Fig. 10.5h) we ensure that the "expected value" is a good approximation of the desired image vector. We have estimated that $r = 0.75$ is an appropriate value for (3.1). This has resulted in Figs. 11.8 and 11.9. According to the picture distance measures (see Table

TABLE 11.1

PICTURE DISTANCE MEASURES AND TIMINGS FOR ART
RECONSTRUCTIONS[a]

		d	r	e	t
	a	0.2397	0.1535	0.1882	919
Fig. 11.2	b	0.1469	0.1003	0.0799	1542
	c	0.1176	0.0806	0.0385	2162
	d	0.1109	0.0748	0.0411	2786
	a	0.3096	0.1564	0.1666	912
Fig. 11.4	b	0.2043	0.0970	0.1183	1528
	c	0.1567	0.0723	0.0952	2145
	d	0.1308	0.0605	0.0807	2762
	a	0.3118	0.1512	0.1703	926
Fig. 11.6	b	0.2039	0.0882	0.1238	1553
	c	0.1540	0.0598	0.0989	2177
	d	0.1257	0.0452	0.0838	2797
	a	0.1068	0.0370	0.0618	1458
Fig. 11.8	b	0.1000	0.0335	0.0574	2065
	c	0.0947	0.0311	0.0542	2661
	d	0.0904	0.0292	0.0514	3256

[a] Timings are accumulative, in each case the first value
of t includes the cost of finding $x^{(0)}$.

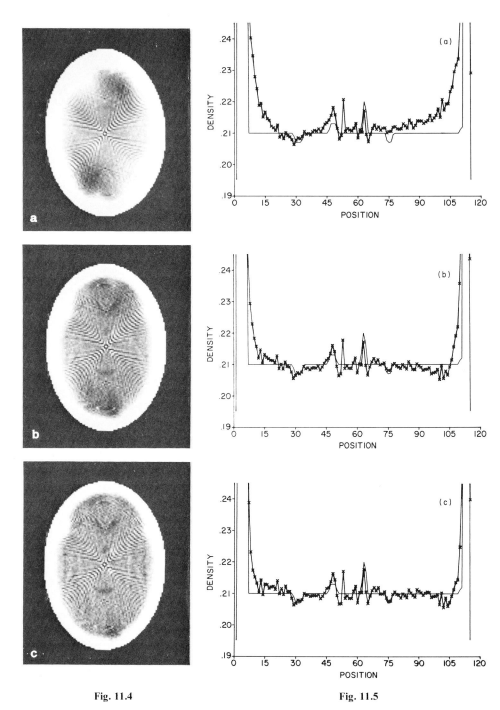

Fig. 11.4   **Fig. 11.5**

Fig. 11.4. Same as Fig. 11.2, except $\lambda^{(k)} = 0.05$, for all k.

Fig. 11.5. Plots of the 63rd columns of the reconstructions in Fig. 11.4.

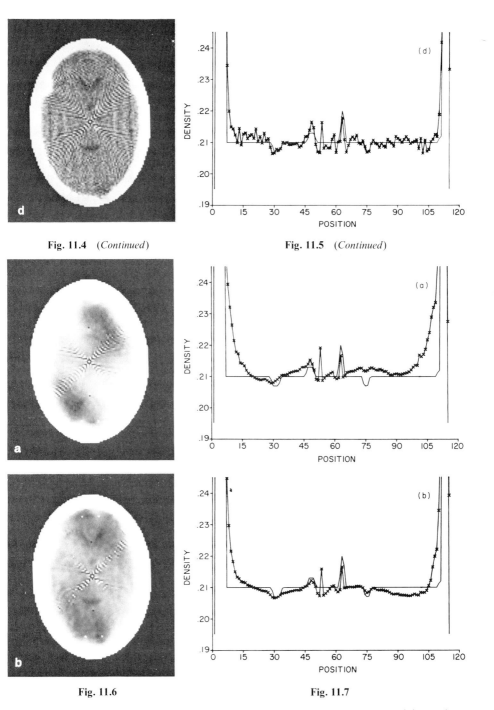

Fig. 11.4 (*Continued*) **Fig. 11.5** (*Continued*)

Fig. 11.6 **Fig. 11.7**

Fig. 11.6. Same as Fig. 11.4, but using the tricks of selective smoothing, constraining, and normalization.

Fig. 11.7. Plots of the 63rd columns of the reconstructions in Fig. 11.6.

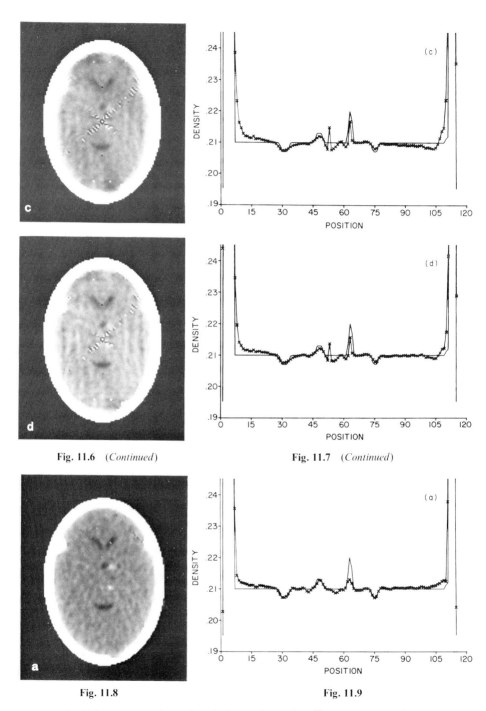

Fig. 11.6 (*Continued*)

Fig. 11.7 (*Continued*)

Fig. 11.8

Fig. 11.9

Fig. 11.8. Reconstructions using (3.13) and (3.14) with $x^{(0)}$ same as Fig. 10.5h, $r = 0.75$, $\lambda^{(k)} = 0.05$ for all k, and using the tricks of selective smoothing, constraining, and normalization.

Fig. 11.9. Plots of the 63rd columns of the reconstructions in Fig. 11.8.

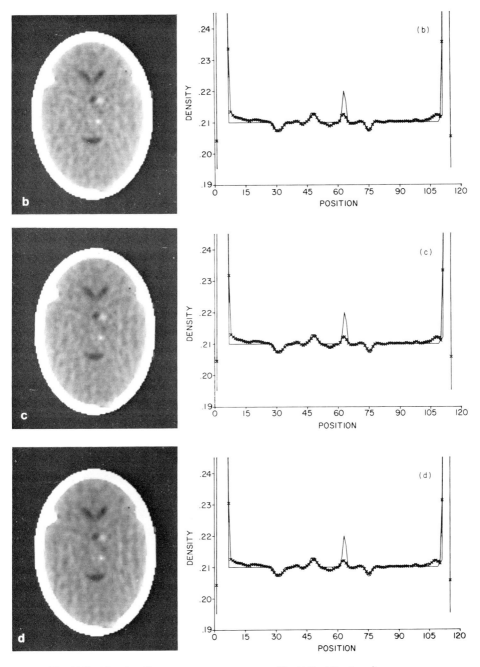

Fig. 11.8 (*Continued*)   Fig. 11.9 (*Continued*)

11.1), successive iterates of this algorithm are improvements on the previous iterates and on the initial vector which is μ_X (see Table 10.2). In fact, these measures imply that the optimization of (3.1), with r and μ_X as described previously, produces reconstructions which are better than anything we have seen so far (or, for that matter, will see later) in this book. We leave the reader to decide whether or not the visual appearance of these reconstructions fulfills the promise of the picture distance measures.

It can be seen from Table 11.1 that each iteration of ART takes approximately 600 sec on our computer, which is of the same order of magnitude as a complete reconstruction using the convolution method. Except in the last of the four cases discussed previously, the extra expense did not result in better reconstructions, and it is dubious that the improvement in the last case is worth the effort. This illustrates that in ordinary x-ray CT ART is not an acceptable alternative to the convolution method. However, in other situations, where the data collection geometry is peculiar or the photon count is rather low, ART may well outperform a convolution method (see Section 14.3).

NOTES AND REFERENCES

ART for image reconstruction was first introduced into the open literature by Gordon, Bender, and Herman (1970). Coincidently, essentially the same method has already been proposed for CT in a patent specification by Hounsfield (1972), originally filed in 1968. In fact, the simple procedure expressed in (1.2) has already been proposed by Kaczmarz (1937) for solving systems of consistent linear equations. A tutorial on ART has been written by Gordon (1974). The methods discussed in this chapter are examples of the so-called *row generation methods* for solving very large sparse systems of equations and inequalities; for a survey, see Censor and Herman (1979).

Our presentation of the relaxation method for solving systems of inequalities and equalities is based on Herman and Lent (1976a) and Herman, Lent, and Lutz (1978). Earlier literature is referenced in those papers. An ART algorithm with a finite convergence property is ART3, described by Herman (1975). The minimum norm theorem is a trivial consequence of what in optimization theory is referred to as the projection theorem (not to be confused by the theorem of the same name in image reconstruction); see, e.g., Luenberger (1969). A relaxational approach to finding the minimum norm solution of systems of inequalities is presented by Lent and Censor (1980). How such an approach translates into an algorithm for image reconstruction is discussed by Herman and Lent (1978).

Our discussion of the Bayesian approach is based on Herman, Hurwitz, Lent, and Lung (1979) and Herman, Hurwitz, and Lent (1978). The former of these two papers gives a detailed discussion of the validity of the assumptions made in the Bayesian approach.

The expression "tricks" was first applied in the literature to the processes described in Section 11.4 by Herman and Lent (1976a). See that paper for earlier references. The algorithm which finds the minimum norm solution of the combined systems (3.15) and (4.5) is described by Herman and Lent (1978). An algorithm for reconstructing objects with only two densities is given by Herman (1973). An interesting demonstration of the power of underrelaxation is given by Herman (1979d), who showed that the trick of using a *complimentary matrix* (not discussed in this book) can be incorporated into ART as a special case of underrelaxation during constraining.

An interesting theoretical study of the order in which views should be treated in ART has been published by Hamaker and Solmon (1978). That paper, and its references, are also of interest, since they use a model for the image reconstruction problem different from anything discussed in this book. The outcome is an iterative procedure, which deals with pictures (as opposed to image vectors). Such procedures have been referred to as *continuous* ART by Herman and Lent (1976a).

For versions of ART for which we did not have space in this book, the reader should consult Gordon (1974) and Herman and Lent (1976a). *Multiplicative* ART is of some particular interest, since it maximizes entropy [see (4.19) of Chapter 6], as has been proved by Lent (1976). Reconstructions using ART and related algorithms from only two or three projections have been reported on by Minerbo and Sanderson (1977).

12

Quadratic Optimization Methods

In this chapter we discuss iterative procedures for minimizing the general quadratic function which incorporates as special cases a number of different optimization criteria discussed in Chapter 4. These iterative procedures are different in nature from ART; they have been referred to in the literature as *SIRT-type* methods.

12.1 MATHEMATICAL BACKGROUND

First we recall some terminology. A matrix M is said to be *symmetric*, if it is a square matrix and $m_{i,j} = m_{j,i}$, for all components $m_{i,j}$ of M. A matrix M is said to be *positive definite*, if it is symmetric and, for every (column) vector x with at least one nonzero component, $x^T M x > 0$. Note that every positive definite matrix M has an inverse M^{-1}. A matrix M is said to be *nonnegative definite* if it is symmetric and, for every vector x, $x^T M x \geq 0$.

The problem we are attempting to solve has the following form. *Given a positive definite matrix D and two nonnegative definite matrices W_1 and W_2, find the x in K which minimizes*

$$\|D^{-1}x\|, \tag{1.1}$$

where

$$K = \{x \mid k(x) \text{ is minimum}\}, \tag{1.2}$$

with

$$k(x) = (y - Rx)^T W_1 (y - Rx) + (x - x_0)^T W_2 (x - x_0). \tag{1.3}$$

Note that the right-hand side of (1.3) is exactly the function (4.14) in

Chapter 6 whose minimization was shown to be the general quadratic optimization criterion, provided that

$$W_1 = aA, \tag{1.4}$$

and

$$W_2 = bB + cC^{-1}. \tag{1.5}$$

In Chapter 6, (4.14) was arrived at as a generalization of (4.8), (4.9), (4.10), (4.12), and (4.13). We now look at the values of W_1, W_2, and x_0 for each of the equations (4.8), (4.9), (4.10), (4.12), and (4.13) of Chapter 6. In the accompanying table U_I and U_J are the identity matrices of the appropriate size, Θ_I and Θ_J are the matrices of appropriate size with zero entries, θ is the vector of all zeros and $\bar{\mathbf{x}}$ is the vector of all $\bar{x}$'s.

	W_1	W_2	x_0
(4.8)	V_F^{-1}	V_X^{-1}	μ_X
(4.9)	U_I	Θ_J	
(4.10)	Θ_I	U_J	$\bar{\mathbf{x}}$
(4.12)	Θ_I	U_J	θ
(4.13)	aU_I	$bB + U_J$	θ

In Chapter 6 we have not discussed in detail the nature of B in (4.13). This is remedied in the following. For now we need only note that B is a nonnegative definite matrix. In view of this, we see that W_2 is positive definite in all cases, except in (4.9), in which case $W_2 = \Theta_J$. In what follows we assume that W_2 in (1.3) is either positive definite or it is the matrix consisting of zeros.

Our basic approach is to translate the quadratic minimization problem into a problem of solving a consistent system of equations. [We have already seen an example of such an approach in Section 11.3. In fact, the function we minimize there is a special case of (1.3), with $W_1 = r^2 U_I$, $W_2 = U_J$, and $x_0 = \mu_X$.] We treat the two cases when W_2 is positive definite and when W_2 consists of zeros separately.

Consider first the case when W_2 is positive definite. We assume that W_2 is defined by (1.5). The reason for writing W_2 in this way is that sometimes C is known, but the optimization criterion refers to C^{-1}. An example of this is (4.8) of Chapter 4, in which $W_2 = V_X^{-1}$, where V_X is the covariance matrix of a multivariate Gaussian distribution. Since C is a large matrix ($J \times J$, where J is the number of basis pictures), we do not wish to invert C if this can be avoided. Rather, we attempt to design algorithms for minimizing $k(x)$ which do not need C^{-1}.

In designing the algorithm, we assume that C is a positive definite matrix, $c > 0$, and B is a nonnegative definite matrix. [It is easy to check that all the examples in the preceding table, except (4.9) where $W_2 = \Theta_J$, satisfy this assumption.] It is a standard result of linear algebra that a nonnegative definite matrix has a *square root*; i.e., that there exists a matrix $C^{1/2}$ such that,

$$C^{1/2}C^{1/2} = C. \tag{1.6}$$

Furthermore, $C^{1/2}$ is also positive definite, and hence has an inverse $C^{-1/2}$, such that $C^{-1/2}C^{-1/2} = C^{-1}$. We do not need to calculate $C^{1/2}$ in the algorithms described in the following, but we need it to describe the rationale behind the algorithms.

We introduce a new vector variable u by

$$u = C^{-1/2}(x - x_0). \tag{1.7}$$

Then

$$x = C^{1/2}u + x_0, \tag{1.8}$$

and, from (1.3), (1.4), and (1.5),

$$
\begin{aligned}
k(x) &= k(C^{1/2}u + x_0) \\
&= a[y - R(C^{1/2}u + x_0)]^T A[y - R(C^{1/2}u + x_0)] \\
&\quad + (C^{1/2}u)^T(bB + cC^{-1})(C^{1/2}u) \\
&= u^T[aC^{1/2}R^T ARC^{1/2} + bC^{1/2}BC^{1/2} + cU_J]u \\
&\quad - 2au^T C^{1/2}R^T A(y - Rx_0) \\
&\quad + a(y - Rx_0)^T A(y - Rx_0).
\end{aligned}
\tag{1.9}
$$

Using the abbreviations

$$P = aC^{1/2}R^T ARC^{1/2} + bC^{1/2}BC^{1/2} + cU_J, \tag{1.10}$$

$$z = aC^{1/2}R^T A(y - Rx_0), \tag{1.11}$$

and

$$h(u) = \tfrac{1}{2}u^T Pu - u^T z, \tag{1.12}$$

we see that, provided (1.8) is satisfied,

$$h(u) = \tfrac{1}{2}k(x) - \tfrac{1}{2}a(y - Rx_0)^T A(y - Rx_0). \tag{1.13}$$

It follows that x^* minimizes $k(x)$ if and only if $x^* = C^{1/2}u^* + x_0$, where u^* minimizes $h(u)$. Thus the problem of finding elements of the set K in (1.2) can be solved by finding u's which minimize h in (1.12).

Consider now the case when $W_2 = \Theta_J$. We assume that $a \neq 0$, for otherwise $W_1 = \Theta_I$, and there is nothing left to minimize. We again introduce a variable u, this time defined by

$$u = D^{-1}x. \tag{1.14}$$

Then

$$x = Du, \qquad (1.15)$$

and, from (1.3) and (1.4),

$$\begin{aligned}
k(x) &= k(Du) \\
&= a(y - RDu)^T A(y - RDu) \\
&= u^T(aDR^T ARD)u - 2au^T DR^T Ay + ay^T Ay.
\end{aligned} \qquad (1.16)$$

Using the abbreviations

$$P = DR^T ARD, \qquad (1.17)$$

$$z = DR^T Ay, \qquad (1.18)$$

and $h(u)$ as defined by (1.12), we see that, provided (1.15) is satisfied,

$$h(u) = (1/2a)k(x) - \tfrac{1}{2}y^T Ay. \qquad (1.19)$$

It follows that x^* minimizes $k(x)$ if and only if $x^* = Du^*$, where u^* minimizes $h(u)$. So in this case also the problem of finding elements of K in (1.2) can be solved by finding u's which minimize h in (1.12).

In both cases, we get from (1.12) to a system of equations by making use of the following result. For any $J \times J$ nonnegative definite matrix P and any J-dimensional vector z, the vector u minimizes (1.12) if and only if

$$Pu = z. \qquad (1.20)$$

Note that this result is applicable to both our cases, since P [defined either by (1.10) or by (1.17)] is nonnegative definite, as it is easily proved by standard techniques of linear algebra.

An interesting consequence of the result is that K is empty, unless (1.20) has a solution. However, in our two cases (1.20) is guaranteed a solution. If P is defined by (1.10), then P is positive definite and so it has an inverse. It is a little more complicated to show, and therefore we omit the details, that (1.20) also has a solution if P and z are defined by (1.17) and (1.18), respectively.

As we have just pointed out, if W_2 is positive definite, then P has an inverse. Therefore there is only one u which is a solution to (1.20), namely $u = P^{-1}z$. Therefore, in this case, there is only one u^* which minimizes $h(u)$ and, consequently, only one x^* which minimizes $k(x)$. This x^* then is the unique element of K, and the secondary optimization criterion expressed by (1.1) is irrelevant.

In case $W_2 = \Theta_J$, let u^* be the minimum norm solution of (1.20). Then among the vectors which minimize $h(u)$, u^* is the one with the smallest norm. Defining $x^* = Du^*$, we see that among the vectors x which minimize

$k(x)$, x^* is the one for which $\|D^{-1}x^*\| = \|u^*\|$ is the smallest. [See comments following (1.19).] Thus, x^* is the vector we set out to find.

In summary, we have done the following. We have shown that the quadratic optimization problem, expressed by (1.1), (1.2), and (1.3), translates into the problem of solving a system of equations (1.20). If W_2 is positive definite, then (1.20) has a unique solution. If $W_2 = \Theta$, then the minimum norm solution of (1.20) is needed. In the next section we discuss a class of algorithms for solving (1.20).

12.2   RICHARDSON'S METHOD FOR SOLVING SYSTEMS OF EQUATIONS

We have already given a method for finding the minimum norm solution of a system of consistent equations in Section 11.2. These are, of course, applicable to (1.20). In this section we discuss an alternative method.

The intuitive motivation for introducing this alternative method in image reconstruction has been the following. If the relaxation method is used with a relaxation parameter 1, then satisfying a single equation may result in a very noticeable stripe along the ray which corresponds to the equation. Repetition of such steps result in noisy looking pictures such as the one shown in Fig. 11.2d. The ART approach takes care of this by the judicious use of relaxation parameters. An alternative approach is to attempt to correct for all rays simultaneously. This is why such methods are called SIRT-like, where SIRT abbreviates *simultaneous iterative reconstruction technique*. (SIRT is a name reserved for a particular one of the SIRT-like methods, whose detailed discussion we omit for reasons of space.)

One way of adjusting an iterate so that errors in all equations are corrected simultaneously is

$$u^{(k+1)} = u^{(k)} + \lambda^{(k)}(z - Pu^{(k)}). \tag{2.1}$$

Note that an iterative step of this type is applicable only if P is a square matrix, since otherwise the dimension of z and $Pu^{(k)}$ would be different from the dimension of $u^{(k)}$. An iterative method whose kth iterative step is of the type expressed in (2.1) is called in numerical analysis a *Richardson's method*. Before discussing the convergence properties of such a method, we investigate its appearance in the two cases discussed in the previous section. This provides an insight to the behavior of a Richardson's method in image reconstruction.

If W_2 is positive definite, then P and z are given by (1.10) and (1.11), respectively. We define, for $k \geq 0$,

$$x^{(k)} = C^{1/2}u^{(k)} + x_0. \tag{2.2}$$

Then, from (2.1), (1.10), and (1.11) we get

$$
\begin{aligned}
x^{(k+1)} &= C^{1/2}u^{(k+1)} + x_0 \\
&= C^{1/2}[u^{(k)} + \lambda^{(k)}(z - Pu^{(k)})] + x_0 \\
&= C^{1/2}u^{(k)} + x_0 + \lambda^{(k)}[C^{1/2}z - C^{1/2}PC^{-1/2}(x^{(k)} - x_0)] \\
&= x^{(k)} + \lambda^{(k)}[aCR^T A(y - Rx_0) \\
&\quad - (aCR^T AR + bCB + cU_J)(x^{(k)} - x_0)],
\end{aligned}
\tag{2.3}
$$

and so

$$
x^{(k+1)} = x^{(k)} + \lambda^{(k)}[aCR^T A(y - Rx^{(k)}) + (bcB + cU_J)(x_0 - x^{(k)})]. \tag{2.4}
$$

It follows from the discussion of the last section, in particular from the remarks following (1.13), that if $u^{(0)}, u^{(1)}, u^{(2)}, \ldots$, converges to a solution of (1.20), then $x^{(0)}, x^{(1)}, x^{(2)}, \ldots$, converges to the unique x^* which minimizes $k(x)$. Note that an algorithm whose iterative step is (2.4) makes no reference to u's; it produces directly a sequence of image vectors $x^{(k)}$ which is supposed to converge to the sought after image vector x^*. Note also that such an algorithm need not evaluate either C^{-1} or $C^{1/2}$, even though the definition of $k(x)$ contains C^{-1} and the mathematical justification made use of $C^{1/2}$.

To give an example of an application of such a procedure in image reconstruction, consider the function $k(x)$ defined by (3.1) of Chapter 11. In this case, $a = r^2$, $b = 0$, $c = 1$, $A = U_I$, $B = \Theta_J$, $C = U_J$ and $x_0 = \mu_X$. In this case, (2.4) yields

$$
x^{(k+1)} = x^{(k)} + \lambda^{(k)}[r^2 R^T(y - Rx^{(k)}) + (\mu_X - x^{(k)})]. \tag{2.5}
$$

This iterative step has a straightforward interpretation in terms of the image reconstruction problem. The present estimate of the image vector, $x^{(k)}$, is changed by the addition of another J-dimensional vector which has two components. The first component is proportional to $R^T(y - Rx^{(k)})$. This is nothing but the discrete backprojection (see Section 7.3) of the difference between the measurement vector and projection data associated with the present estimate. By backprojecting this difference we get a J-dimensional vector which can be used to correct the present estimate so that its projection data are nearer to the measured projection data. The second component is $\mu_X - x^{(k)}$. This is nothing but the difference between the mean vector of the a priori distribution and the present estimate, and so it can be used to bring the present estimate nearer to the expected value of the image vector prior to the measurements. The relative importance given to the two components is determined by r, whose physical interpretation has been discussed in Section 11.3. Hence we see that Richardson's method leads in this case to an iterative step which operates in an intuitively reasonable fashion.

If $W_2 = \Theta_J$, then P and z are given by (1.17) and (1.18), respectively. We define, for $k \geq 0$,

$$x^{(k)} = Du^{(k)}. \tag{2.6}$$

Then, from (2.1), (1.17), and (1.18), we get

$$
\begin{aligned}
x^{(k+1)} &= Du^{(k+1)} \\
&= D[u^{(k)} + \lambda^{(k)}(z - Pu^{(k)})] \\
&= Du^{(k)} + \lambda^{(k)}(D^2R^{\mathrm{T}}Ay - D^2R^{\mathrm{T}}ARDu^{(k)}), \tag{2.7}
\end{aligned}
$$

and so

$$x^{(k+1)} = x^{(k)} + \lambda^{(k)}D^2R^{\mathrm{T}}A(y - Rx^{(k)}). \tag{2.8}$$

It follows from the discussion of the last section that if $u^{(0)}, u^{(1)}, u^{(2)}, \ldots,$ converges to the minimum norm solution of $h(u)$, then $x^{(0)}, x^{(1)}, x^{(2)}, \ldots,$ converges to the x^*, which minimizes $k(x)$ and which is such that, for any other x which minimizes $k(x)$, $\|D^{-1}x^*\| \leq \|D^{-1}x\|$. Note that in this case also, an algorithm whose iterative step is (2.8) makes no reference to u's; it produces directly a sequence of image vectors $x^{(k)}$ which is supposed to converge to the sought after image vector x^*.

Now that we have seen the realizations of Richardson's method in image reconstruction, we must return to the all important question: Can the initial vector $u^{(0)}$ and the sequence of relaxation parameters $\lambda^{(k)}$ be chosen so that (2.1) produces a sequence of vectors which converges to the minimum norm solution of $Pu = z$?

There are a number of ways of choosing the $\lambda^{(k)}$ to ensure the convergence of (2.1) to a solution of (1.20). Here we describe a simple method, since the underlying mathematics of some of the more complicated methods is beyond the scope of this book. At the end of the section we discuss a slightly more complex way of choosing the $\lambda^{(k)}$'s, but one which is claimed to lead to a better approximation to the solution in a limited number of steps.

A real number ρ is called a *proper value* of the matrix P if there exists a nonzero vector u such that

$$Pu = \rho u. \tag{2.9}$$

It is easily seen that a nonnegative definite matrix has only nonnegative proper values. We use $\rho_{\max}P$ and $\rho_{\min}P$ to denote the largest and smallest positive proper values of the matrix P. There are standard methods for estimating $\rho_{\max}P$ and $\rho_{\min}P$ for any given nonnegative definite matrix P.

The following is the case. For any $u^{(0)}$, the algorithm of (2.1) produces a sequence $u^{(0)}, u^{(1)}, u^{(2)}, \ldots,$ which converges to a solution of (1.20), provided that, for all $k \geq 0$,

$$\lambda^{(k)} = \lambda, \tag{2.10}$$

where

$$0 < \lambda < 2/(\rho_{max} P). \tag{2.11}$$

Furthermore, an "optimal" choice for λ is

$$\lambda = 2/(\rho_{max} P + \rho_{min} P). \tag{2.12}$$

This result, in conjunction with the minimum norm theorem in Section 11.2, shows that provided $u^{(0)}$ is chosen to be a linear combination of columns of P, Richardson's algorithm with $\lambda^{(k)}$ defined by (2.10) and (2.11) converges to the minimum norm solution of $Pu = z$.

Some more sophisticated ways of choosing the $\lambda^{(k)}$ involve knowing ahead of time how many iterations we want to carry out. For example, if we know that the total number of iterations is four, then the following sequence of $\lambda^{(k)}$'s is likely to give a better result than the constant value in (2.12):

$$\lambda^{(k)} = 2/[\rho_{max} P + \rho_{min} P - (\rho_{max} P - \rho_{min} P)\cos(\pi(2p(k) - 1)/8)], \quad (2.13)$$

where $p(0) = 1$, $p(1) = 4$, $p(2) = 2$, and $p(3) = 3$.

12.3 SMOOTHING MATRICES

In practice, the matrices B and C in (1.5) are what we call *smoothing matrices*. In this section we define these matrices and explain how they arise in image reconstruction.

Note that B and C are both $J \times J$ matrices, and so they map image vectors into image vectors. Let us assume that the image vectors represent $n \times n$ digitized pictures, i.e., that the values of the components represent densities in pixels. Consider now the process of selective smoothing described in Section 11.4, except that the threshold is assumed to be infinitely high. In such a case, the density in each pixel is replaced by a weighted average of itself and the density in the neighboring pixels. The smoothing is determined by three smoothing weights which are denoted by w_1, w_2, and w_3 in Section 11.4.

More mathematically, let, for $1 \leq j \leq J$, E_j denote the set of indices of the pixels which have exactly one edge in common with the jth pixel and let V_j denote the set of indices of pixels which have exactly one vertex in common with the jth pixel in the $n \times n$ digitization. If x denotes the image vector before smoothing and x' denotes the image vector after smoothing then

$$x' = Sx, \tag{3.1}$$

where S is a $J \times J$ matrix whose (j, k)th component $s_{j,k}$ is defined by

$$s_{j,k} = \begin{cases} w_1 & \text{if} \quad k = j, \\ w_2 & \text{if} \quad k \in E_j, \\ w_3 & \text{if} \quad k \in V_j, \\ 0 & \text{otherwise.} \end{cases} \tag{3.2}$$

Such a matrix S is called the *basic smoothing matrix associated with* (w_1, w_2, w_3).

Note that a basic smoothing matrix is symmetric.

A particular case which gives rise to a basic smoothing matrix in image reconstruction is the Bayesian optimization criterion expressed in (4.8) of Chapter 6. There V_X is the covariance matrix associated with the a priori probability function p_X [see (4.6) of Chapter 6]. If the samples of X are image vectors, it is reasonable to assume that x_j and x_k are not correlated unless the pixels have at least an edge or a vertex in common, and that the covariance of x_j and x_k is determined by whether they have an edge or a vertex in common. Clearly, such a V_X is a basic smoothing matrix.

An associated notion which also occurs in image reconstruction is the *modified smoothing matrix*, which we now define.

Let N denote the set of indices of pixels which are not on the border of the $n \times n$ digitization. Let Z be the $J \times J$ diagonal matrix, whose (j, j)th element is defined by

$$z_{j,j} = \begin{cases} 1 & \text{if} \quad j \in N, \\ 0 & \text{otherwise} \end{cases} \tag{3.3}$$

Clearly, if x is an image vector, then Zx is an image vector representing the same digitized picture as x, except that the densities in the border pixels have been set to zero. The *modified smoothing matrix* S' *associated with* (w_1, w_2, w_3) is defined by

$$S' = SZS, \tag{3.4}$$

where S is the basic smoothing matrix associated with (w_1, w_2, w_3).

An example of how modified smoothing matrices occur in image reconstruction is the following. Suppose that we desire a solution of the discrete image reconstruction problem in which the values x_j assigned to neighboring pixels should be close to one another on the average. Such a condition can be expressed mathematically by requiring that

$$\sum_{j \in N} \left(x_j - \frac{1}{8} \sum_{k \in N_j} x_k \right)^2 \tag{3.5}$$

should be as small as possible, where

$$N_j = E_j \cup V_j, \tag{3.6}$$

for $1 \le j \le J$; i.e., N_j is the set of indices of pixels neighboring the jth pixel.

Let S be the basic smoothing matrix associated with $(1, -\frac{1}{8}, -\frac{1}{8})$, and let s_j denote the transpose of the jth row of S. It is easy to check that

$$\left(x_j - \frac{1}{8}\sum_{k \in N_j} x_k\right)^2 = (s_j^T x)^2 = x^T s_j s_j^T x. \tag{3.7}$$

Therefore

$$\sum_{j \in N}\left(x_j - \frac{1}{8}\sum_{k \in N_j} x_k\right)^2 = x^T B x, \tag{3.8}$$

where

$$B = \sum_{j \in N} s_j s_j^T. \tag{3.9}$$

So far we have succeeded in showing that minimizing (3.5) is in fact minimizing the quadratic form $x^T B x$. Clearly, B is symmetric, and in view of (3.8), it is nonnegative definite. We are now going to show that B is a modified smoothing matrix.

Define T by

$$T = SZ, \tag{3.10}$$

where S is the basic smoothing matrix associated with $(1, -\frac{1}{8}, -\frac{1}{8})$ and Z is the diagonal matrix defined by (3.3). Then the (j, k)th component of T is

$$t_{j,k} = \begin{cases} s_{j,k} & \text{if } k \in N, \\ 0 & \text{otherwise.} \end{cases} \tag{3.11}$$

Hence, the (i, j)th element of SZS is

$$(SZS)_{i,j} = (SZS)_{j,i} = \sum_{k=1}^{J} t_{j,k} s_{k,i} = \sum_{k \in N} s_{j,k} s_{k,i} = \sum_{k \in N} (s_k s_k^T)_{i,j} = B_{i,j}, \tag{3.12}$$

where $B_{i,j}$ denotes the (i, j)th element of B. This proves that

$$B = SZS \tag{3.13}$$

is the modified smoothing matrix associated with $(1, -\frac{1}{8}, -\frac{1}{8})$.

In general, multiplication of a J-dimensional vector x by a $J \times J$ matrix S requires J^2 scalar multiplications. However, if the vector is an image vector representing an $n \times n$ digitization ($J = n^2$) and the matrix is a smoothing matrix, then the number of scalar multiplications required to evaluate Sx is approximately kJ, where $k = 3$ for a basic smoothing matrix and $k = 6$ for a modified smoothing matrix. This is easily seen by looking at the smoothing mechanism described by (4.3) of Chapter 11.

In our application, with J typically over 10,000, there is a very significant difference between the computational requirements for the evaluation of Sx when S is a general matrix and when S is a smoothing matrix. Observing the table in Section 12.1 we see that it is reasonable to assume that both B and C of (1.5) are smoothing matrices.

The iterative step of Richardson's algorithm as applied to the image reconstruction problem is described by (2.4) and (2.8). In both cases, the iterative step requires the evaluation of

$$R^T A(y - Rx^{(k)}). \tag{4.1}$$

This appears at first sight to be quite a difficult computational task. We now show that under an acceptable assumption, the evaluation of (4.1) is not nearly as expensive as the size of the matrices imply.

The assumption we make is that A is a diagonal matrix. The reasonableness of this assumption in our application area follows from the fact that in the table in Section 12.1 the only case when A is not a diagonal is provided by the Bayesian estimation, for which $A = V_E^{-1}$. But V_E is the covariance matrix of the random variable whose samples are the error vectors in the measurements. The assumption that A (and hence V_E) is diagonal is equivalent to assuming that the errors in the physical estimation of $\langle r_i, x \rangle$ (r_i^T is the ith row of the projection matrix R) are not correlated with each other. Physical and simulation experiments confirm that this is not an unreasonable assumption.

If A is a diagonal with entries $a_{i,i}$, then

$$R^T A(y - Rx^{(k)}) = \sum_{i=1}^{I} a_{i,i}(y_i - \langle r_i, x^{(k)} \rangle) r_i. \tag{4.2}$$

The right-hand side of (4.2) can be evaluated in I stages, adding at each stage an extra term to the accumulating sum. The computational process at each stage is very similar to a single iterative step of ART (see Section 11.1). At any given stage only one row of the matrix R is needed, and only the nonzero components of this row need to be used explicitly. The only essential difference between this process of evaluating (4.2) in this way and I steps of ART is that while in ART the image vector is updated at each step (and hence only one J-dimensional vector need to be stored), in evaluating (4.2) we need to keep two J-dimensional vectors: $x^{(k)}$ and the sum we are evaluating.

If we assume that D is a smoothing matrix (in practice D is usually a diagonal matrix, see Section 6.4), then all other operations in (2.4) and (2.8) are either a multiplication of a J-dimensional vector by a smoothing matrix, or a multiplication of a J-dimensional vector by a scalar, or an addition of two J-dimensional vectors. All these are likely to be computationally even less expensive than the evaluation of (4.2). Thus, the total computation of one iterative step of Richardson's method takes about as long as I iterative steps of ART. Since a SIRT-type method takes all the I measurements into consideration during one iterative step (while ART only uses one) this is to be expected. One disadvantage of Richardson's method is the additional storage requirement.

Since Richardson's method is an iterative process, the discussion on tricks in Section 11.4 applies with only minor alterations.

12.5 PRACTICAL USE OF RICHARDSON'S METHOD

We illustrate Richardson's method on two reconstructions of our standard projection data.

For the first reconstruction, we have chosen the following values for the parameters in (1.3). x_0 is the output of the discrete backprojection method with multiplicative normalization (see Fig. 7.5b). W_1 is U_I and W_2 is $B + U_J$, where B is the modified smoothing matrix associated with $(1, -\frac{1}{8}, -\frac{1}{8})$; see Section 12.3. We chose $x^{(0)} = x_0$ [justified by (2.2) if $u^{(0)}$ is the zero vector] and applied four iterations of (2.4) with $\lambda^{(k)} = \lambda$ chosen according to (2.12). The tricks of constraining and normalization were used after each iteration. The results are reported in Figs. 12.1 and 12.2 and Table 12.1.

The most important thing to note about this reconstruction is that the iterative process is nowhere near its limit after the fourth iteration. The values of $\|z - Pu^{(k)}\|^2$ for $k = 1, 2, 3$, and 4 are 1316, 848, 594, and 442, respectively. Since the algorithm is supposed to converge to a solution of $Pu = z$ [with P, u, and z defined by (1.10), (1.7), and (1.11), respectively], we see that probably many more iterations are needed before we can consider $x^{(k)}$ to be a good approximation to the sought after minimizing vector. This is a general problem with the quadratic optimization methods; their rate of convergence is slow and therefore many iterations may be necessary before acceptable reconstructions are obtained. These iterations can be expensive, on our computer each iteration took over five minutes.

An artifact, similar to what can be seen in Fig. 11.4, is noticeable in the reconstructions in Fig. 12.1, as well. This is to some extent due to using multiplicative normalized discrete backprojection (Fig. 7.5b) as the initial vector in both cases, but more importantly it reflects a strong discretization error resulting from our choice of pixels as basis functions combined with our divergent geometry of data collection.

For the second reconstruction, we have selected the parameters so that the sought after vector is the Bayesian estimate x which minimizes (1.3) with $W_1 = r^2 U_I$, $W_2 = U_J$, and $x_0 = \mu_X$. This makes the $k(x)$ of (1.3) to be the same as (3.1) of Chapter 11. In fact, we have used for μ_X and r the same values as in Section 11.5; namely, μ_X is the selectively smoothed output of the convolution method based on a generalized Hamming window with $\alpha = 0.8$ (see Fig. 10.5h) and $r = 0.75$. The tricks of selective smoothing, constraining, and normalization have been used, with exactly the same values for the

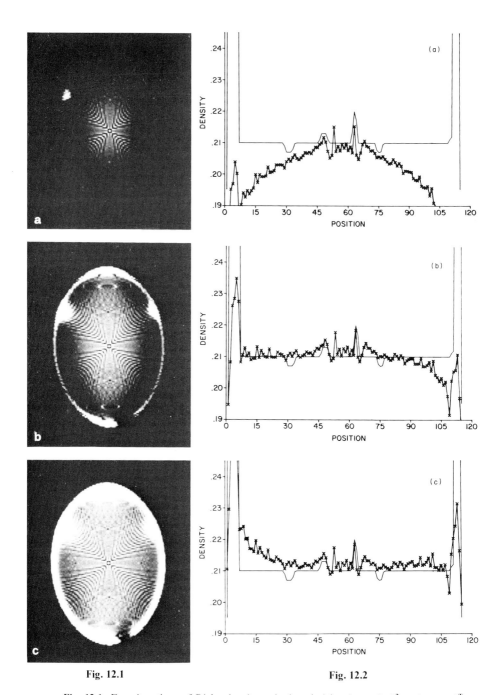

Fig. 12.1   Fig. 12.2

Fig. 12.1. Four iterations of Richardson's method optimizing $\|y - Rx\|^2 + (x - x_0)^T$
$(B + U_J)(x - x_0)$, with $x^{(0)} = x_0$ (the output of discrete backprojection with multiplicative
normalization) and B is the modified smoothing matrix associated with $(1, -\frac{1}{8}, -\frac{1}{8})$. (a) $x^{(1)}$,
(b) $x^{(2)}$, (c) $x^{(3)}$, (d) $x^{(4)}$.

Fig. 12.2. Plots of the 63rd columns of the reconstructions in Fig. 12.1.

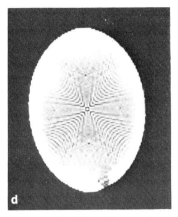

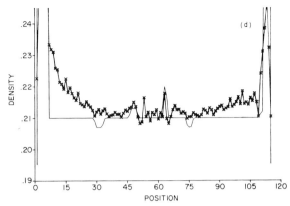

Fig. 12.1 (*Continued*)   **Fig. 12.2** (*Continued*)

parameters as in Section 11.5. The results are reported in Figs. 12.3 and 12.4. They should be compared with Figs. 11.8 and 11.9, which report on the ART reconstruction aimed at optimizing the same function using the same tricks. Note that I iterations of the ART algorithm correspond to one iteration of the Richardson's method, in the sense that all ray sums are used exactly once in both cases. Again, the slow convergence of the quadratic optimization algorithm is in evidence. It is especially noticeable by looking at the values in Table 12.1 as compared to the corresponding values in Table 11.1.

The comments at the end of Section 11.5 regarding the efficacy of ART as opposed to the convolution method apply nearly verbatim to the efficacy

TABLE 12.1

PICTURE DISTANCE MEASURES AND COMPUTER TIMES
FOR THE QUADRATIC OPTIMIZATION ALGORITHMS[a]

		d	r	e	t
Fig. 12.1	a	0.6765	0.4267	0.2490	638
	b	0.5926	0.3359	0.2351	979
	c	0.5331	0.2863	0.2214	1319
	d	0.4874	0.2579	0.2089	1659
Fig. 12.3	a	0.1148	0.0418	0.0673	1196
	b	0.1141	0.0413	0.0668	1540
	c	0.1134	0.0409	0.0662	1884
	d	0.1128	0.0405	0.0657	2229

[a] Times are accumulative, in each case the first value of t includes the cost of finding $x^{(0)}$.

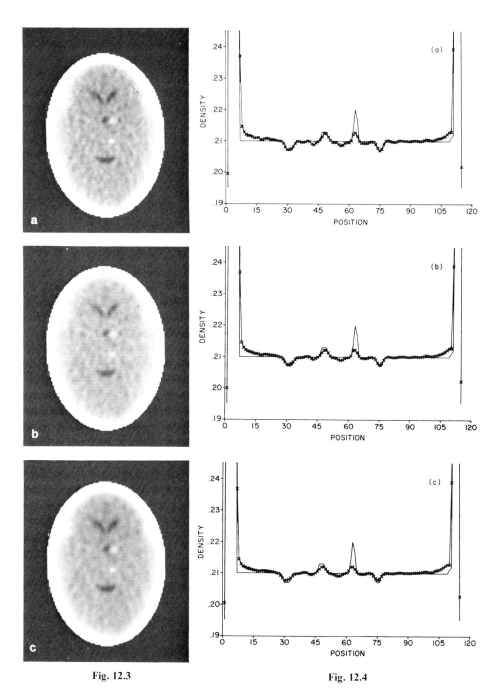

Fig. 12.3   Fig. 12.4

Fig. 12.3. Four iterations of Richardson's method optimizing $(0.75)^2 \, \|y - Rx\|^2 + \|x - \mu_X\|^2$, with $x^{(0)} = \mu_X$ (the selectively smoothed output of the convolution method based on the generalized Hamming window with $\alpha = 0.8$). (a) $x^{(1)}$, (b) $x^{(2)}$, (c) $x^{(3)}$, (d) $x^{(4)}$.

Fig. 12.4. Plots of the 63rd columns of the reconstructions in Fig. 12.3.

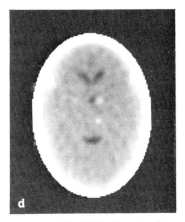

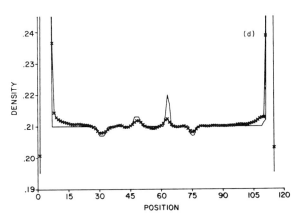

Fig. 12.3 (*Continued*)   Fig. 12.4 (*Continued*)

of quadratic optimization as opposed to the convolution method. As far as comparing ART with quadratic optimization is concerned, we find that ART requires less storage and gets much further in a single cycle through the data. On the other hand, a larger selection of quadratic functionals can be optimized within the framework of quadratic optimization algorithms than with ART, and (although this is unlikely to be of great significance) an iterative step of Richardson's method takes somewhat less computer time than I iterations of ART.

NOTES AND REFERENCES

The reason for calling the methods described in this chapter SIRT-type is that the first method of this type proposed for image reconstruction is the simultaneous iterative reconstruction technique (SIRT) of Gilbert (1972). For recent results about SIRT, see Lakshminarayanan and Lent (1979).

Definitions and results of linear algebra that we have used can be found in such standard texts as Halmos (1958). Our derivation of the appropriate forms for P and z follows Herman and Lent (1976b). That paper can be used to fill in the few gaps in our discussion. A recent follow-up to that work is Artzy *et al.* (1979), which discusses (2.13) and smoothing matrices, as well as two non-Richardson type methods for solving the system $Pu = z$, namely the *conjugate gradient method* and *Chebyshev semi-iteration*. We use the term "Richardson's method" in the general sense, as has been done, for example, by Young (1971), which gives background references, as well as the derivation of (2.13).

Further information regarding quadratic optimization and SIRT-type methods can be obtained from the papers just referred to and their references.

13

Noniterative Series Expansion Methods

The series expansion methods for image reconstruction discussed in the last two chapters are based on iterative procedures: the relaxation method and Richardson's method. While these techniques are applicable to any set of basis pictures, much of the discussion in the last two chapters was oriented towards the basis pictures produced by digitization. While in principle it is possible to apply noniterative methods to the systems of equations which arise in the image reconstruction problem when pixels provide the basis pictures, the enormous size of the system combined with the lack of any observable structure in the location of the nonzero coefficients make iterative techniques just about the only choice from the point of view of practical computational feasibility.

In this chapter we discuss alternative ways of choosing the basis pictures. For certain choices, the resulting system of equations turns out sufficiently simple that iterative methods are not necessary for their solution.

13.1 ANNULAR HARMONIC DECOMPOSITION

Prior to introducing the basis pictures we first discuss the property of the projection matrix R towards which we are aiming.

Consider the quadratic optimization criterion of Section 12.1, with $W_1 = U_I$ and $W_2 = \Theta_J$. [This is exactly the least squares criterion stated in (4.9) of Chapter 6.] For the sake of simplicity of discussion we also assume that $D = U_I$, although, as the reader can easily check, the method we describe would retain all its essential properties for any invertible diagonal matrix D. As it is shown in Section 12.1, the solution x^* we seek is the minimum norm solution of

$$R^T R x = R^T y; \tag{1.1}$$

see (1.17), (1.18), and (1.20) of Chapter 12. The consistent set of equations (1.1) is called the *normal equations* associated with the problem of minimizing $\|y - Rx\|^2$.

The matrix $R^{\mathsf{T}}R$ is a $J \times J$ matrix. Even when it is invertible, its inversion in general is a very large problem. Matrix inversion of a $J \times J$ matrix by a standard technique (such as *Gaussian elimination*) requires approximately $J^3/3$ computer multiplications and multiplying a vector (such as $R^{\mathsf{T}}y$) by the $J \times J$ inverse matrix requires J^2 multiplications. These are formidable problems in our application area (J in our standard phantom is 13,225); this is why in the last two sections we used iterative methods, which achieved acceptable solutions in a reasonable time by making essential use of the fact that most entries of R are zero.

In the present section we use an alternative approach. We choose the basis functions in such a way that (for reasonable modes of data collection) the matrix $R^{\mathsf{T}}R$ has a simple structure which we can exploit to our advantage.

Suppose that there exist $U \times U$ matrices, $P_{-V}, P_{-V+1}, \ldots, P_{V-1}, P_V$ [where $J = U(2V + 1)$; the choice of notation becomes clearer in the following] such that $R^{\mathsf{T}}R$ can be written as a *block diagonal matrix*

$$\begin{bmatrix} P_{-V} & \Theta_U & \cdots & \Theta_U \\ \Theta_U & P_{-V+1} & \cdots & \Theta_U \\ \vdots & \vdots & \ddots & \vdots \\ \Theta_U & \Theta_U & \cdots & P_V \end{bmatrix}, \tag{1.2}$$

where Θ_U is the $U \times U$ zero matrix. Then the inverse of $R^{\mathsf{T}}R$ (if it exists) is

$$\begin{bmatrix} P_{-V}^{-1} & \Theta_U & \cdots & \Theta_U \\ \Theta_U & P_{-V+1}^{-1} & \cdots & \Theta_U \\ \vdots & \vdots & \ddots & \vdots \\ \Theta_U & \Theta_U & \cdots & P_V^{-1} \end{bmatrix}. \tag{1.3}$$

So inversion can be achieved by inverting each of the P_v's separately, which requires a total of $(2V + 1)U^3/3$ multiplications. If U is approximately $\sqrt{J}$, this is a very considerable saving. Furthermore, multiplication of a vector by the inverse of $R^{\mathsf{T}}R$ requires only $(2V + 1)U^2$ multiplications, and can be done separately block by block. This can be summarized by saying that if $R^{\mathsf{T}}R$ is of the form shown in (1.2), then the problem can be decomposed into $2V + 1$ smaller problems resulting in a considerable saving in computational cost. We have used Gaussian elimination to demonstrate this point, but its validity is not dependent on the method chosen to solve (1.1).

For the method that we now describe, aimed at obtaining an $R^{\mathsf{T}}R$ of the form shown in (1.2), not only do the basis pictures have to be chosen carefully, but also the method of data collection must satisfy some conditions. Briefly stated, the conditions are that views are taken at equal angular increments and the rays in each view can be obtained by rotation of the rays in the first view around the center of rotation. (All modes of two-dimensional data collection described in Section 3.4 satisfy these conditions.) More precisely, assume that there are positive integers M and N such that

$$I = M(2N + 1) \tag{1.4}$$

and

$$\mathcal{R}_i f = [\mathcal{R}f](\ell_n, \theta_{n,m}), \tag{1.5}$$

where

$$\theta_{n,m} = \theta_{n,0} + m(2\pi/M), \tag{1.6}$$

and n and m are the unique integers such that

$$-N \leq n \leq N, \qquad 0 \leq m \leq M - 1, \tag{1.7}$$

and

$$i = m + nM + NM + 1. \tag{1.8}$$

[Compare (1.8) of Chapter 6.]

At last we are in position to discuss our choice of the basis pictures. Digitization provided us with basis pictures whose value is zero outside a single pixel. In this section we discuss basis pictures whose value is zero outside a single annulus. For each annulus there is a number of basis pictures with nonzero values in that annulus; they are all harmonic functions of the angle ϕ. (See Section 8.4, for a discussion of harmonic functions.)

More precisely, let d be a positive real number (the width of the annuli) and let U and V be positive integers (the number of annuli and the number of harmonic frequencies, respectively). We choose U so that $Ud \geq E$; see (1.1) of Chapter 6. Let the number of basis pictures be defined by

$$J = U(2V + 1). \tag{1.9}$$

For $1 \leq j \leq J$, there is a unique u in the range $0 \leq u \leq U - 1$ and a unique v in the range $-V \leq v \leq V$, such that

$$j = u + vU + VU + 1. \tag{1.10}$$

We define, for $1 \leq j \leq J$, the basis picture b_j by

$$b_j(r, \phi) = R_u(r)T_v(\phi), \tag{1.11}$$

where, for $0 \leq u \leq U - 1$,

$$R_u(r) = \begin{cases} 1 & \text{if } ud \leq r < (u + 1)d, \\ 0 & \text{otherwise,} \end{cases} \tag{1.12}$$

and, for $-V \le v \le V$,

$$T_v(\phi) = \begin{cases} \sin(v\phi) & \text{if} \quad v > 0, \\ \cos(v\phi) & \text{if} \quad v \le 0, \end{cases} \tag{1.13}$$

and u and v are determined from j using (1.10).

Why is this a reasonable set of basis pictures? We need to convince ourselves that any picture in which we are likely to be interested can be approximated by a linear combination of the b_j. Note, first of all, that if d is chosen small enough, it is reasonable to assume that for all ϕ and for $0 \le u \le U - 1$, if $ud \le r < (u + 1)d$, then $f(r, \phi)$ is approximately equal to

$$f_u(\phi) = f((u + \tfrac{1}{2})d, \phi). \tag{1.14}$$

In words this says that in a thin enough annulus f may be assumed to have a constant value along radial lines. Thus, in the uth annulus we may assume that f is equal to the function f_u, which is a function of ϕ alone. Using (1.12) this yields that for $0 \le r < E$,

$$f(r, \phi) \simeq R_u(r) f_u(\phi). \tag{1.15}$$

Furthermore, f_u is a periodic function of period 2π. Hence, provided it satisfies some physically reasonable conditions, it has a *Fourier series expansion*; i.e., it can be expressed as an (infinite) linear combination of functions of the form T_v as defined by (1.13). Truncating this Fourier series so that only terms with $-V \le v \le V$ are retained gives an approximation to f_u. Combining the approximations provided by expressing $f(r, \phi)$ as in (1.15) and expressing f_u by its truncated Fourier series gives us an approximation to f as a linear combination of the basis pictures b_j defined by (1.11).

It is necessary in some of the discussion that follows to use, for any integer j such that $1 \le j \le J$, the notation u_j and v_j to denote the unique integers such that $0 \le u_j \le U - 1$, $-V \le v_j \le V$, and (1.10) is satisfied if $u = u_j$ and $v = v_j$. When there is no possible confusion, we drop the subscript j.

In order to determine the entries $r_{i,j}$ of the projection matrix R, we need to evaluate $\mathcal{R}b_j$ at all points $(\ell_n, \theta_{n,m})$. To simplify notation, we introduce, for $-N \le n \le N$, a function α_n, defined by

$$\alpha_n(z) = \begin{cases} \tan^{-1}(z/\ell_n) & \text{if} \quad \ell_n \ne 0, \\ \pi/2 & \text{if} \quad \ell_n = 0 \quad \text{and} \quad z \ge 0, \\ -\pi/2 & \text{if} \quad \ell_n = 0 \quad \text{and} \quad z < 0. \end{cases} \tag{1.16}$$

Using this notation we get, see (1.4) of Chapter 6,

$$[\mathcal{R}b_j](\ell_n, \theta_{n,m}) = \int_{-\infty}^{\infty} R_u(\sqrt{\ell_n^2 + z^2}) T_v(\theta_{n,m} + \alpha_n(z)) \, dz. \tag{1.17}$$

Let, for $-N \leq n \leq N, 0 \leq u \leq U$,

$$z_{n,u} = \begin{cases} \sqrt{(ud)^2 - \ell_n^2} & \text{if } \ell_n < ud, \\ 0 & \text{if } ud \leq \ell_n. \end{cases} \qquad (1.18)$$

Using (1.12) and (1.18), we can rewrite (1.17) as

$$[\mathscr{R}b_j](\ell_n, \theta_{n,m}) = \int_{-z_{n,u+1}}^{-z_{n,u}} T_v(\theta_{n,m} + \alpha_n(z)) \, dz$$

$$+ \int_{z_{n,u}}^{z_{n,u+1}} T_v(\theta_{n,m} + \alpha_n(z)) \, dz. \qquad (1.19)$$

However, (1.19) can be simplified further in a way which is very significant for our development. We claim that

$$[\mathscr{R}b_j](\ell_n, \theta_{n,m}) = 2T_v(\theta_{n,m}) \int_{z_{n,u}}^{z_{n,u+1}} \cos(v\alpha_n(z)) \, dz. \qquad (1.20)$$

The significance of (1.20) is better seen by defining for $0 \leq u \leq U - 1$, $-V \leq v \leq V$, and $-N \leq n \leq N$,

$$G_{u,v}(n) = 2 \int_{z_{n,u}}^{z_{n,u+1}} \cos(v\alpha_n(z)) \, dz. \qquad (1.21)$$

Then, (1.20) can be rewritten as

$$r_{i,j} = T_{v_j}(\theta_{n,m})G_{u_j,v_j}(n). \qquad (1.22)$$

So the (i, j)th entry of the projection matrix can be written as the product of two terms. One is determined by i and v (but not by u), the other is determined by j and n (but not by m).

The proof that (1.19) implies (1.20) has to be done separately for the case $v > 0$ and $v \leq 0$. We give details only for the case $v > 0$; the other case has a similar proof.

$$\int_{z_{n,u}}^{z_{n,u+1}} \sin(v\theta_{n,m} + v\alpha_n(z)) \, dz = \sin(v\theta_{n,m}) \int_{z_{n,u}}^{z_{n,u+1}} \cos(v\alpha_n(z)) \, dz$$

$$+ \cos(v\theta_{n,m}) \int_{z_{n,u}}^{z_{n,u+1}} \sin(v\alpha_n(z)) \, dz. \qquad (1.23)$$

Similarly, and noting that $\alpha_n(-z) = -\alpha_n(z)$,

$$\int_{-z_{n,u+1}}^{-z_{n,u}} \sin(v\theta_{n,m} + v\alpha_n(z)) \, dz = \sin(v\theta_{n,m}) \int_{z_{n,u}}^{z_{n,u+1}} \cos(v\alpha_n(z)) \, dz$$

$$- \cos(v\theta_{n,m}) \int_{z_{n,u}}^{z_{n,u+1}} \sin(v\alpha_n(z)) \, dz. \qquad (1.24)$$

Our claim in (1.20) now follows by adding (1.23) and (1.24).

Having found an expression, (1.22), for the general component $r_{i,j}$ of the projection matrix R, we are now in position to evaluate a general component $(R^T R)_{p,q}$ of the matrix $R^T R$.

$$
(R^T R)_{p,q} = \sum_{m=0}^{M-1} \sum_{n=-N}^{N} T_{v_p}(\theta_{n,m}) G_{u_p,v_p}(n) T_{v_q}(\theta_{n,m}) G_{u_q,v_q}(n)
$$

$$
= \sum_{n=-N}^{N} G_{u_p,v_p}(n) G_{u_q,v_q}(n) \left(\sum_{m=0}^{M-1} T_{v_p}(\theta_{n,m}) T_{v_q}(\theta_{n,m}) \right). \quad (1.25)
$$

Now we are at the moment of truth, provided by the following "orthogonality" result, the elementary (but tedious) proof of which is omitted.

Let W be any positive integer and γ be any real number. We define, for any integer w, γ_w by

$$
\gamma_w = \gamma + w(2\pi/W). \quad (1.26)
$$

Let L be any integer and a and b be nonnegative integers such that $a + b < W$. Then

$$
\sum_{w=L}^{L+W-1} \sin a\gamma_w \cos b\gamma_w = 0, \quad (1.27)
$$

$$
\sum_{w=L}^{L+W-1} \cos a\gamma_w \cos b\gamma_w = \begin{cases} 0 & \text{if } a \neq b, \\ \tfrac{1}{2}W & \text{if } a = b \text{ and } a \neq 0, \\ W & \text{if } a = b = 0, \end{cases} \quad (1.28)
$$

and

$$
\sum_{w=L}^{L+W-1} \sin a\gamma_w \sin b\gamma_w = \begin{cases} 0 & \text{if } a \neq b \text{ or } a = b = 0, \\ \tfrac{1}{2}W & \text{otherwise.} \end{cases} \quad (1.29)
$$

It easily follows from this result that if $M \geq 2V + 1$, then, for $-V \leq v \leq V$,

$$
\sum_{m=0}^{M-1} (T_v(\theta_{n,m}))^2 = h_v M, \quad (1.30)
$$

where $h_v = \tfrac{1}{2}$ if $v \neq 0$ and $h_v = 1$ if $v = 0$. For $-V \leq v_p \neq v_q \leq V$,

$$
\sum_{m=0}^{M-1} T_{v_p}(\theta_{n,m}) T_{v_q}(\theta_{n,m}) = 0. \quad (1.31)
$$

It follows that $R^T R$ is of the form (1.2), provided only that the number of views M is not less than the number of harmonics $2V + 1$. For $-V \leq v \leq V$, the matrix P_v in (1.2) is a $U \times U$ matrix, whose (k, ℓ)th component is

$$
(P_v)_{k,\ell} = h_v M \sum_{n=-N}^{N} G_{k-1,v}(n) G_{\ell-1,v}(n). \quad (1.32)
$$

Calculating all the coefficients $(P_v)_{k,\ell}$ is quite a formidable one time cost for a realistic choice of U, V, M, and N. There are, however, certain savings. The P_v are symmetric, $G_{u,v}(n) = G_{u,-v}(n)$ [see (1.21)], etc. In any case, we have succeeded in replacing the original problem (1.1) of solving a system of J equations in J unknowns by a problem of solving independently $2V + 1$ systems of U equations in U unknowns.

13.2   POLYNOMIAL DECOMPOSITION

The essential mathematical results which allowed us to bring $R^T R$ into a block diagonal form is (1.31). This has been referred to as an *orthogonality* result, since one way of stating it is the following. For a fixed v and n, let $V_{v,n}$ be the M-dimensional vector with components $T_v(\theta_{n,m})$. Then (1.31) says that if $v_p \neq v_q$, then $V_{v_p,s}$ and $V_{v_q,t}$ are orthogonal for any s and t, in the sense that their inner product is zero.

Consider (1.25) and (1.32). Suppose for now that the sum

$$\sum_{n=-N}^{N} G_{u_p,v_p}(n)G_{u_q,v_q}(n) \tag{2.1}$$

also satisfied some orthogonality-type theorem. More particularly, suppose that whenever $v_p = v_q$, the value of (2.1) is zero unless $u_p = u_q$. If such a result were true, then $R^T R$ would be a diagonal matrix, and its inversion would be a totally trivial task. In this section we discuss a way of choosing the basis pictures which leads exactly to a result of this type.

Unfortunately, the mathematical background required for following the details is beyond the scope of this book. We give only an outline of the argument. We attempt to keep the discussion as similar to the discussion of the last section as possible.

Let U and V be positive integers. V is the number of harmonic frequencies (as previously), but the meaning of U becomes clear only in the following. The number J of basis functions is $U(2V + 1)$ and u and v (more precisely u_j and v_j) are determined from j according to (1.10). We define, for $1 \leq j \leq J$, the basis picture b_j by

$$b_j(r, \phi) = R_{u,v}(r)T_v(\phi), \tag{2.2}$$

where, for $0 \leq u \leq U - 1$ and $-V \leq v \leq V$, T_v is defined by (1.13) and

$$R_{u,v}(r) = \begin{cases} (r/E)^{|v|}Q_{|v|,u}((r/E)^2) & \text{if } r \leq E, \\ 0 & \text{otherwise}, \end{cases} \tag{2.3}$$

where $Q_{|v|,u}$ is a polynomial of degree u. For completeness, we now state a precise form of $Q_{|v|,u}$, but since we are omitting the details in the derivation, we have no further occasion to use this definition in this book.

$$Q_{|v|,u}(t) = \sum_{w=0}^{u} (-1)^{u-w} \binom{u}{w} \binom{|v| + u + w}{u} t^w. \tag{2.4}$$

The basis pictures of (2.2) differ from those of (1.11) in the choice of the radial component. In (1.12), R_u is a "box" function, its value is 1 for a small interval and zero elsewhere. In (2.3), $R_{u,v}$ is a polynomial of degree $|v| + 2u$. Although we do not prove this, the reader should be aware of the fact that any function f of two polar variables that can be expressed as a polynomial of degree w in $r \cos \phi$ and $r \sin \phi$ is a linear combination of those b_j's for which $|v| + 2u \leq w$. We can restate this by saying that the b_j's provide us with polynomial approximations to the picture functions f. This shows that the b_j form a reasonable set of basis pictures from the point of view of approximating an arbitrary picture.

For our purpose, it is equally significant that the Radon transforms of the b_j's satisfy an orthogonality theorem, provided that the data are collected in an appropriate fashion. It is this result that we discuss next.

For any ℓ, such that $-E \leq \ell \leq E$,

$$[\mathscr{R}b_j](\ell, \theta) = (2E/(|v| + 2u + 1))(1 - (\ell/E)^2)^{1/2} U_{|v|+2u}(\ell/E) T_v(\theta), \tag{2.5}$$

where, for any nonnegative integer w, U_w is the wth *Chebyshev polynomial of the second kind*, defined by

$$U_w(\cos \phi) = (\sin(w + 1)\phi)/\sin \phi. \tag{2.6}$$

We do not derive (2.5), but wish to emphasize that for our discussion the only significance of the definition of $Q_{|v|,u}$ in (2.4) is that it leads to (2.5).

At first sight, it is not clear why (2.5) is a desirable formula in the sense that it leads to an orthogonality condition being satisfied. However, observing (2.6) gives us an indication that if the ℓ_n are carefully selected, then the right-hand side of (2.5) can be significantly simplified.

For example, choose, for $-N \leq n \leq N$,

$$\ell_n = E \cos \gamma_n, \tag{2.7}$$

where γ_n is defined by (1.26) with $W = 2N + 1$ and γ arbitrary. Then

$$[\mathscr{R}b_j](\ell_n, \theta) = (2E/(|v| + 2u + 1))\sin((|v| + 2u + 1)\gamma_n)T_v(\theta). \tag{2.8}$$

Evaluating (2.8) for the values of θ provided by $\theta_{n,m}$ ($-N \leq n \leq N$, $0 \leq m \leq M - 1$), we get exactly (1.22), but with $G_{u,v}$ now defined by

$$G_{u,v}(n) = (2E/(|v| + 2u + 1))\sin((|v| + 2u + 1)\gamma_n). \tag{2.9}$$

Following the argument given in the last section, we find that (R^TR) is of the form (1.2), provided only that the number of views M is not less than the number of harmonics $2V + 1$. For $-V \le v \le V$, the matrix P_v in (1.2) is a $U \times U$ matrix, whose (k, ℓ)th component is given by (1.32) with $G_{u,v}$ as defined by (2.9).

However, this time (1.32) can be considerably simplified. Substituting (2.9) into (1.32) we get

$$(P_v)_{k,\ell} = \frac{4h_v ME^2}{(|v| + 2k - 1)(|v| + 2\ell - 1)}$$

$$\times \sum_{n=-N}^{N} \sin((|v| + 2k - 1)\gamma_n)\sin((|v| + 2\ell - 1)\gamma_n). \quad (2.10)$$

Now, if in (1.29) we let $W = 2N + 1$, $L = -N$, $a = |v| + 2k - 1$, where $1 \le k \le U$, and $b = |v| + 2\ell - 1$, where $1 \le \ell \le U$, then we see that

$$\sum_{n=-N}^{N} \sin((|v| + 2k - 1)\gamma_n)\sin((|v| + 2\ell - 1)\gamma_n)$$

$$= \begin{cases} 0 & \text{if } \ell \ne k, \\ (2N + 1)/2 & \text{if } \ell = k, \end{cases} \quad (2.11)$$

provided that $2|v| + 2k + 2\ell - 2 < 2N + 1$. Combining this result with (2.10) gives that, provided $V + 2U - 1 \le N$,

$$(P_v)_{k,\ell} = \begin{cases} 0 & \text{if } k \ne \ell, \\ 2h_v M(2N + 1)E^2/(|v| + 2k - 1)^2 & \text{if } k = \ell. \end{cases} \quad (2.12)$$

Combining the results of this and the previous section, we can say in summary the following. If data are collected along rays $(\ell_n, \theta_{n,m})$, where ℓ_n satisfies (2.7) and $\theta_{n,m}$ satisfies (1.6), with total number of rays $I = M(2N + 1)$, and if the $J = U(2V + 1)$ basis pictures are given by (2.2), (2.3), and (1.13), then, provided $2V + 1 \le M$ and $V + 2U - 1 \le N$, R^TR is a diagonal matrix whose jth diagonal entry (for $1 \le j \le J$) is

$$(R^TR)_{j,j} = 2h_{v_j} IE^2/(|v_j| + 2u_j + 1)^2, \quad (2.13)$$

where u_j and v_j are determined from j by (1.10).

We now discuss the reasonableness of choosing ℓ_n according to (2.7).

One possibility is to choose γ to be $-\pi/2$. In that case $\gamma_0 = -\pi/2$ and so $\ell_0 = 0$. In general, we have, for $-N \le n \le N$,

$$\ell_n = E \sin[n2\pi/(2N + 1)]. \quad (2.14)$$

Since the values of ℓ_n first decrease, then increase, and then decrease again as n ranges from $-N \le n \le N$, the arrangement of the rays in any one view is not obvious at first sight. To understand this better we define a set of distances d_k, such that

$$0 = d_0 < d_1 < \cdots < d_N < E, \tag{2.15}$$

and, for $1 \leq k \leq N$,

$$d_{-k} = -d_k, \tag{2.16}$$

and the set of d_k's is the same as the set of ℓ_n's; in symbols:

$$\{d_k | -N \leq k \leq N\} = \{\ell_n | -N \leq n \leq N\}. \tag{2.17}$$

Such a set of d_k's is defined by

$$d_k = E \sin[k\pi/(2N + 1)], \tag{2.18}$$

for $-N \leq k \leq N$. That these d_k's satisfy (2.15) and (2.16) is obvious from elementary properties of the sine function. Noting that

$$\sin \alpha = \sin(\pi - \alpha), \tag{2.19}$$

it is easy to derive [by setting $\alpha = (2N + 1 - 2n)\pi/(2N + 1)$] that, for $-N \leq n \leq N$,

$$\sin[(2N + 1 - 2n)\pi/(2N + 1)] = \sin[n2\pi/(2N + 1)]. \tag{2.20}$$

From (2.14) and (2.20) we have that, for $1 \leq n \leq N$,

$$\ell_n = d_k, \tag{2.21}$$

where

$$k = \begin{cases} 2n & \text{if} \quad 1 \leq n \leq N/2, \\ 2N + 1 - 2n & \text{if} \quad N/2 < n \leq N. \end{cases} \tag{2.22}$$

Note that as n ranges from 1 to N, k also ranges from 1 to N. The validity of (2.17) now follows from (2.16) and the fact that $\ell_{-n} = -\ell_n$.

Thus, defining ℓ_n by (2.14) provides us with a set of distances which covers the interval $-E$ to E reasonably well. In fact, looking at the sine curve, it is easy to see that

$$0 < (E - d_N) < (d_N - d_{N-1}) < \cdots < d_2 - d_1 < d_1 - d_0 < (\pi/(2N + 1))E. \tag{2.23}$$

It follows that, even though the sample points ℓ_n are not uniformly placed in the interval $-E$ to E, the distance between two neighboring sample points is never more than $\pi/2$ times (≈ 1.57) the distance that would be achieved by uniform sampling using the same number of points.

If for a particular machine it is difficult to collect data for the values of ℓ_n as defined by (2.14), the collected data can be rebinned (see Section 10.5) so that the method derived in this section can be applied.

In particular the divergent mode of data collection leads naturally to ℓ_n as defined by (2.7). In the divergent mode data are collected for rays $(\ell_n, \theta_{n,m}) = (D \sin n\lambda, m\Delta + n\lambda)$ where $\Delta = 2\pi/M$; see (5.1) of Chapter 10. If λ is chosen by

$$\lambda = \pi/(2N + 1), \tag{2.24}$$

for some suitably large N, then we see that for these rays $\theta_{n,m}$ satisfies (1.6) (with $\theta_{n,0} = n\lambda$) and ℓ_n satisfies (2.18), provided that we assume that $E = D$. In other words, if we assume that the reconstruction region occupies the whole interior of the circle in which the source moves (see Fig. 5.2) we end up with ℓ_n of the type we needed for our theory stated previously.

However, this is not necessarily the best approach. First, by setting E equal to D, we lose the important a priori information that the picture function is zero outside the original (small) reconstruction region. Second, awkwardness arises since the N in (2.24) and the N in Fig. 5.2 are not the same. Using N' to denote the N in Figure 5.2 we see that $N > N'$. In order to apply the algorithm of the present section we have to assume that the ray sums for the additional rays are zero.

13.3 IMPLEMENTATION OF THE NONITERATIVE SERIES EXPANSION METHOD

When implementing the annular harmonic decomposition method, a reasonable alteration to the algorithm as described in Section 13.1 is to make the number of harmonics dependent on the annulus. That is, for $0 \le u \le U - 1$, we define a positive integer V_u, and use the basis pictures b_j, as defined by (1.11), only if $- V_u \le v \le V_u$. (This is equivalent to setting the coefficient x_j to zero if $|v_j| > V_{u_j}$.) The reasoning behind such an approach is that the areas of smaller annuli are smaller, and there is no need to have as high frequency harmonics as in the larger annuli.

Similarly, when implementing the polynomial decomposition method, a reasonable alteration to the algorithm as described in Section 13.2 is to use all polynomials $R_{u,v}$ up to degree $2U$. The degree of $R_{u,v}$ as defined by (2.3), is $|v| + 2u$. Hence, here again we define, for $0 \le u \le U - 1$, a positive integer V_u [namely, $V_u = (2U - 2u)$] and use the basis functions b_j, as defined by (2.2), only if $- V_u \le v \le V_u$.

Implementation of the methods described in this chapter can be done in three stages.

  (i) calculate $R^T y$,
  (ii) solve the normal equations (1.1), and
  (iii) evaluate the picture based on the solution of the normal equations [see (3.9) of Chapter 6].

We discuss these stages one by one.

In principle, the multiplication of y by R^T is the multiplication of an I-dimensional vector by a $J \times I$ matrix, and so seems to require $J \times I$ multiplications. However, note that $r_{i,j}$ is given by (1.22) and so

$$(R^T y)_j = \sum_{n=-N}^{N} \left(G_{u_j, v_j}(n) \sum_{m=0}^{M-1} T_{v_j}(\theta_{n,m}) p_{n,m} \right), \tag{3.1}$$

where

$$p_{n,m} = y_i \tag{3.2}$$

denotes the measured ray sum for the ray $(\ell_n, \theta_{n,m})$. For a fixed n, the calculation of the inner sum

$$\sum_{m=0}^{M-1} T_v(\theta_{n,m}) p_{n,m} \tag{3.3}$$

for $-V \leq v \leq V$ can be considerably speeded up by the use of fast Fourier transform (FFT, see Section 9.2). The details are beyond the scope of this book. In the case of the polynomial expansion method, where the $G_{u,v}$'s are also defined in terms of harmonic functions, see (2.9), the outer summation of (3.1) can also be speeded up using the FFT.

The whole approach of the last two sections has been motivated by the desire to simplify the solution of the normal equations, and we say no more about the second stage of implementation.

The third stage is something we did not have to worry about when our basis pictures were based on digitization. This is because in that case the output is a digitized picture, immediately suitable for display as an image or for reporting on the estimated relative attenuations at individual points. The situation is quite different now. In the polynomial expansion method, each of the basis pictures contributes to each of the points in the reconstruction region, and the calculation of $f^*(r, \phi)$ for a number of different values of (r, ϕ) can become quite expensive. The situation is slightly better from this point of view in the case of the annular harmonic decomposition, since only $2V + 1$ basis functions contribute to the value of $f^*(r, \phi)$ for a fixed point (r, ϕ). It is customary to evaluate $f^*(r, \phi)$ first on points which lie on a set of circles concentric around the origin, and then interpolate to get a digitized picture. This allows us to use the FFT once more in speeding up what otherwise may be a very time consuming procedure.

We now illustrate the method described in Section 13.2 on the standard projection data. This has been done by the use of additional rays (with zero ray sums) as described in the last paragraphs of Section 13.2. In fact, since in the standard geometry D is very much larger than E, the number of rays used was $2N + 1 = 1631$ (of which the central 165 had the measured ray sums and the rest had zero ray sums). Since the number of views in the standard projection data is $M = 288$, the limitation on the size of V implies (see

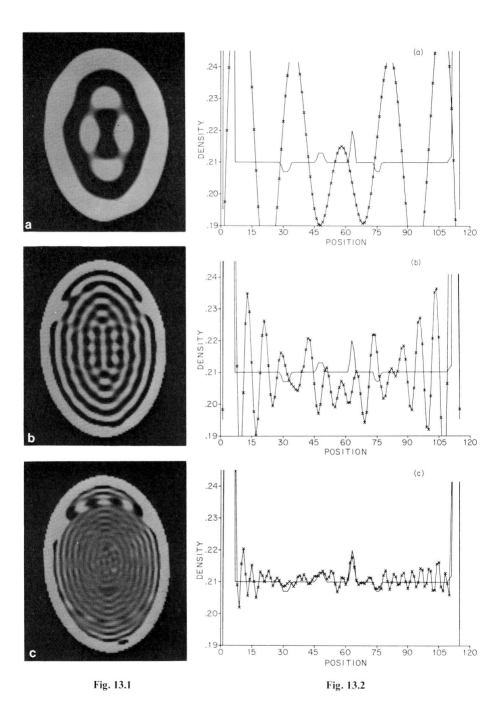

Fig. 13.1   Fig. 13.2

Fig. 13.1. Reconstructions from the standard projection data using the polynomial decomposition method, with different degree G polynomials. (a) $G = 143$, (b) $G = 429$, (c) $G = 815$, (d) $G = 1630$.

Fig. 13.2. Plots of the 63rd columns of the reconstructions in Fig. 13.1.

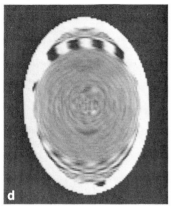

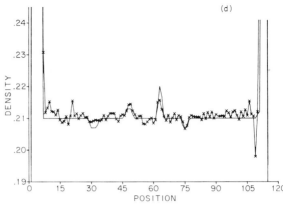

Fig. 13.1. (*Continued*)   **Fig. 13.2.** (*Continued*)

just before (2.13)) that $V \leq 143$. We used $V = 143$. Also, in each of our experiments we have used all permissible polynomials $R_{u,v}$ up to a certain degree. That is, we have selected a degree G and then used all values of u and v which satisfy

$$0 \leq u, \qquad -143 \leq v < 143, \qquad \text{and} \qquad |v| + 2u \leq G. \qquad (3.4)$$

Since a polynomial is fitted to the whole of the interior of the circle of source positions of radius D (rather than just to the reconstruction region), it is not surprising that large values of G are needed for accurate reconstruction.

In Fig. 13.1 we show four reconstructions using the polynomial decomposition method with the G of (3.4) equal to 143, 429, 815, and 1630, respectively. Note that the last value seems to be too large based on the theory presented in this chapter, but its use can be justified by appeal to a stronger orthogonality result than stated in (1.29). Line plots along the 63rd column are shown in Fig. 13.2 and picture distance measures are presented in Table 13.1. Note that the rather curious artifact in the higher degree approximations is emphasized by our choice of black and white levels; the overall

Table 13.1

PICTURE DISTANCE MEASURES FOR THE
RECONSTRUCTIONS IN FIG. 13.1

Degree G	d	r	e	t
143	0.5564	0.3545	0.2374	542
429	0.2413	0.1315	0.1415	725
815	0.1772	0.0769	0.1020	953
1630	0.1586	0.0650	0.0926	1452

reconstructions are reasonably accurate, as is indicated by the picture distance measures. A problem with the approach taken here is that accuracy outside the reconstruction region is also insured (the reconstructed values are near zero, right up to the circle of source positions), but this is not reflected in the pictures (and distance measures) which show (and evaluate) only the reconstruction region.

NOTES AND REFERENCES

The earliest published work proposing a noniterative series expansion approach to image reconstruction is Cormack (1963). The pioneering nature of this work was acknowledged by the award of the 1979 Nobel prize in medicine to A. M. Cormack (jointly with G. N. Hounsfield). A recent work, with many references on the intervening literature is Lewitt and Bates (1978).

The annular harmonic decomposition section is based on the work of Perry *et al.* (1975), which can be consulted for implementational details (see also Herman and Rowland, 1978). The particular set of basis pictures have been adopted from Altschuler and Perry (1972), who used similar basis pictures for the three-dimensional reconstruction of the solar corona. The indexing scheme and data collection scheme is based on the work of Altschuler and Herman (1977).

For a discussion of Gaussian elimination and other standard techniques for solving systems of equations see, e.g., Ralston and Rabinowitz (1978). Fourier series expansions are discussed in many books on analysis, see, e.g., Apostol (1957), or Courant and Hilbert (1953). The latter work may also be consulted for background on Chebyshev and other special polynomials.

The polynomial decomposition section is based on Marr (1974), which may be consulted for details we left out. Note, in particular, that the polynomials $Q_{|v|, u}$ of (2.4) are shifted special cases of the classical *Jacobi polynomials*. Precise implementational details can be found in Herman and Rowland (1978).

14

Truly Three-Dimensional Reconstruction

If we wish to reconstruct a three-dimensional body by the methods discussed in the previous chapters, the only option available to us is to reconstruct the body cross section by cross section and then stack the cross sections to form the three-dimensional distribution. This may cause a number of problems, the most important of which are associated with time requirements. During the time needed to collect all the data, the patient may move, causing a disalignment between the cross sections. More basically, in moving organs such as the lungs (and even more so, the heart), changes in the organ over time are unavoidable, and it is desirable to collect data for all cross sections simultaneously.

Sometimes, it is actually the change in the object over time which is the desired information. If we wish to see cardiac wall motion or the spread of radiopaque dye in a part of the circulatory system, then it is essential that we reconstruct the whole three-dimensional object at short time intervals. One may consider this as four-dimensional (spatio-temporal) reconstruction.

Of all the scanning modes discussed in Section 3.4 it is only the fifth one (see Fig. 3.3e) which is capable of producing the data required. In this chapter we discuss reconstruction algorithms for data collected by such a device.

14.1 THREE-DIMENSIONAL SERIES EXPANSION

We use *cylindrical coordinates* to describe three-dimensional space. That is, a point is represented by a triple of numbers (r, ϕ, z). It is assumed that there is a z axis (an infinite straight line) along which z is measured. The set of points (r, ϕ, z_0), with (r, ϕ) varying and z_0 fixed, forms the plane perpendicular to the z axis, crossing the z axis at z_0. We specify points in this plane by considering (r, ϕ) to be polar coordinates in the plane with origin at the intersection of the plane with the z axis.

Note that this coordinate system is rather natural when we look upon a three-dimensional body as a stack of cross-sectional slices. Each cross section is a plane for a fixed value of z, and the value of the three-dimensional function restricted to this plane is a function of the two polar variables (r, ϕ).

We assume that all the objects we wish to reconstruct are of a limited physical size. More precisely, we assume that there exist constants E and F such that

$$f(r, \phi, z) = 0 \qquad \text{if} \quad |r| \geq E \quad \text{or} \quad |z| \geq F, \tag{1.1}$$

where $f(r, \phi, z)$ is the value at the point (r, ϕ, z) of the object we wish to reconstruct.

In this book we discuss only series expansion methods for truly three-dimensional reconstructions. Just as in the case of two-dimensional reconstruction, we assume a fixed set of J basis objects $\{b_1, \ldots, b_J\}$, whose linear combinations give us an adequate approximation to any object f we may wish to reconstruct.

An example of such an approach which corresponds to $n \times n$ digitization is the following. Let c be a positive real number and W be an integer such that

$$(W + \tfrac{1}{2})c \geq \max\{E, F\}. \tag{1.2}$$

A cube, whose center is at the origin $(0, 0, 0)$ of the cylindrical coordinate system with four edges parallel to the z axis and whose sides are $(2W + 1)c$ long, properly encloses the region of space within which f has nonzero value. We divide this cube into $(2W + 1) \times (2W + 1) \times (2W + 1)$ little cubes (all of size $c \times c \times c$), which we call voxels (see Section 2.4). Let

$$J = (2W + 1)^3. \tag{1.3}$$

We number the voxels from 1 to J, and define

$$b_j(r, \phi, z) = \begin{cases} 1 & \text{if } (r, \phi, z) \text{ is inside the } j\text{th voxel,} \\ 0 & \text{otherwise.} \end{cases} \tag{1.4}$$

Our approximation $\hat{f}$ to f is the object defined by

$$\hat{f}(r, \phi, z) = \sum_{j=1}^{J} x_j b_j(r, \phi, z), \tag{1.5}$$

where x_j is the average value of f inside the jth voxel.

An alternative way of choosing basis objects, based on the annular harmonic expansion of Section 13.1, is the following. Let c and d be positive real numbers and U, V, W be positive integers such that

$$(W + \tfrac{1}{2})c \geq F \qquad \text{and} \qquad Ud \geq E. \tag{1.6}$$

Let

$$J = U(2V + 1)(2W + 1). \tag{1.7}$$

For $1 \leq j \leq J$, there is a unique u in the range $0 \leq u \leq U - 1$, a unique v in the range $-V \leq v \leq V$, and a unique w in the range $-W \leq w \leq W$ such that

$$j = u + (w + v(2W + 1))U + (W + V(2W + 1))U + 1. \tag{1.8}$$

We use u_j, v_j, and w_j to denote the u, v, and w defined by (1.8), but we sometimes omit the subscripts when this is unlikely to lead to confusion.

We define, for $1 \leq j \leq J$, the basis object b_j by

$$b_j(r, \phi, z) = R_u(r)T_v(\phi)S_w(z), \tag{1.9}$$

where R_u and T_v are defined by (1.12) and (1.13) of Chapter 13 and

$$S_w(z) = \begin{cases} 1 & \text{if } |z - wc| < c/2, \\ \frac{1}{2} & \text{if } |z - wc| = c/2, \\ 0 & \text{otherwise.} \end{cases} \tag{1.10}$$

(Note that the definition in case $|z - wc| = c/2$ is a bit of mathematical pedantry, which does not affect any of the following.)

Each of the basis objects as defined by (1.9) have zero value outside a slab of thickness c. Inside that slab they are analogous to the basis pictures used in the annular harmonic decomposition. As long as the values of the objects we are interested in are unlikely to change substantially as z changes by c or less, the argument given in Section 13.1 to justify the claim that a picture can be approximated by an annular harmonic expansion can be extended to justify the claim that an object of interest can be approximated by a linear combination of the functions defined in (1.9).

Just as in the two-dimensional case, the basis objects defined by (1.4) are more suitable for reporting and displaying the results, while the basis objects defined by (1.9) lead to a system of normal equations with computationally advantageous properties. We give details of the latter in the next section.

Following the development in Section 6.3 we assume that we have a set of I linear continuous functions $\mathcal{R}_i$ which map objects into real numbers. Denoting by R the $I \times J$ matrix whose (i, j)th element is $\mathcal{R}_i b_j$, we end up with

$$y = Rx + e \tag{1.11}$$

[same as (3.8) of Chapter 6], where y is an I-dimensional *measurement vector* whose ith component is the measured value of $\mathcal{R}_i f$, x is the J-dimensional *image vector* which we wish to find so that we can use it in (1.5) for estimating the object *f*, and *e* is an *I*-dimensional *error vector*. The problem is again of the form:

given the data *y*, **estimate** the image vector *x*.

In CT, the $\mathscr{R}_i$ are usually defined as follows. We assume that there are *I* straight lines connecting source and detector positions in three-dimensional space. We refer to these lines as rays, and number them from 1 to *I*. For any object *f*, $\mathscr{R}_i f$ is the line integral of *f* along the *i*th ray. (The comment in Section 6.3 about the continuity assumption not always being satisfied by such $\mathscr{R}_i$ is valid here as well.)

All methods previously discussed for solving (1.11) are in principle applicable in the three-dimensional case as well. However, problems of size are even greater now than they were before, since the values of *I* and *J* are likely to be 10 to 100 times larger in the three-dimensional case than they are in the two-dimensional case. In the next section we discuss a particular approach. At the time of writing there has been very little work done in comparing various series expansion approaches for truly three-dimensional reconstruction; hence, the method in the next section is given as an example, rather than as a recommendation.

14.2   SOLVING THE NORMAL EQUATIONS FOR A SPECIAL GEOMETRY

The particular approach we take here is the minimization of the norm of the error vector, in other words the use of the least squares criterion. As it is shown in Section 12.1, the image vector *x* we seek is the one which satisfies the normal equations $R^{\mathsf{T}} R x = R^{\mathsf{T}} y$.

Similar to the approach in Chapter 13, we attempt to select the set of basis objects and the method of data collection in such a way that $R^{\mathsf{T}} R$ has a relatively simple structure. Following Section 13.1, we choose the basis objects according to (1.9) and a data collection method in which the rays in each view can be obtained by rotation of the rays in the first view around the center of rotation.

More precisely, we assume that there are *M* source positions all equally spaced on a circle of radius *D* in the plane for which $z = 0$, with the coordinates of the *m*th source position S_m at $(D, m(2\pi/M) + \pi/2, 0)$. Note that this can be achieved by the fifth scanner mode as shown in Fig. 3.3e only by rotation of the whole apparatus around the patient. For each of the *M* source positions there are a number of rays for which we collect ray sums. For consistency of notation with previous chapters we assume that for each source position there are $2N + 1$ such rays, numbered from $-N$ to N. We assume that for $-N \leq n \leq N$, there are two angles τ_n and σ_n such that, for $0 \leq m \leq M - 1$, the nth ray from the mth source position makes an angle τ_n with the $z = 0$ plane, and the projection of the nth ray from the mth source position onto the $z = 0$ plane makes an angle σ_n with the line from the mth source position to the origin (see Fig. 14.1).

We are now in position to work out the cylindrical coordinates of an arbitrary point on the nth ray in the mth view. We do this in terms of a parameter t, which measures distance along the ray. The value $t = 0$ is at the point Q in Fig. 14.1. This point is chosen so that the line OP, drawn from the origin perpendicular to the projection (in the $z = 0$ plane) of the nth ray, meets the projection $S_m P$ at the point P, which is the projection of Q. If we define

$$\ell_n = D \sin \sigma_n \qquad (2.1)$$

and

$$\theta_{n,m} = \sigma_n + m(2\pi/M), \qquad (2.2)$$

we see that P has cylindrical coordinates $(\ell_n, \theta_{n,m}, 0)$ and Q has cylindrical

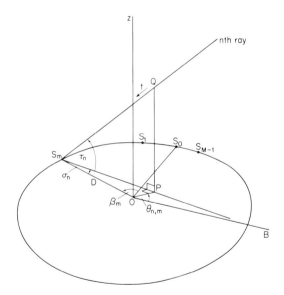

Fig. 14.1. Geometry of data collection using cone beams of x rays from a source situated on a circle in the $z = 0$ plane. $S_0, S_1, \ldots, S_{M-1}$ denote the M source positions. The nth ray $(S_m Q)$ from the mth source position makes an angle τ_n with the $z = 0$ plane, and the projection $(S_m P)$ of this ray onto the $z = 0$ plane makes an angle σ_n with the line $S_m O$ where O is the origin of the coordinate system. The points P and Q are selected so that the angles $\angle OPS_m$ and $\angle S_m PQ$ are both $90°$.

coordinates $(\ell_n, \theta_{n,m}, D \cos \sigma_n \tan \tau_n)$. A point at a distance t from Q (in direction of S_m) has coordinates

$$(\sqrt{\ell_n^2 + (t \cos \tau_n)^2}, \theta_{n,m} + \alpha_n(t \cos \tau_n), D \cos \sigma_n \tan \tau_n - t \sin \tau_n), \quad (2.3)$$

where α_n is defined by (1.16) of Chapter 13. If we now index all the rays from 1 to I according to (1.7) and (1.8) of Chapter 13, we see that, for $1 \le i \le I$, the ith ray sum for an object f is an approximation to

$$\mathcal{R}_i f = \int_{-\infty}^{\infty} f(\sqrt{\ell_n^2 + (t \cos \tau_n)^2}, \theta_{n,m} + \alpha_n(t \cos \tau_n),$$

$$D \cos \sigma_n \tan \tau_n - t \sin \tau_n) \, dt. \quad (2.4)$$

Fortunately when f is one of the basis objects defined by (1.9), the evaluation of the integral (2.4) is not as complex as the appearance of the integrand might imply. This is because the only effect of the R_u and S_w terms in (1.9) is the restriction of b_j to an annular ring, i.e., a region of space surrounded by the two planes $z = w(c - \frac{1}{2})$ and $z = w(c + \frac{1}{2})$, and by the two cylinders $r = ud$ and $r = (u + 1)d$; see Fig. 14.2. The ith ray may miss this annular ring altogether (in which case $\mathcal{R}_i b_j = 0$), or it may intersect it in either one or two separate line segments.

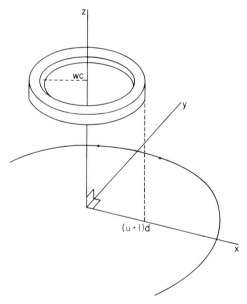

Fig. 14.2. The basis function $b_j (r, \phi, z)$ defined by (1.9) has value zero outside the annular ring of height c and width d with location as indicated in the figure. Inside the annular ring its value is a harmonic function of ϕ. (The figure uses rectangular coordinates, x, y, and z, only to ease the three-dimensional perception of the drawing).

In any case, let $L_{n,u,w}$ be the set of values of t which corresponds to the points on the ith ray which lie in the annular ring associated with the jth basis function. More precisely,

$$L_{n,u,w} = \{t \,|\, ud \le \sqrt{\ell_n^2 + (t \cos \tau_n)^2} < (u + 1)d \text{ and}$$

$$|D \cos \sigma_n \tan \tau_n - t \sin \tau_n - wc| \le \tfrac{1}{2}c\}. \quad (2.5)$$

The indices chosen reflect that $L_{n,u,w}$ depends on n (the ray position) but not on m (the source position), on u and w (the annulus and the cross section) but not on v (the harmonic). Independence from m is of course an immediate consequence of the way the data collection geometry has been set up. Using this notation, we can write

$$\mathcal{R}_i b_j = \int_{L_{n,u,w}} T_v(\theta_{n,m} + \alpha_n(t \cos \tau_n)) \, dt, \quad (2.6)$$

where either the value of the integral is zero (if $L_{n,u,w}$ is empty) or it is equal to the integral of the same integrand over one or two connected intervals of values of t.

Using the well-known formulas for the cosine and sine of sums of two angles, we get that

$$r_{i,j} = T_v(\theta_{n,m}) G_{u,v,w}(n) + T_{-v}(\theta_{n,m}) H_{u,v,w}(n), \quad (2.7)$$

where

$$G_{u,v,w}(n) = \int_{L_{n,u,w}} \cos(v\alpha_n(t \cos \tau_n)) \, dt, \quad (2.8)$$

and

$$H_{u,v,w}(n) = \int_{L_{n,u,w}} \sin(|v|\alpha_n(t \sin \tau_n)) \, dt \quad (2.9)$$

[cf (1.21) and (1.22) of Chapter 13].

It follows that the general component $(R^T R)_{p,q}$ of the matrix $R^T R$ is [see (1.25) of Chapter 13],

$$(R^T R)_{p,q} = \sum_{n=-N}^{N} G_{u_p, v_p, w_p}(n) G_{u_q, v_q, w_q}(n) \left(\sum_{m=0}^{M-1} T_{v_p}(\theta_{n,m}) T_{v_q}(\theta_{n,m}) \right)$$

$$+ \sum_{n=-N}^{N} G_{u_p, v_p, w_q}(n) H_{u_q, v_q, w_q}(n) \left(\sum_{m=0}^{M-1} T_{v_p}(\theta_{n,m}) T_{-v_q}(\theta_{n,m}) \right)$$

$$+ \sum_{n=-N}^{N} H_{u_p, v_p, w_p}(n) G_{u_q, v_q, w_q}(n) \left(\sum_{m=0}^{M-1} T_{-v_p}(\theta_{n,m}) T_{v_q}(\theta_{n,m}) \right)$$

$$+ \sum_{n=-N}^{N} H_{u_p, v_p, w_q}(n) H_{u_q, v_q, w_q}(n) \left(\sum_{m=0}^{M=1} T_{-v_p}(\theta_{n,m}) T_{-v_q}(\theta_{n,m}) \right).$$

$$(2.10)$$

Now recall the orthogonality theorem of Section 13.1. In particular, look at (1.26)–(1.31) of Chapter 13. We see that if $M \geq 2V + 1$, then for $1 \leq p \leq J$ and $1 \leq q \leq J$,

$$(R^T R)_{p,q} = \begin{cases} h_{v_p} M \sum\limits_{n=-N}^{N} (G_{u_p, v_p, w_p}(n) G_{u_q, v_q, w_q}(n) \\ \qquad\qquad + H_{u_p, v_p, w_p}(n) H_{u_q, v_q, w_q}(n) & \text{if } v_p = v_q, \\ \dfrac{M}{2} \sum\limits_{n=-N}^{N} (H_{u_p, v_p, w_p}(n) G_{u_q, v_q, w_q}(n) \\ \qquad\qquad + G_{u_p, v_p, w_p}(n) H_{u_q, v_q, w_q}(n)) & \text{if } v_p = -v_q, \\ 0 \quad \text{otherwise,} \end{cases}$$

(2.11)

where h_{v_p} is as defined after (1.30) of Chapter 13. This means that $R^T R$ has the form

$$\begin{bmatrix} P_{-V} & \Theta_{U(2W+1)} & \cdots & \Theta_{U(2W+1)} & Q_{-V} \\ \Theta_{U(2W+1)} & P_{-V+1} & \cdots & Q_{-V+1} & \Theta_{U(2W+1)} \\ \vdots & \vdots & \vdots & \vdots & \vdots \\ \Theta_{U(2W+1)} & Q_{V-1} & \cdots & P_{V-1} & \Theta_{U(2W+1)} \\ Q_V & \Theta_{U(2W+1)} & \cdots & \Theta_{U(2W+1)} & P_V \end{bmatrix},$$

(2.12)

where, for $-V \leq v \leq V$, P_v and Q_v are $U(2W + 1) \times U(2W + 1)$ matrices. We note that the form of (2.12) is *not* block diagonal, and so it cannot be inverted (as it presently stands) in the simple fashion discussed in Section 13.1. We delay correcting this until after we have discussed the nature of the individual P_v's and Q_v's.

For $-V \leq v \leq V$, P_v can be written as

$$P_v = \begin{bmatrix} P_v^{(-W, -W)} & P_v^{(-W, -W+1)} & \cdots & P_v^{(-W, W)} \\ P_v^{(-W+1, -W)} & P_v^{(-W+1, -W+1)} & \cdots & P_v^{(-W+1, W)} \\ \vdots & \vdots & \vdots & \vdots \\ P_v^{(W, -W)} & P_v^{(W, -W+1)} & \cdots & P_v^{(W, W)} \end{bmatrix},$$

(2.13)

where, for $-W \leq w' \leq W$ and $-W \leq w'' \leq W$, $P_v^{(w', w'')}$ is a $U \times U$ matrix whose (k, ℓ)th element is

$$(P_v^{(w', w'')})_{(k, \ell)} = h_v M \sum_{n=-N}^{N} (G_{k-1, v, w'}(n) G_{\ell-1, v, w''}(n) H_{k-1, v, w'}(n) H_{\ell-1, v, w''}(n)).$$

(2.14)

In particular, it follows from (2.8) and (2.9) that $P_{-v} = P_v$, for $-V \leq v \leq V$.

Now note the definitions of $G_{u,v,w}$ and $H_{u,v,w}$ in (2.8) and (2.9). If the mth ray does not enter the wth cross section (i.e., $L_{n,u,w}$ is empty for $0 \leq u \leq U - 1$), then both $G_{u,v,w}(n)$ and $H_{u,v,w}(n)$ are zero. If w' and w'' are such that no ray enters both the cross sections indexed by w' and w'', then $(P_v^{(w',w'')})_{(k,\ell)} = 0$ for $1 \leq k \leq U$ and $1 \leq \ell \leq U$. Examples of such w' and w'' are easily given: If $w' > 0$ and $w'' < 0$, then clearly no ray can enter both cross sections (see Figs. 14.1 and 14.2).

In general, there exists a positive integer Ω (which is usually smaller than W), such that whenever $|w' - w''| > \Omega$, no ray enters both the cross sections indexed by w' and w''. This and the previous discussion implies that

$$P_v^{(w',w'')} = \Theta_u \qquad \text{if} \quad |w' - w''| > \Omega. \tag{2.15}$$

A matrix P_v of this form is said to be *block polydiagonal*. While inversion of block polydiagonal matrices is not quite as simple as of block diagonal matrices, there exist algorithms which achieve inversion of block polydiagonal matrices faster than can be done by general inversion routines.

Now we look at the Q_v's in (2.12). For $-V \leq v \leq V$, Q_v can be written as

$$Q_v = \begin{bmatrix} Q_v^{(-W,-W)} & Q_v^{(-W,-W+1)} & \cdots & Q_v^{(-W,W)} \\ Q_v^{(-W+1,-W)} & Q_v^{(-W+1,-W+1)} & \cdots & Q_v^{(-W+1,W)} \\ \vdots & \vdots & \vdots & \vdots \\ Q_v^{(W,-W)} & Q_v^{(W,-W+1)} & \cdots & Q_v^{(W,W)} \end{bmatrix}, \tag{2.16}$$

where, for $-W \leq w' \leq W$ and $-W \leq w'' \leq W$, $Q_v^{(w',w'')}$ is a $U \times U$ matrix whose (k,ℓ)th element is

$$(Q_v^{(w',w'')})_{(k,\ell)} = \frac{M}{2} \sum_{n=-N}^{N} (H_{k-1,v,w'}(n)G_{\ell-1,v,w''}(n)$$
$$+ G_{k-1,v,w'}(n)H_{\ell-1,v,w''}(n)). \tag{2.17}$$

Note that it follows from (2.8) and (2.9) that $Q_{-v} = Q_v$, for $-V \leq v \leq V$, and that $Q_0 = \Theta_U$.

By an argument identical to the one given following (2.14) we can show that the Q_v's are also block polydiagonal.

Finally we note that reordering the rows and columns in the matrix (2.12)—this is equivalent to using an alternative indexing scheme to (1.8)—we can bring the matrix into a block diagonal form with $V + 1$ blocks, one of size $U(2W + 1)$ (this is essentially P_0) and all others of size $2U(2W + 1)$ (these are essentially combinations of P_v, P_{-v}, Q_v, and Q_{-v}). Furthermore each of the blocks on the diagonal can be made into a block polydiagonal matrix. It does therefore appear that it is feasible to attempt the solution of the normal equations associated with the truly three-dimensional reconstruction problem.

In summary, by an appropriate indexing of the basis objects [somewhat different from the indexing in (1.8)], the $R^T R$ in the normal equations is a block diagonal matrix with blocks $P_0, R_1, \ldots, R_V$. The block P_0 is a block polydiagonal matrix defined by (2.13), with its blocks $P_0^{(w',\,w'')}$ defined by (2.14). The blocks R_v (for $1 \le v \le V$) are block polydiagonal matrices of the form

$$
R_v = \left[\begin{pmatrix} R_v^{(-W,\,-W)} & R_v^{(-W,\,-W+1)} & \cdots & R_v^{(-W,\,W)} \\ R_v^{(-W+1,\,W)} & R_v^{(-W+1,\,-W+1)} & \cdots & R_v^{(-W+1,\,W)} \\ \vdots & \vdots & & \vdots \\ R_v^{(W,\,-W)} & R_v^{(W,\,-W+1)} & \cdots & R_v^{(W,\,W)} \end{pmatrix} \right]. \qquad (2.18)
$$

For $-W \le w' \le W$ and $-W \le w'' \le W$,

$$
R_v^{(w',\,w'')} = \begin{bmatrix} P_v^{(w',\,w'')} & Q_v^{(w',\,w'')} \\ Q_v^{(w',\,w'')} & P_v^{(w',\,w'')} \end{bmatrix}, \qquad (2.19)
$$

where $P_v^{(w',\,w'')}$ and $Q_v^{(w',\,w'')}$ are defined by (2.14) and (2.17), respectively.

In particular, $R_v^{(w',\,w'')}$ is the zero matrix Θ_{2U} if $|w' - w''| > \Omega$; see (2.15).

14.3   GENERATION OF DYNAMICALLY CHANGING THREE-DIMENSIONAL PHANTOMS AND THEIR PROJECTIONS

In order to test algorithms which are to be used for "four-dimensional" (spatio-temporal) reconstructions, we need the capability of generating appropriate phantoms and projection data. Similar methodology has been discussed for the two-dimensional case; in this section we discuss and illustrate a four-dimensional extension. While there are a number of applications, we restrict our discussion to a particular device.

The dynamic spatial reconstructor (DSR) is a device constructed at the Biodynamics Research Unit of the Mayo Clinic for (among other things) the visualization of the beating heart inside the intact thorax. The device consists of 28 x-ray sources arranged on a circular arc at $6°$ intervals (total span $162°$) and a matching set of 28 imaging systems. The whole thorax of the patient is projected onto the two-dimensional screen of the imaging systems by cone beams of x-rays from the sources. All of the x-ray sources are switched on and off within a total period of 10 msec. This process is repeated at the rate of 60 times a second. The apparatus continuously rotates at one revolution per four seconds (approximately four heartbeats), during which time a total of 240 positions are occupied by each of the x-ray sources. See Fig. 14.3 for a photograph of a model of the DSR.

In order to test an algorithm to be used by the DSR, we need the capability of generating the type of data expected from the DSR on known objects.

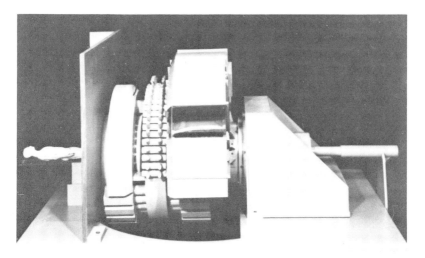

Fig. 14.3. A model of the dynamic spatial reconstructor (DSR). In this view the array of 28 x-ray tubes is in the upper half and the opposing semicircular fluorescent screen and associated 28 video imaging chains are in the lower half of the circular gantry. (Illustration provided by Dr. E. L. Ritman.)

Computer software has been developed for mathematically describing a dynamically changing three-dimensional object and then simulating the process of x-ray projection taking by the DSR.

In this software, phantoms are described as collections of ellipsoids. An ellipsoid is determined by ten parameters: three for the location of its centroid in space, three for the length of its axes, three for its orientation in space, and one for its "density." The "density" of the phantom at any point at any time is defined as the sum of the densities of all of the ellipsoids which contain the point in question. The parameters defining the ellipsoids are given as harmonic functions of time. In this fashion, a time varying three-dimensional density distribution is defined.

For our illustration, we have designed a phantom of the human thorax using 19 ellipsoids, all but two of them stationary. The two dynamically changing ellipsoids represent the myocardium and the left ventricular cavity. Cross sections and projections of this phantom are shown in the following at appropriate places.

Projection taking is done by integrating the density of the phantom along lines between the x-ray source position and points on the detector screen. It is assumed that for every source position, data are collected for 127 equally spaced sample positions in each of 63 rows on the screen. (This matches the proposed DSR data collection method.) For any time instant the data are collected simultaneously for the 28 sources. (In fact, data collection takes 100 msec on the DSR, but organ motion is negligible in such a short period of time.) Here 132 time instants at 1/60-sec intervals are simulated, with the DSR gantry moving 1.5° from instant to instant. This way the angular distance between the locations of the "first" x-ray source at the first time instant and of the "last" x-ray source at the last time instant is also 1.5° (see Fig. 14.4). In other words, all 240 positions, which can be occupied by an

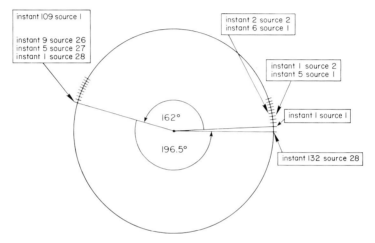

Fig. 14.4. Data collection by the DSR. At any given instant the 28 x-ray sources subtend a 162° angle at the center, with 6° between two consecutive sources. From instant to instant, the apparatus moves by 1.5°.

x-ray source at all, are occupied during our simulation at least once by one of the 28 x-ray sources. The total length of DSR operation that was simulated is 2.1833 sec. During this time, integrals of the density are collected for 29,571,696 lines (132 time instants × 28 x-ray sources × 63 rows × 127 samples). Each of these integrals are calculated by using the positions of the ellipsoids at the appropriate times. To simulate the statistical nature of x-ray data collection, "noise" has been added to the line integrals from a zero mean Gaussian distribution.

The goal of a reconstruction algorithm for the DSR is to estimate the time varying density distribution from its cone beam x-ray projections collected over time.

Figure 14.5 shows projections of the phantom at a given instant from four different source positions. Figure 14.6 shows projections of the phantom from a fixed source position at four different instants.

For our experiments we generated two data sets from all the calculated

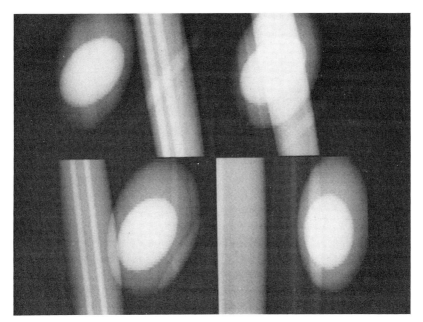

Fig. 14.5. Projections of the thorax phantom by four different x-ray sources at the same instant. Note that the thorax is so large that only part of it is projected onto the field of the imaging system.

line integrals. We refer to these as Data A (A for Average) and Data I (I for Instantaneous).

Data A contains 240 time averaged cone beam projections. During the simulation period every one of the 240 potential source positions (see Fig. 14.4) is occupied by at least one and at most 28 of the x-ray sources (although at different time instants). In creating Data A, for each source position we calculated a single average projection (127 samples in each of 63 rows) by averaging over all the projections taken with an x-ray source in that position. Thus Data A consists of 1,920,240 items (240 source positions × 63 rows × 127 samples).

Data I is the data collected at a particular instant of time. It consists of 224,028 items (28 x-ray sources × 63 rows × 127 samples).

In view of the well-demonstrated success of the fan beam convolution algorithm (see Chapter 10), it would be pleasant to apply this algorithm to Data I. Unfortunately, the geometry of the DSR data collection at a single time instant fails to satisfy the assumptions which were made in the design of the fan beam convolution reconstruction algorithms in the following three ways.

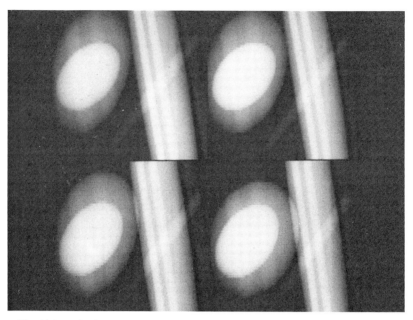

Fig. 14.6. Projections of the thorax phantom from a fixed source position at four different instants.

(i)   The x-ray beam is *cone beam*, rather than fan beam: x rays do not travel parallel to the circle of source positions.

(ii)   At any given time instant, the x-ray source positions lie on a 162° arc (rather than all the way around the 360° circle). That is, we have a *limited range of views*. (Note that this condition also violates the assumptions in Section 14.2.)

(iii)   Due to the size of the imaging system, parts of the body fall outside the cone beam of x rays. (This can be observed in Figs. 14.5 and 14.6.) That is, we have a *limited field of views*.

The combined effect of these inconsistencies between the data collection geometry and the assumptions in the algorithm is that for DSR data of stationary objects the reconstructions produced by the fan beam convolution algorithm are not quite as good as those generally achieved using single cross-section CT devices. This is further aggravated by the fact that for a single time instant the DSR uses only 28 source positions, while the single cross-section devices rotate so that the x-ray source occupies as many as 288 or more positions to obtain the input data for the reconstruction algorithm.

In Figure 14.7 we indicate how a cone beam projection may be interpreted as a series of fan beam projections. The quality of output by applying the fan beam algorithm to Data I is illustrated in the following.

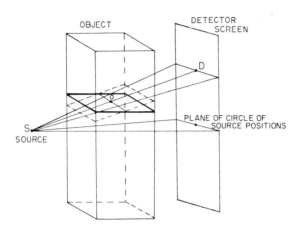

Fig. 14.7. The relationship between cone and fan beam projections. In the DSR, from a given x-ray source S a cone beam of x rays project the object onto the detector screen. A line on the screen which is parallel to the circle of source positions (containing the point D at its center) determines a cross section in the object (indicated by broken lines), which is oblique; i.e., it is *not* parallel to the circle of source positions. Points in this cross-section project onto the line containing D. For a different source position, a *different* oblique plane would project onto the same level of the detector screen. However, all these planes go through the same point O, which lies on the axis of rotation of the gantry. Consider the cross section parallel to the circle of source positions which contains O (indicated by the heavy line). As a first approximation, it may be assumed that all data collected on the screen at the level of D are fan beam data of the cross section containing O parallel to the circle of source positions. Reconstructions based on such an assumption may in places be blurred in the direction perpendicular to the plane of the circle of source positions.

14.4   A Three-Dimensional Algorithm Based on Bayesian Optimization

We now discuss a reconstruction algorithm whose derivation does not require untrue (or only approximately true) assumptions about the DSR geometry. We make essential use of Section 11.3 which describes a similar algorithm for cross-sectional reconstruction, namely, the additive ART algorithm for obtaining the Bayesian estimate which minimizes (3.1) of Chapter 11.

Consider the three-dimensional object to be reconstructed at a particular instant of time. We use f to denote this object. In this section we use the basis objects defined by (1.4). Thus, f is represented by the J-dimensional image vector x, with x_j equal to the average value of f inside the jth voxel.

In order for this representation to be useful the voxels should be small, and so the number of components in x has to be large. For our phantom, we have used layers of voxels parallel to the plane of the circle of source positions. In each layer we have 127×127 voxels to include the whole thorax, and 63 layers were necessary to contain the myocardium. In our work we used only the central 39 layers (which contained most of the left ventricular cavity). Thus our vector x has 629,031 components (39 layers of 127×127 voxels) for any instant of time. The purpose of the reconstruction algorithm is then to estimate x from the given data. To reconstruct a complete heart-beat, this would have to be done for about 60 successive time instants!

It has been shown in Section 11.3 that under certain assumptions the algorithm described by (3.13) and (3.14) of Chapter 11 produces a sequence of vectors which converges to the Bayesian estimate x^*. The same algorithm can, in principle, be applied to the cone beam problem.

The important thing to observe is that despite the enormous size of the problem (in our case x has over half a million components), the algorithm is implementable even on a minicomputer by making use of our understanding of the underlying geometry of the problem. We omit the computational details, but warn the reader that the practical feasibility of the algorithm is very much dependent on the organization of the data sets containing $x^{(k)}$, y, and $u^{(k)}$. (R is not stored at all: its components are calculated as and when needed.) In fact, in order to reduce the number of disk accesses, we have used a slightly altered version of the algorithm.

We note that this algorithm treats the cone beam nature of data collection, and its use is justified by the theory even though the sources lie only on a 162° arc and parts of the body fall outside the cone beam of x rays. On the other hand, the theory is based on assumptions regarding the Gaussian nature of the random variables $X - \mu_X$ and E (see Section 11.3), which are likely to be violated in practice. However, even if these assumptions are violated, the resulting estimator has some mathematically desirable properties.

An important question which has been left open so far is how to select the expected value μ_X and the r in (3.1) of Chapter 11.

The image vector x is a sample of a random variable whose expected value is μ_X. Data A is obtained by averaging projections over time. This justifies the use of a reconstruction from Data A as the vector μ_X.

Data A contains 240 cone beam projections for source positions situated all around a circle. Hence, the objection concerning limited range of views is not applicable to Data A. Using a fan beam algorithm for the cone beams results in a slice-to-slice blurring (see Fig. 14.7), not unreasonable for an expected value image. The only remaining objection to using a fan beam convolution reconstruction algorithm is that the data are of limited field of view.

Fortunately, there are effective algorithms to preprocess limited field of view data so that it becomes appropriate for a fan beam convolution reconstruction algorithm. The one we have chosen to use operates as follows.

For each source position, the divergent beam projection data are padded by ray sums for additional rays on both sides so that the two extreme rays (after padding) properly enclose the reconstruction region. The ray sum for a newly added ray is calculated to be the line integral (along the ray) of a circular disk of uniform density, centered at the origin. The diameter of the disk is selected to be such that it neither encloses the whole of the body cross section to be reconstructed, nor is it enclosed by it. The density of the disk is separately calculated for both ends of the extended projection. Its value for one end of a projection is chosen so that it fits best (in the least squares sense) the actually measured ray sums for the five originally extreme rays at that end. As we demonstrate in the following, even such a crude extension leads to useful reconstructions.

Organizing our cone beam Data A into sets of fan beam data as described in the legend of Fig. 14.7, and extending each set of fan beam data so that it is no longer of limited field of view, we can produce μ_X layer by layer, by applying the divergent beam convolution algorithm of Section 10.1.

The value of r can be estimated by using a phantom (or phantoms) x similar to what we are trying to reconstruct and defining $r = t/s$, where t is the standard deviation of the components of $x - \mu_X$, and s is the standard deviation of the components of $y - Rx$.

14.5   A DEMONSTRATION

We used Data A and Data I to produce reconstructions.

First we used 39 subsets of Data A to produce μ_X. Each subset is determined by a single layer of the object to be reconstructed. For each of the 240 source positions, we selected the samples from the appropriate row, as described in Fig. 14.7. Thus μ_X was produced by 39 separate limited field of view fan beam convolution reconstruction algorithms. In each one of these, the values of μ_X at 16,129 points (127×127 voxel centers) were calculated from 30,480 data items (240 source positions, 127 samples of each).

We have estimated that the value $r = 0.8$ is appropriate for the type of object and error that we have in this example. Now that we had μ_X and r, "all" we had to do was to find the x^* which minimizes (3.1) of Chapter 11, using Data I as the measurement vector y. The reader should bear in mind though that the sizes of x and y are 629,031 and 224,028, respectively.

Nevertheless, the algorithm of the last section was implemented and applied. We have chosen the constant value 0.5 for the relaxation parameter $\lambda^{(k)}$. We have run the algorithm for three complete cycles through the data. The difference between the estimates of the object at the ends of the second and third cycles was negligible, so it seemed reasonable to terminate the algorithm at this point.

We now report on our results.

Figure 14.8 shows a projection with two lines on it. These lines are two alternative locations for the line whose center is marked by D in Fig. 14.7. In the succeeding figures we report on the corresponding cross sections in the object. The corresponding cross section in Fig. 14.7 is the one parallel to the circle of source positions, with its center O (it is marked by the heavy line). Corresponding to the lines in Fig. 14.8, we get the 22nd and 42nd of the original 63 layers of our digitization. These are located approximately 3 cm above and below, respectively, the circle of source positions.

Figures 14.9–14.12 report on these cross sections. In each case (a) contains the original phantom, (b) contains the object produced from Data I with an unaltered divergent beam convolution algorithm, (c) contains the object μ_X produced from Data A using the limited field of view fan beam convolution algorithm, and (d) contains the output of the Bayesian method (using Data I) at the end of the third cycle. In what we call the "unaltered divergent beam convolution algorithm," the limited range of views is taken care of in the simplest possible way: the "missing" views are ignored. This has the same effect as assuming that ray sums for these views are all zeros and then applying the formulas of Section 10.1. The result of this process is multiplicatively normalized, by a number which is the ratio of the number of views if there were

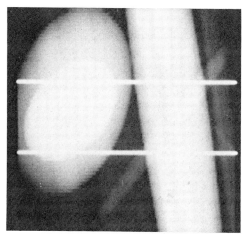

Fig. 14.8. Projection of the thorax phantom, indicating the 22nd and 42nd of the 63 rows on the screen.

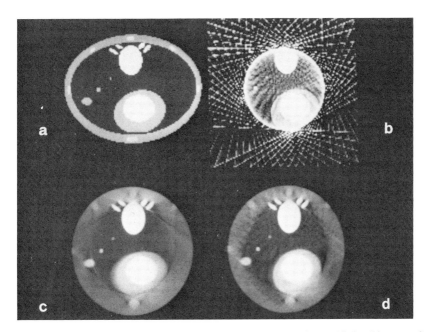

Fig. 14.9. The 22nd level of the phantom (a) and reconstructions. This level is approximately 3 cm above the circle of source positions. (b) is the unaltered divergent beam convolution method reconstruction from Data I, (c) is reconstruction from Data A, and (d) is the ART reconstruction from Data I.

none missing, in our case 60, and the actual number of views, in our case 28. Each cross section is reconstructed separately from a subset of Data I, selected according to the method described in the legend of Fig. 14.7.

In Figs. 14.9 and 14.11 we show the visual appearance of the 22nd and 42nd layers, respectively. For the phantom, the value assigned to a voxel is the value of the phantom at the center of the voxel. In the divergent beam convolution method reconstruction on Data I, the bright circle is an artifact due to the limited field of view. Its location indicates the field of view in the data. This artifact is essentially removed by the limited field of view reconstruction algorithm from Data A, but we find instead blurring of the moving ellipsoids representing the heart. The Bayesian reconstruction starting from this blurred image, μ_X, essentially removes the blurring by making use of the instantaneous Data I.

The same is illustrated more quantitatively in Figs. 14.10 and 14.12. Plots are drawn of the values in the 67th (out of a total of 127) column of the pictures shown in Figs. 14.9 and 14.11, respectively.

This demonstration supports our claim regarding the versatility of series expansion methods such as ART. The mathematical development of Section

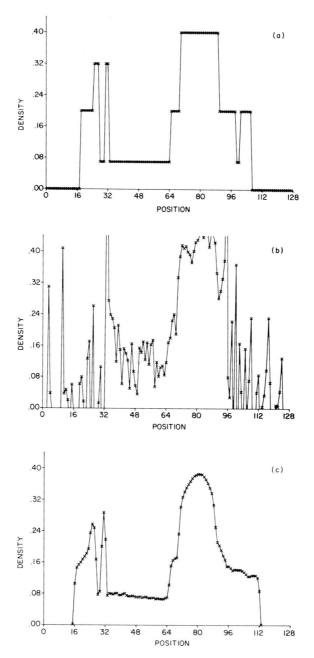

Fig. 14.10. Plots of the 67th columns of the phantom and reconstructions shown in Fig. 14.9. Positions 34–94 lie within the limited field of view for which data have been collected.

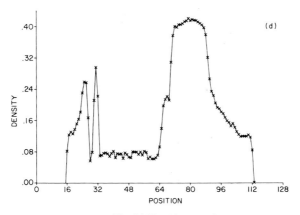

Fig. 14.10   (*Continued*)

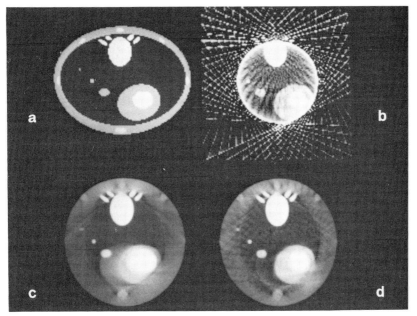

Fig. 14.11. The 42nd level of the phantom and reconstructions. This level is approximately 3 cm below the circle of source positions. Arrangement is the same as in Fig. 14.9.

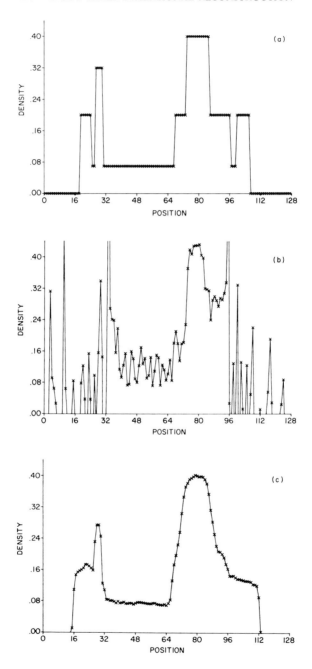

Fig. 14.12. Plots of the 67th columns of the phantom and reconstructions shown in Fig. 14.11. Positions 34–94 lie within the limited field of view for which data have been collected.

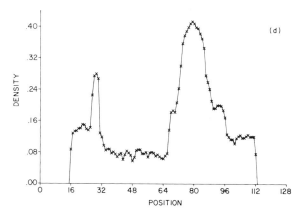

Fig. 14.12   (*Continued*)

11.3 (originally designed for two-dimensional reconstruction) was adopted without any change to truly three-dimensional reconstruction. Despite the extreme size of the three-dimensional problems, implementation on a mini-computer is feasible. In fact, the reconstructions shown in Figs. 14.9 and 14.11 were all produced on a minicomputer (the Eclipse S/200).

NOTES AND REFERENCES

There have been a number of methods proposed for truly three-dimensional reconstruction. For a brief survey, see Altschuler, Censor, *et al.* (1979). The same paper also surveys approaches to reconstruction from both limited range of view data and from limited field of view data. In particular, that survey mentions the work of Bracewell and Wernecke (1975), Chang (1979), Colsher (1977), Hinderling *et al.* (1979), Huang, *et al.* (1977), Kowalski (1977), and Minerbo (1979b) but was written too early to include the work of Denton *et al.* (1979).

The method described in Section 14.2 is based on Altschuler and Herman (1977).

The phantom and projection data generation is based on the work of Altschuler, Chang, and Chu (1979), who have described an earlier (not dynamically changing) version of this system. For a detailed description of the DSR, as well as a discussion of its applications in physiology and medicine, see Wood *et al.* (1979).

The algorithm based on Bayesian optimization is taken from Altschuler *et al.* (1980). Our method for extending the limited field of view data is based on the work of Lewitt (1979). For a detailed discussion of an extremely rapid hardward implementation for the DSR of what we called the "un-altered divergent beam convolution algorithm" see Gilbert *et al.* (1979).

15

Three-Dimensional Display of Organs

In the last chapter we discussed methods which can be used to produce a three-dimensional array of numbers, each number representing the average density (relative linear attenuation) in a voxel at an appropriate location. Even if two-dimensional reconstruction techniques are used, from a sequence of computed tomograms of two-dimensional transverse slices one can build up a three-dimensional array of numbers containing spatial rather than cross-sectional information.

Given such an array, it is easy to display the saggital and coronal sections of the body (see Fig. 2.2). Using linear interpolation one can calculate densities at arbitrary points inside the body, and thus produce displays of a slice at any desired orientation through the object. Such techniques are simple in conception (although they may require clever implementation when dealing with large arrays on a minicomputer), and we do not discuss them in detail in this book.

We concentrate instead on methods which, based on the three-dimensional array of densities, display what a particular organ would look like if it were removed from the body. This is done by a computer technique that first detects the surface of the organ of interest and then displays this surface on a screen. The combination of computerized tomography with such display techniques has been aptly named as "noninvasive vivisection."

15.1   THE BASIC APPROACH

We assume that the region of interest is subdivided into voxels, in a manner similar to the three-dimensional digitization approach of Section 13.1. Each voxel has a CT number associated with it, these are the x_j's of (1.5) in Chapter 14.

We also assume that in the resulting three-dimensional array of numbers an organ can be distinguished from its surrounding in the following way. There exists a range $\mathcal{O}$ of values such that the CT number of a voxel just inside the organ is in $\mathcal{O}$ and the CT number of a voxel just outside the organ is not in $\mathcal{O}$. Note that we assume that a voxel is either entirely within or entirely outside the organ, and so our accuracy of organ representation is limited by the size of the voxels. It follows that the surface of (our approximation to) the organ consists of faces which separate two voxels that are respectively inside and outside the organ.

An example of this is given in Fig. 15.1a which shows corresponding parts of three CT cross sections of the human head containing part of the ventricular system. The range $\mathcal{O}$ has been selected so that voxels inside the ventricles have CT numbers in $\mathcal{O}$, while voxels just outside the ventricles have CT numbers not in $\mathcal{O}$. In Fig. 15.1b, the voxels with CT numbers in $\mathcal{O}$ are shown bright and the other voxels are shown dark.

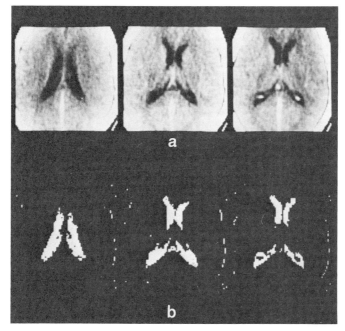

Fig. 15.1. (a) Ventricles in the CT slices appear darker than the surrounding brain. In (b) all pixels which have CT numbers similar to the CT numbers of ventricles are white, all other pixels are black.

In this manner we define a subset B of voxels, which contains all the voxels whose value is in the range $\mathcal{O}$. Our intuitive idea is that an "organ" is a subset of B which is in some sense "connected." In the next section we define such notions precisely, and discuss an algorithm for finding a boundary of an organ. Note that an organ may have multiple boundary surfaces. For example, the heart muscle has an exterior surface and several interior surfaces, one for each of the chambers.

15.2   BOUNDARY DETECTION

As previously, we use J to denote the number of voxels, and we index the voxels with integers j, $1 \leq j \leq J$. Given two different voxels j and k, we use the notation $f(j, k)$ if j and k have a face in common, and the notation $e(j, k)$ if j and k have an edge in common but they do not have a face in common. If $f(j, k)$, we call the pair of voxels (j, k) a *face*. We say that the pair of voxels (j, ℓ) is an *edge of the face* (j, k) if $e(j, \ell)$ and $f(k, \ell)$, see Fig. 15.2. If $f(j, k)$,

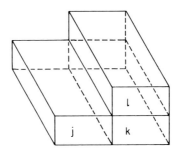

Fig. 15.2. The pair (j,k) is a face of the voxel j. The pair (j,l) is an edge of the face (j,k).

we also say that (j, k) is a face of j. Clearly, each voxel has six faces and each of these faces has four edges. Note that we do *not* identify the face (j, k) with the face (k, j). Reasons for this become clear later.

Let B and W be two disjoint sets of voxels. The *boundary* $P(B, W)$ between B and W is defined to be the set of faces between voxels one of which is in B and the other one of which is in W. Mathematically,

$$P(B, W) = \{(b, w) | b \in B, w \in W \text{ and } f(b, w)\}. \tag{2.1}$$

We are not particularly interested in boundaries between arbitrary sets of voxels. We restrict our attention to boundaries between "organs" and their "coorgans." We now define these concepts.

In these definitions we refer to a set Q. Intuitively, the reader should think of Q as a set of voxels whose CT numbers fall in the range $\mathcal{O}$ (see Section 15.1). For example, if Q contains all the voxels which have the same density as heart muscle (which, for the sake of argument, we assume to be different from the density of blood), the heart muscle would be an organ in Q and each of its chambers (as well as a connected part of its exterior) would be coorgans of Q. We place certain restrictions on the sets Q in which we are interested. First, Q has to be nonempty. Second, Q must not contain any of the border voxels (i.e., Q has to be a subset of the set of interior voxels, which in the two-dimensional case is denoted by N in Section 12.3). In what follows we refer to a set of voxels satisfying these two conditions as an *interior set*. The reason for the second restriction is that in our definition of a boundary, (2.1), we need voxels on both sides of boundary faces. The second condition can always be achieved by padding out the array of voxels by an additional layer of voxels on all sides and assigning them CT numbers which are not in $\mathcal{O}$.

Let Q be an interior set and let B be a nonempty subset of Q. In such a case, we say that B is an *organ* of Q if

(i)   whenever j and k are distinct elements of B, then there exists a sequence $\ell^1, \ldots, \ell^u$ of voxels in B such that $\ell^1 = j$, $\ell^u = k$, and, for $1 \leq v < u$, either $f(\ell^v, \ell^{v+1})$ or $e(\ell^v, \ell^{v+1})$, and

(ii) B is not a proper subset of any subset of Q which satisfies (i).

In less mathematical terms, an organ B of Q is determined by any one of its elements j in the following way. B consists of all the voxels k, which can be reached from j by going through faces and edges of voxels which are in Q. In Fig. 15.3 we illustrate this definition.

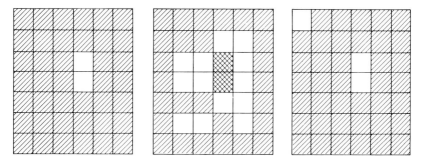

Fig. 15.3. Illustration of the concepts of organ and coorgan. Parts of three consecutive layers in the array are shown. Elements of Q are those voxels which are represented by blank squares. We assume that all voxels not shown in the illustration are in $\bar{Q}$. In this case Q has two organs. One consists of a single voxel in the top left corner of the part of the array shown on the right. The other contains all of the rest of the elements of Q. Q has two coorgans. The one consists of two voxels cross-hatched in the central level; the other consists of the rest of the elements of $\bar{Q}$.

Let Q be an interior set and let W be a nonempty set of voxels which does not contain any element of Q. In other words, W is a subset of the complement $\bar{Q}$ of Q. In such a case, we say that W is a *coorgan* of Q, if

(i)   whenever j and k are distinct elements of W, then there exists a sequence $\ell^1, \ldots, \ell^u$ of voxels in W such that $\ell^1 = j$, $\ell^u = k$, and $1 \leq v < u$, $f(\ell^v, \ell^{v+1})$, and

(ii) B is not a proper subset of any subset of $\bar{Q}$ which satisfies (i).

In less mathematical terms, a coorgan W of Q is determined by one of its elements j in the following way. W consists of all the voxels k, which can be reached from j by going through faces of voxels which are not in Q. This definition also is illustrated in Fig. 15.3.

Note that coorgans are defined so that they have to be connected in a "stronger" sense than organs: connectedness through edges is not allowed. The reason for this is that we wish the surface that we produce to be a *Jordan surface*, that is, a surface which divides three-dimensional space into two regions of which it is the common boundary, called the *interior* and *exterior* region, respectively. [In our work, the surface elements are pairs of voxels (b, w), where b is in the interior and w is in the exterior. Note that the intended meaning of interior is "interior to the organ." Quite possibly the interior of the surface may enclose the exterior of the surface, as is the case between the heart muscle and the chamber.] Furthermore, each point in space which is not on the Jordan surface must belong either to the interior or the exterior. Any two points in the interior (or exterior) can be joined by a curve which does not contain any points in the surface. Any curve that joins a point of the interior and a point of the exterior must contain at least one point of the surface. In particular, a half-line starting at a point in the exterior of the surface cannot enter the interior without passing through the surface. We make essential use of this property later on.

Our aim in this section is the following: Find an algorithm which for any interior set Q and for any element (b, w) of $P(Q, \bar{Q})$ provides us with all the elements of $P(B, W)$, where B is the organ of Q which contains b and W is the coorgan of Q which contains w. More loosely speaking, the algorithm finds all faces in the (part of the) boundary of an organ which contains the given face.

Suppose we had a method which, for any interior set Q, for any organ B of Q, for any coorgan W of Q, and for any face r in the boundary $P(B, W)$, produces two other faces $f_1(r)$ and $f_2(r)$ in the boundary $P(B, W)$ so that the following is true: whenever p and q are distinct faces in $P(B, W)$, then there exists a sequence $r^1, \ldots, r^u$ of faces in $P(B, W)$ such that $r^1 = p$, $r^u = q$, and, for $1 \leq v < u$, either $r^{v+1} = f_1(r^v)$ or $r^{v+1} = f_2(r^v)$. Such a method can be utilized in an algorithm for boundary surface detection, which we now explain.

The algorithm produces a "list" L of faces, and it makes use of a "pool" P of faces. We assume that (b, w) is the given face in $P(Q, \bar{Q})$. The following are the steps of the algorithm.

(i)   Put (b, w) into both L and P.
(ii)   Remove an element r from P.
(iii) If $f_1(r)$ is not in L, put $f_1(r)$ into both L and P.
(iv)   If $f_2(r)$ is not in L, put $f_2(r)$ into both L and P.
(v)   If P is empty, STOP. If P is not empty, go to step (ii).

We now look at the behavior of this algorithm. First of all, we assumed the existence of the method which produces $f_1(r)$ and $f_2(r)$ for any r in $P(B, W)$. The r obtained in step (ii) is in $P(B, W)$, since it is in P, and it is easy to see that at any time during the execution of the algorithm all elements of P are in $P(B, W)$. Similarly, all elements of L are in $P(B, W)$, and due to the nature of f_1 and f_2, any element which is in $P(B, W)$ is sooner or later put into L. From that time on, P gets depleted by continued use of step (ii), and does *not* get enlarged due to steps (iii) or (iv), and so eventually becomes empty. At this point the algorithm stops with L containing all elements of $P(B, W)$ and nothing else.

Thus the algorithm performs the task for which it is designed. The only thing we left unexplained is how $f_1(r)$ and $f_2(r)$ are to be calculated from r. Although this detail is essential, a general discussion is omitted from this book because of its technical difficulty. We give a simple illustration using an organ of three voxels.

In Fig. 15.4, the three voxels which are drawn are assumed to be in Q, all other voxels are assumed to be in $\bar{Q}$. We label all the faces in $P(B, W)$ by the numbers 1 through 14, and we assume that the given face is the face labeled 1. The functions f_1 and f_2 are defined by the graph in Fig. 15.4b; each face r is connected to the face $f_1(r)$ by a solid arrow and to the face $f_2(r)$

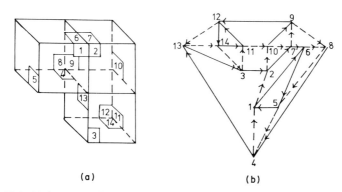

(a)   (b)

Fig. 15.4. (a) An organ of three voxels and (b) the associated functions f_1 (solid arrow) and f_2 (broken arrow) mapping faces into faces.

by a broken arrow. It is straightforward, but somewhat tedious, to check that these functions f_1 and f_2 have the required properties.

We now illustrate the algorithm in the accompanying tabulation. Lines indicate successive values of r, P, and L at step (v) of the algorithm.

r	P	L
1	{6,2}	{1,6,2}
6	{2,5,8}	{1,6,2,5,8}
2	{5,8,7,10}	{1,6,2,5,8,7,10}
5	{8,7,10,4}	{1,6,2,5,8,7,10,4}
8	{7,10,4}	{1,6,2,5,8,7,10,4}
7	{10,4,9}	{1,6,2,5,8,7,10,4,9}
10	{4,9}	{1,6,2,5,8,7,10,4,9}
4	{9,13}	{1,6,2,5,8,7,10,4,9,13}
9	{13,12}	{1,6,2,5,8,7,10,4,9,13,12}
13	{12,3,14}	{1,6,2,5,8,7,10,4,9,13,12,3,14}
12	{3,14}	{1,6,2,5,8,7,10,4,9,13,12,3,14}
3	{14,11}	{1,6,2,5,8,7,10,4,9,13,12,3,14,11}
14	{11}	{1,6,2,5,8,7,10,4,9,13,12,3,14,11}
11	ϕ	{1,6,2,5,8,7,10,4,9,13,12,3,14,11}

In practice, it may become unacceptably time consuming to check, in steps (iii) and (iv), whether or not $f_1(r)$ and $f_2(r)$ are in L. This is because $P(B, W)$ may contain well over 10,000 elements (we see an example in Section 15.5), and eventually L is of the same size. There are techniques to avoid most of this work, but except for one of them we do not discuss them here.

One technique for reducing the work load, for checking whether a face is already in L, is to divide L into several smaller lists depending on some properties of its members. Then for each new face r only one of the groups need to be checked. For example, all faces point in one of six possible directions [i.e., for the face (j, k) the vector from the center of voxel j to the center of voxel k has one of six possible values]. We can make use of this fact to reduce the work involved in checking membership in L by a factor of six. Also, dividing L into six groups according to this criterion is also helpful in the display of the surface, as we see in the next section.

15.3   HIDDEN SURFACE REMOVAL

As it is discussed in the previous section, the boundary detection algorithm produces a list L of faces. A face is represented as an ordered pair of voxels, but it is best thought from now on as a square shaped surface element which lies in one of six possible orientations (three mutually perpendicular pairs of opposing directions).

For the sake of simplifying our discussion, we assume that the exterior of the surface encloses the interior. (This can usually be achieved for any surface of interest by an appropriate choice of the range of the CT numbers which defines Q.) We assume that there is a display screen which is placed in a fixed position in space, so that the plane of the screen is entirely in the exterior of the surface. Our display of the surface is a projection of the appearance of the surface onto the screen.

In displaying surfaces we use *orthogonal projections*. That is, we assume that a point P on the screen displays the point Q on the surface which is such that

(i)   the line segment QP is perpendicular to the screen,

(ii) the interior of the line segment QP does not contain any point of the surface.

See Figure 15.5.

Note that such a method does not make any use of perspective. Organs being fairly small objects, an orthogonal projection gives a realistic appearance, which is not improved noticeably by the introduction of perspective.

There are two separate questions involved in the display method just described. The first is: By what intensity should the point Q on the surface be

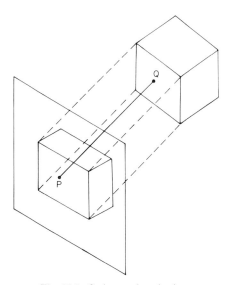

Fig. 15.5. Orthogonal projection.

displayed at the point P on the screen? The second is: If there are several points on the surface which lie on the line perpendicular to the screen at the point P, how should the correct point Q be selected? In this section we deal with the latter question, which is the problem of "hidden surface removal" or equivalently "visible surface display." We leave the discussion of the first question until the next section.

There are many techniques for hidden surface removal. Here we discuss one which appears to be particularly appropriate for the environment in which we are working. This method is generally referred to as the *Z-buffer algorithm*.

With each point (raster element) P on the display screen we associate two numbers: *brightness* $b(P)$ and *distance from the screen* $d(P)$. Initially, for each point we assign zero (dark) to the brightness and a very large number (essentially infinity) to the distance from the screen. If a face α is such that it is perpendicular to the screen, then it is not displayed. All other faces making up our surface are displayed one by one, according to the following procedure.

For each face α, we locate all the points P on the screen that would be used if that face alone were to be displayed. These points then are treated one by one as follows.

For each point P we find the point Q on the face α such that PQ is perpendicular to the screen. Let $\bar{d}(Q)$ be the distance of Q from the screen (i.e., the distance from P to Q) and let $\bar{b}(Q)$ be the brightness that would be assigned to P if the face α alone were to be displayed. If $\bar{d}(Q)$ is less than $d(P)$, then we change the value of $b(P)$ to that of $\bar{b}(Q)$ and the value of $d(P)$ to that of $\bar{d}(Q)$. However, if $\bar{d}(Q)$ is not less than $d(P)$, we do not change the values of $b(P)$ and $d(P)$.

In this fashion, by the time we have dealt with all the faces, brightnesses are displayed for the visible faces, and the hidden faces (or parts of faces) do not influence the display.

There are three ways that the general Z-buffer algorithm, as just described, can be made to work faster in our special environment.

First, we can make use of the following result, whose somewhat messy proof we omit. If neither of the faces α and β are perpendicular to the display screen, if A is a point inside α (i.e., on α but not on an edge of α) and B is a point inside β such that the line AB is perpendicular to the screen, then $\bar{d}(A) < \bar{d}(B)$ if, only if, $\bar{d}(C(\alpha)) < \bar{d}(C(\beta))$, where $C(\alpha)$ and $C(\beta)$ denote the center points on the faces α and β, respectively. This result tells us that we can approximate, for any point Q on α, $\bar{d}(Q)$ by $\bar{d}(C(\alpha))$ in the Z-buffer algorithm, and yet end up with the same display.

Second, since each of the faces is small, we may also assume that all points on the face would be displayed by the same brightness, and so approximate for any point Q on α, $\bar{b}(Q)$ by $\bar{b}(C(\alpha))$.

Third, half the faces need not be displayed at all. At most three of the six sublists discussed in the last section need to be considered for any fixed orientation of the screen. The faces in the other three are sure to be hidden, as can be seen by recalling the fact that our surfaces are Jordan surfaces.

A series of such displays can be obtained by moving the position of the screen.

15.4 SHADING

We desire to display the visible part of a detected surface on a cathode-ray tube in such a way that its appearance resembles the appearance of the surface of the original object in the same orientation. This three-dimensional appearance in a raster graphics device is attempted by "shading," i.e., by assigning different gray levels to the display points on the screen. A number of depth and shape cues exists. Here we discuss only two of them: Z distance and orientation.

The underlying assumption in this simple case is that light travels in parallel rays perpendicular to the screen from a plane source which is parallel to the screen. The intensity assigned to a point P on the screen, which is displaying a point Q on a surface element in three-dimensional space, depends on the distance of Q from the light source and on the angle between the normal to the surface element at Q and the direction of the light.

Computationally, cube shaped voxels are very appropriate for such calculations. Since each surface element is a square in one of three orientations, only three normals need to be calculated. Since the surface elements are small, one may assume, without appreciably affecting the output, that all points on a surface element α are at the same Z distance, namely the Z distance $\bar{d}(C(\alpha))$ of its center, which has already been established during the hidden surface removal process.

In practice, something further has to be done, because of the limited number of orientations of the faces of the detected surface. The original surface is likely to have been quite smooth, but the displayed surface often looks jagged.

We list three techniques that have been proposed and used to overcome this, either individually or in combination with each other. (i) Put the final image through a low-pass filter in order to smooth its appearance (i.e., convolve it with a function which has no high frequency components). (ii) Assume a virtual display screen of higher resolution than the actual screen and display on the actual screen by averaging the values on the virtual screen. (iii) Make the influence of the angle between the light and surface normal unimportant as compared to the Z distance.

None of these solutions is entirely satisfactory. The third one essentially removes the important depth cue provided by the angle between the direction of light and the surface normal. The other two do nothing to resolve the type of difficulty which we now describe.

Consider a part of the surface of the original object which is flat and is perpendicular to the light. If the orientation of two voxel faces is also perpendicular to the light, then the above-mentioned flat surface is approximated by faces of voxels all parallel to each other (and perpendicular to the light direction). In this case, at every point, the normal to the detected surface makes an angle zero with the direction of light, and the surface will appear uniformly very bright. If the orientation of the voxels happens to be chosen at $\pi/4$ to the flat part of the surface of the original object, then the flat surface is approximated by faces of voxels which make an angle $\pi/4$ with the flat face (and hence an angle $\pi/4$ with the light direction). In this case, at every point, the normal to the detected surface makes an angle $\pi/4$ with the direction of light, and the surface will appear uniformly lit, but not as bright as in the previous case.

This is a serious drawback of our model. It can be overcome either by determining shading based on the orientation of a face *and* its neighbors, or by using surface elements more complex than squares. However, as is demonstrated in the next section, in practice excellent quality three-dimensional displays can be obtained using the Z distance as the major depth cue, and then applying low-pass filtering to the image so formed.

15.5   EXPERIMENTAL RESULTS

Our first illustration involves the ventricular system of the human brain. We were provided with a set of eight contiguous 8 mm-thick slices containing parts of the ventricular system of a patient. Figure 15.1 shows (on top) an 80×80 pixel part of three of these eight slices. The same 80×80 pixel part was extracted from each slice. The ventricles were entirely within this part in each of the eight slices. Since the pixels in the slices are 1.5×1.5 mm, the corresponding voxels in the original slices are $1.5 \times 1.5 \times 8$ mm. We would like to have cube shaped voxels for the procedures described in the previous sections. For this purpose we used linear interpolation to estimate the appearance of thirty-eight contiguous 1.5 mm-thick slices. This resulted in an $80 \times 80 \times 38$ array of numbers, representing the average density in an array of cube shaped voxels.

The reason why the ventricles in Fig. 15.1 appear darker than the surrounding tissue is that they contain cerebrospinal fluid which has a slightly lower linear attenuation coefficient than brain (see Table 4.1). Hence the range $\mathcal{O}$ of values referred to in Section 15.1 has to be such that its upper limit is greater than the linear attenuation coefficient of cerebrospinal fluid and less than that of the brain. This means that all voxels filled with spinal fluid have CT numbers in the range $\mathcal{O}$. Thus the set Q of voxels whose CT numbers are in the range $\mathcal{O}$ (see Section 15.2) contains not only the ventricles, but also other systems filled by spinal fluid, and even some voxels which do not contain spinal fluid, but happen to have CT numbers in the range $\mathcal{O}$ due to other reasons (noise in data, reconstruction artifact, etc.). The voxels which are in the set Q are indicated as bright in the lower part of Fig. 15.1. An anatomical drawing of the relevant part of the ventricular system (indicating the position of the corpora quadragemina as well) is shown in Fig. 15.6.

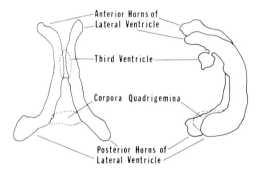

Fig. 15.6. Anatomical drawing of part of the ventricular system of the human brain.

The boundary detection, hidden surface removal, and shading procedures described in the last three sections were applied to produce the three-dimensional displays of the ventricular system shown in Fig. 15.7. The number of detected boundary faces for the ventricular system is 8,970. Detection of this surface from the $80 \times 80 \times 38$ array of voxels required less than half a minute computer time on a minicomputer (Eclipse S/200).

The next illustration is on displaying the spine of a patient suffering from dysraphism. Dysraphism is a disease in which the spinal cord does not develop normally. In Fig. 15.8 we show a CT cross section of this patient in which the bony spicule that divides the spinal chord is clearly visible.

In Fig. 15.8 we indicate a 96×96 pixel frame which encloses the spinal column. Each pixel is 0.8×0.8 mm. From a sequence of 8 contiguous 1.5 mm-thick patient slices, we have produced (using linear interpolation) a three-dimensional array of numbers, representing the average densities in a $96 \times 96 \times 14$ array of $0.8 \times 0.8 \times 0.8$ mm voxels. We specified a range of CT numbers which should distinguish voxels filled with bone from the rest.

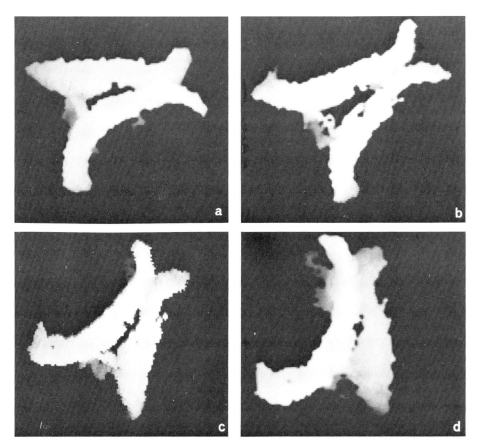

Fig. 15.7. Three-dimensional displays of the detected surface of the ventricular system.

The result, for two consecutive layers in the $96 \times 96 \times 14$ array is shown in Fig. 15.9.

The problem with 1.5 mm-thick slices is that one needs many of them to cover a significant part of the spine. The same patient has been scanned using a sequence of ten contiguous 5 mm-thick slices. From this we have produced another three-dimensional array of numbers, this time representing a $96 \times 96 \times 57$ array of $0.8 \times 0.8 \times 0.8$ mm voxels. Layers approximately corresponding to those in Fig. 15.9 are shown in Fig. 15.10.

Note that there is one significant difference between Fig. 15.9 and 15.10. The CT numbers associated with the bony spicule are lower in Fig. 15.10, so much so that in the right picture of (b) the spicule does not seem to totally separate the spinal chord. This is an illustration of the partial volume effect discussed in Section 3.3. The spicule is too thin to fill the voxels in the 5 mm-thick slices and so the CT values in these slices do not correctly reflect the

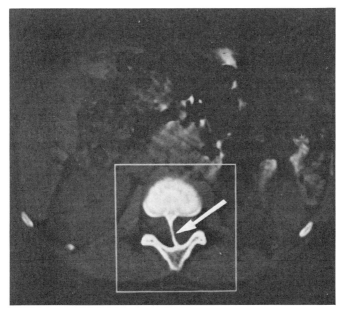

Fig. 15.8. Cross section of a patient with dysraphism. Location of bony spicule indicated by arrow. A 96 × 96 voxel area enclosing the spine is shown.

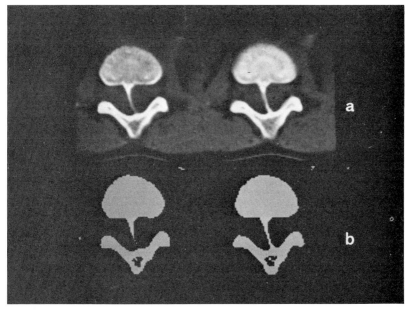

Fig. 15.9. Two consecutive 0.8 mm-thick slices produced from 1.5 mm slices by interpolation. (a) Display corresponding to the 96 × 96 region shown in Fig. 15.8. (b) Pixels with "high" CT numbers are shown bright ("high" selected to include bone).

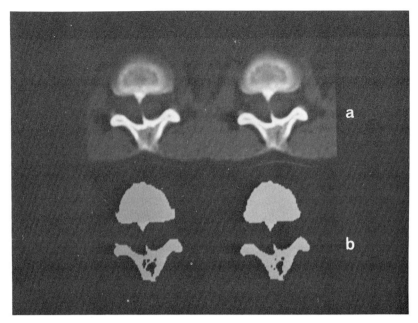

Fig. 15.10. Two consecutive 0.8 mm-thick slices, produced from the 5 mm slices by interpolation. The arrangement matches that of Fig. 15.9. The spicule is not totally reproduced in (b) due to the partial volume effect.

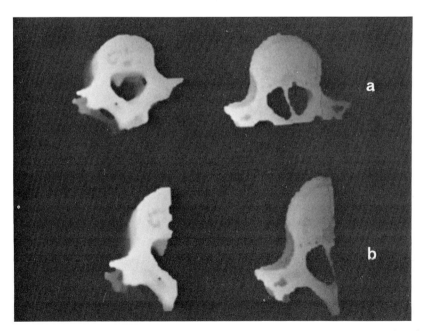

Fig. 15.11. Displays of four detected surfaces of the spine. (a) Using the 96 × 96 work area (whole spine). (b) Using a 48 × 96 work area (half spine). Left: Based on the ten 5 mm slices. Right: Based on the eight 1.5 mm slices.

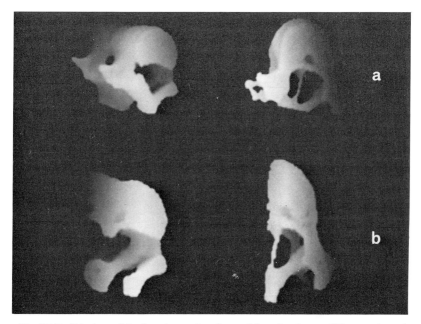

Fig. 15.12. Displays of the four detected surfaces of the spine from a different orientation. The arrangement is the same as in Fig. 15.11.

linear attenuation coefficient of the bony spicule tissue. On the other hand, the 1.5 mm slices, on which Fig. 15.9 is based, are thin enough to provide us with accurate CT values, and so the whole of the spicule is correctly identified.

This is further indicated in Figs. 15.11 and 15.12. In both figures, the displays on the left are based on the ten 5 mm slices and the pictures on the right are based on the eight 1.5 mm-thick slices. In (a) we show displays based on Figs. 15.8–15.10, in which a 96 × 96 pixel frame was used to identify the whole spinal column. In (b) we show displays of half of the spinal column, which have been created by the use of 48 × 96 frames occupying the left half of the original 96 × 96 frames. This way one can simultaneously observe both the inside and the outside structure of the spinal column from different orientations. By the way, Figs. 15.11 and 15.12 are just two stills from a movie which has been made to show the four synchronously rotating aspects of the spine of this patient.

NOTES AND REFERENCES

The phrase "noninvasive vivisection" has been used by Wood (1977) in describing the potential of such techniques for the study of structural and functional dynamics of the heart, lungs and circulation.

A particular method for displaying arbitrary sections through the body based on a sequence of computed tomograms of transverse sections is described by Herman and Liu (1977). That paper also gives references to earlier literature both on sectional display and three-dimensional boundary detection and display, using methods which are in some cases quite different from what has been described in this chapter. An alternative source of information on the literature is the survey by Altschuler *et al.* (1979), which includes such diverse references as Fuchs *et al.* (1977), Glenn *et al.* (1975), Greenleaf *et al.* (1970), Harris *et al.* (1978), Ledley and Park (1977), Liu (1977) and Mazziota and Huang (1976).

The material in the present chapter closely follows Herman (1979c), Artzy and Herman (1978), and Herman and Liu (1979), which may be consulted for relevant earlier references.

Patient data were provided by Dr. W. Kinkel (Dent Neurologic Institute, Millard Filmore Hospital, Buffalo, New York) and Drs. D. C. Hemmny, V. M. Haughton, and A. L. Williams (Medical College of Wisconsin, Milwaukee, Wisconsin).

16

Mathematical Background

Throughout the previous chapters we have repeatedly omitted proofs of mathematical claims, since we did not want such proofs to interfere with the flow of the main argument. In this chapter we fill in some of these gaps, in the order in which they appear in the previous text.

In order to do this in not too excessive space we occasionally have to assume greater mathematical knowledge than what was assumed until now.

16.1 THE DIMENSIONALITY OF THE LINEAR ATTENUATION COEFFICIENT

In Section 2.4 the claim is made that the linear attenuation coefficient has to be measured in units of inverse length; that is, its dimensionality is inverse length (see also Section 7.1). We now justify this claim.

Let $\mu_e(z)$ denote the linear attenuation coefficient at energy e at the point z between the source ($z = z_s \leq 0$) and the detector ($z = z_d \geq D$). Let $p_e(z)$ denote the probability that a photon of energy e which leaves the source in the direction of the detector gets as far as the point z without being removed from the beam. Let $q_e(z, \Delta z)$ denote the probability that a photon of energy e which made it as far as a distance z from the source is removed before it gets to a distance $z + \Delta z$ from the source. As can be easily worked out, the relationship between $p_e(z)$ and $q_e(z, \Delta z)$ is given by

$$p_e(z + \Delta z) = p_e(z) - p_e(z)q_e(z, \Delta z). \tag{1.1}$$

More importantly, we now show that

$$\mu_e(z) = \lim_{\Delta z \to 0} q_e(z, \Delta z)/\Delta z. \tag{1.2}$$

In order to prove (1.2) let us use $v_e(z)$ to denote the right-hand side of the equation. Observe that $v_e(z)$ is a property of the tissue t occupying the point, and so may be written as v_e^t. Thus our aim is to prove that, for any tissue t, $\mu_e^t = v_e^t$.

From (1.1) it follows that

$$\frac{p_e(z + \Delta z) - p_e(z)}{\Delta z} \frac{1}{p_e(z)} = -\frac{q_e(z, \Delta z)}{\Delta z}. \tag{1.3}$$

Taking the limit as $\Delta z \to 0$, we get

$$p_e'(z)/p_e(z) = -v_e(z). \tag{1.4}$$

Integration of both sides from z_s to z_d (source to detector) leads to

$$\ln p_e(z_d) - \ln p_e(z_s) = -\int_{z_s}^{z_d} v_e(z)\, dz. \tag{1.5}$$

Recalling the definition of $p_e(z)$, we see that $p_e(z_s) = 1$ [hence $\ln p_e(z_s) = 0$], and so

$$-\ln p_e(z_d) = \int_{z_s}^{z_d} v_e(z)\, dz. \tag{1.6}$$

Now we show that $v_e(z) = \mu_e(z)$ for whatever tissue t occupies the position z along the line L.

Suppose that the object between the source and detector is a uniform slab of unit thickness of the tissue t and that the line L is perpendicular to the face of the slab (see Fig. 1.21). In this case $\int_{z_s}^{z_d} v_e(z)\, dz = v_e^t$ [since $v_e(z) = 0$ at points not occupied by the slab]. Using (1.6) we see that $v_e^t = -\ln p_e(z_d)$, where $p_e(z_d)$ is the probability that a photon at energy e which approaches the slab along the line L will not get removed from the line before exiting through the other side of the slab. Hence, by the definition of the linear attenuation coefficient $v_e^t = \mu_e^t$.

Since the probability $q_e(z, \Delta z)$ is dimensionless, and Δz is a length, the validity of (1.2) justifies our claim that the linear attenuation coefficient is measured in units of inverse length.

16.2   THE LINE INTEGRAL OF THE RELATIVE LINEAR ATTENUATION

In this section we prove that

$$-\ln \frac{\rho_a}{\rho_c} = \int_0^D \mu_{\bar{e}}(x, y)\, dz, \tag{2.1}$$

where, based on Fig. 2.8, ρ_a is the transmittance along the line L during the monochromatic actual measurement, ρ_c is the transmittance along L during the monochromatic calibration measurement, and the right-hand side of (2.1) is the line integral along L of the relative linear attenuation. Equation (2.1) is exactly (1.5) of Chapter 3. Using (1.4) of Chapter 3, (2.1) also gives rise to (6.1) of Chapter 2.

To prove (2.1), let $\mu_{\bar{e}}^a(z)$ and $\mu_{\bar{e}}^c(z)$ be the linear attenuation coefficients along the line L (see Fig. 2.8) during the actual and calibration measurements, respectively. We know that

$$\mu_{\bar{e}}^a(z) = \mu_{\bar{e}}^c(z), \qquad \text{if} \quad z < 0 \quad \text{or} \quad z > D, \tag{2.2}$$

and

$$\mu_{\bar{e}}(x, y) = \mu_{\bar{e}}^a(z) - \mu_{\bar{e}}^c(z), \qquad \text{if} \quad 0 \leq z \leq D, \tag{2.3}$$

where (x, y) are the coordinates of the point z along the line L. Hence, we get (2.1) from

$$\int_0^D \mu_{\bar{e}}(x, y) \, dz = \int_{z_s}^{z_d} (\mu_{\bar{e}}^a(z) - \mu_{\bar{e}}^c(z)) \, dz$$

$$= -\ln \rho_a + \ln \rho_c, \tag{2.4}$$

where the last step follows from (1.6).

16.3   THE RADON INVERSION FORMULA

The most important single fact for image reconstruction by transform methods is that there exists a closed formula which expresses a function in terms of its Radon transform. In this section we derive such a formula.

In fact there are two different formulations of the Radon inversion formula that appear in the earlier text. One is in (6.2) of Chapter 2 and the other is in (2.2) of Chapter 6. We prove the validity of both of them.

We follow closely Radon's original proof. We do this both because of its historical interest and because it uses only basic calculus. The only objection that can be reasonably raised against it is that the same result can be proved using less restrictive assumptions, but such considerations are beyond the scope of this book.

In this section we assume that the picture function f is continuous and bounded. Recall also that $f(r, \phi) = 0$, if $r \geq E$.

For any point (r, ϕ) in the picture region (in particular, $|r| < E$), we define a function $\bar{F}_{(r, \phi)}$ of one variable by

$$\bar{F}_{(r, \phi)}(q) = \frac{1}{2\pi} \int_0^{2\pi} [\mathcal{R}f](r \cos(\theta - \phi) + q, \theta) \, d\theta. \tag{3.1}$$

Note that, for $q > 0$, the right-hand side of (3.1) is an integral on a circle of radius q around the point (r, ϕ). Since $[\mathscr{R}f](l, \theta) = 0$, if $|l| \geq E$, we have that, for $|r| < E$,

$$\bar{F}_{(r, \phi)}(q) = 0, \qquad \text{if} \quad q \geq 2E. \tag{3.2}$$

Radon proved the following.

$$f(r, \phi) = \frac{1}{\pi} \lim_{\varepsilon \to 0} \left[\frac{1}{\varepsilon} \bar{F}_{(r, \phi)}(\varepsilon) - \int_{\varepsilon}^{\infty} \frac{1}{q^2} \bar{F}_{(r, \phi)}(q) \, dq \right]. \tag{3.3}$$

We are interested in the validity of this result for all (r, ϕ)'s in the picture region. Prior to giving the proof, we show how the formulas used in the previous chapters can be derived from (3.3). For this we have to make an additional assumption, namely that $\mathscr{R}f$ has a continuous first derivative; i.e., that $\mathscr{D}_Y \mathscr{R}f$ exists and is continuous in its first variable [see (2.3) of Chapter 6 for definition of $\mathscr{D}_Y$]. In what follows we make repeated use of (3.2).

$$\int_{\varepsilon}^{\infty} \frac{1}{q^2} \bar{F}_{(r, \phi)}(q) \, dq$$

$$= \int_{\varepsilon}^{2E} \frac{1}{q^2} \left(\frac{1}{2\pi} \int_{0}^{2\pi} [\mathscr{R}f](r \cos(\theta - \phi) + q, \theta) \, d\theta \right) dq$$

$$= \frac{1}{2\pi} \int_{0}^{2\pi} \left(\int_{\varepsilon}^{2E} \frac{1}{q^2} [\mathscr{R}f](r \cos(\theta - \phi) + q, \theta) \, dq \right) d\theta. \tag{3.4}$$

Using integration by parts, we get

$$\int_{\varepsilon}^{2E} \frac{1}{q^2} [\mathscr{R}f](r \cos(\theta - \phi) + q, \theta) \, dq$$

$$= \left[-\frac{1}{q} [\mathscr{R}f](r \cos(\theta - \phi) + q, \theta) \right]_{q = \varepsilon}^{q = 2E}$$

$$- \int_{\varepsilon}^{2E} -\frac{1}{q} [\mathscr{D}_Y \mathscr{R}f](r \cos(\theta - \phi) + q, \theta) \, dq. \tag{3.5}$$

Substituting this into (3.4), we obtain

$$\int_{\varepsilon}^{\infty} \frac{1}{q^2} \bar{F}_{(r, \phi)}(q) \, dq$$

$$= \frac{1}{\varepsilon} \bar{F}_{(r, \phi)}(\varepsilon) + \frac{1}{2\pi} \int_{0}^{2\pi} \int_{\varepsilon}^{2E} \frac{1}{q} \lfloor \mathscr{D}_Y \mathscr{R}f \rfloor (r \cos(\theta - \phi) + q, \theta) \, dq \, d\theta. \tag{3.6}$$

Changing the order of integration in the second term and substituting into (3.3), we get

$$f(r, \phi) = -\frac{1}{2\pi^2} \lim_{\varepsilon \to 0} \int_{\varepsilon}^{\infty} \frac{1}{q} \int_{0}^{2\pi} [\mathscr{D}_Y \mathscr{R}f](r \cos(\theta - \phi) + q, \theta) \, d\theta \, dq, \tag{3.7}$$

which is (6.2) of Chapter 2, but with polar coordinates instead of rectangular coordinates.

Next we derive (2.2) of Chapter 6 from (3.7). First note that, for all ℓ and θ,

$$[\mathscr{D}_Y \mathscr{R} f](\ell, \theta) = -[\mathscr{D}_Y \mathscr{R} f](-\ell, \theta - \pi). \tag{3.8}$$

Using this fact and the change of variables $\theta' = \theta - \pi$ and $q' = -q$, we get

$$\int_\varepsilon^\infty \frac{1}{q} \int_\pi^{2\pi} [\mathscr{D}_Y \mathscr{R} f](r \cos(\theta - \phi) + q, \theta)\, d\theta\, dq$$

$$= \int_{-\varepsilon}^{-\infty} -\frac{1}{q'} \int_0^\pi [\mathscr{D}_Y \mathscr{R} f](-r \cos(\theta' - \phi) - q', \theta' + \pi)\, d\theta'(-dq')$$

$$= \int_{-\infty}^{-\varepsilon} \frac{1}{q} \int_0^\pi [\mathscr{D}_Y \mathscr{R} f](r \cos(\theta - \phi) + q, \theta)\, d\theta\, dq. \tag{3.9}$$

Substituting into (3.7) provides

$$f(r, \phi) = -\frac{1}{2\pi^2} \lim_{\varepsilon \to 0} \left[\int_{-\infty}^{-\varepsilon} \frac{1}{q} \int_0^\pi [\mathscr{D}_Y \mathscr{R} f](r \cos(\theta - \phi) + q, \theta)\, d\theta\, dq \right.$$

$$\left. + \int_\varepsilon^\infty \frac{1}{q} \int_0^\pi [\mathscr{D}_Y \mathscr{R} f](r \cos(\theta - \phi) + q, \theta)\, d\theta\, dq \right]$$

$$= -\frac{1}{2\pi^2} \int_0^\pi \lim_{\varepsilon \to 0} \left[\int_{-\infty}^{-\varepsilon} \frac{1}{q} [\mathscr{D}_Y \mathscr{R} f](r \cos(\theta - \phi) + q, \theta)\, dq \right.$$

$$\left. + \int_\varepsilon^\infty \frac{1}{q} [\mathscr{D}_Y \mathscr{R} f](r \cos(\theta - \phi) + q, \theta)\, dq \right] d\theta, \tag{3.10}$$

where the last step is justified by the assumed continuity of $\mathscr{D}_Y \mathscr{R} f$ in its first variable. The integrand of the outer integral can also be written as an improper integral from $-\infty$ to ∞ (equivalently from $-2E$ to $2E$) which is to be evaluated in its Cauchy principle value sense. By changing the variable, $q = \ell - r \cos(\theta - \phi)$, we get

$$f(r, \phi) = \frac{1}{2\pi^2} \int_0^\pi \int_{-E}^{E} \frac{1}{r \cos(\theta - \phi) - \ell} [\mathscr{D}_Y \mathscr{R} f](\ell, \theta)\, d\ell\, d\theta, \tag{3.11}$$

which is (2.2) of Chapter 6.

All that is left is to prove (3.3). First note that it is sufficient to prove (3.3) for the case $r = 0$ and $\phi = 0$, since its validity in the general case then follows by shifting the origin of the coordinate system. We denote $\bar{F}_{(0,0)}$ by $\bar{F}$, i.e.,

$$\bar{F}(q) = \frac{1}{2\pi} \int_0^{2\pi} [\mathscr{R} f](q, \theta)\, d\theta. \tag{3.12}$$

We also define $\bar{f}$ by

$$\bar{f}(r) = \frac{1}{2\pi} \int_0^{2\pi} f(r, \phi) \, d\phi. \tag{3.13}$$

The following basic relationship between $\bar{F}$ and $\bar{f}$ is essential to our proof. For any $q > 0$,

$$\bar{F}(q) = 2 \int_q^\infty \frac{r\bar{f}(r)}{\sqrt{r^2 - q^2}} \, dr. \tag{3.14}$$

The proof of (3.14) is by the following sequence of steps which makes use of a change of variables $s = \sqrt{r^2 - q^2}$.

$$\bar{F}(q) = \frac{1}{2\pi} \int_0^{2\pi} \int_{-\infty}^\infty f(\sqrt{q^2 + s^2}, \theta + \tan^{-1}(s/q)) \, ds \, d\theta$$

$$= \frac{1}{2\pi} \int_{-\infty}^\infty \int_0^{2\pi} f(\sqrt{q^2 + s^2}, \theta) \, d\theta \, ds$$

$$= 2 \int_0^\infty \bar{f}(\sqrt{q^2 + s^2}) \, ds$$

$$= 2 \int_q^\infty \frac{r}{\sqrt{r^2 - q^2}} \bar{f}(r) \, dr. \tag{3.15}$$

Substituting (3.14) into the right-hand side of (3.3) we get

$$\frac{2}{\pi} \lim_{\varepsilon \to 0} \left[\frac{1}{\varepsilon} \int_\varepsilon^\infty \frac{r\bar{f}(r)}{\sqrt{r^2 - \varepsilon^2}} \, dr - \int_\varepsilon^\infty \frac{1}{q^2} \int_q^\infty \frac{r\bar{f}(r)}{\sqrt{r^2 - q^2}} \, dr \, dq \right]. \tag{3.16}$$

The last double integral simplifies as follows.

$$\int_\varepsilon^\infty \frac{1}{q^2} \int_q^\infty \frac{r\bar{f}(r)}{\sqrt{r^2 - q^2}} \, dr \, dq = \int_\varepsilon^\infty \int_\varepsilon^r \frac{r\bar{f}(r)}{q^2\sqrt{r^2 - q^2}} \, dq \, dr$$

$$= \int_\varepsilon^\infty r\bar{f}(r) \left[-\frac{\sqrt{r^2 - q^2}}{r^2 q} \right]_{q=\varepsilon}^{q=r} \, dr$$

$$= \frac{1}{\varepsilon} \int_\varepsilon^\infty \frac{\sqrt{r^2 - \varepsilon^2}}{r} \bar{f}(r) \, dr. \tag{3.17}$$

Substituting this into (3.16) we get that

$$\frac{2}{\pi} \lim_{\varepsilon \to 0} \left[\varepsilon \int_\varepsilon^\infty \frac{1}{r\sqrt{r^2 - \varepsilon^2}} \bar{f}(r) \, dr \right] \tag{3.18}$$

is equal to the right-hand side of (3.3). To complete our proof we need to show that (3.18) is equal to $f(0, 0)$.

First note that $\bar{f}(r)$ is continuous and $\bar{f}(0) = f(0, 0)$. Hence, for any $\eta > 0$, there exists a $\delta > 0$ such that

$$|\bar{f}(r) - f(0, 0)| < \eta, \qquad \text{if} \quad r \leq \delta. \tag{3.19}$$

Also,

$$\frac{2}{\pi} \lim_{\varepsilon \to 0} \varepsilon \int_{\varepsilon}^{\delta} \frac{1}{r\sqrt{r^2 - \varepsilon^2}} \, dr = \frac{2}{\pi} \lim_{\varepsilon \to 0} \cos^{-1} \frac{\varepsilon}{\delta} = 1. \tag{3.20}$$

Combining (3.19) and (3.20) we get that, for an arbitrary $\eta > 0$,

$$\left| \frac{2}{\pi} \lim_{\varepsilon \to 0} \left[\varepsilon \int_{\varepsilon}^{\infty} \frac{1}{r\sqrt{r^2 - \varepsilon^2}} \bar{f}(r) \, dr \right] - f(0, 0) \right|$$

$$\leq \left| f(0, 0) \left(\frac{2}{\pi} \lim_{\varepsilon \to 0} \left[\varepsilon \int_{\varepsilon}^{\delta} \frac{1}{r\sqrt{r^2 - \varepsilon^2}} \, dr \right] - 1 \right) \right|$$

$$+ \left| \eta \frac{2}{\pi} \lim_{\varepsilon \to 0} \left[\varepsilon \int_{\varepsilon}^{\delta} \frac{1}{r\sqrt{r^2 - \varepsilon^2}} \, dr \right] \right|$$

$$+ \left| \frac{2}{\pi} \lim_{\varepsilon \to 0} \left[\varepsilon \int_{\delta}^{\infty} \frac{\bar{f}(r)}{r\sqrt{r^2 - \varepsilon^2}} \, dr \right] \right|$$

$$\leq \eta. \tag{3.21}$$

This completes the proof of the Radon inversion formula.

16.4   A PICTURE IS NOT UNIQUELY DETERMINED
BY A FINITE NUMBER OF ITS VIEWS

In the previous section it is shown that, if the picture function f is continuous, then it is uniquely determined by its Radon transform $\mathscr{R}f$. In practice we only have available to use estimates of $[\mathscr{R}f](\ell, \theta)$ for a finite number of values of ℓ and θ. In this section we show that the finiteness of the data alone is a source of a fundamental nondeterminacy. We prove the following result.

Let M and K be any positive integers. For $1 \leq k \leq K$, let (r_k, ϕ_k) be arbitrary distinct points in the interior of the picture region and let L_k be arbitrary real numbers. Then there exists a continuous picture function e such that, for $1 \leq k \leq K$,

$$e(r_k, \phi_k) = L_k, \tag{4.1}$$

and, for $0 \leq m \leq M - 1$ and for all ℓ,

$$[\mathscr{R}e](\ell, m\pi/M) = 0. \tag{4.2}$$

The significance of this result is the following. For any continuous picture function f, there exists another continuous picture function, $f + e$, such that f and $f + e$ have the same line integrals for all lines which lie in one of the given M equally spaced directions, and yet f and $f + e$ may differ from each other in an arbitrary fashion at each of an arbitrary large finite set of given points. We first prove this result and then further discuss its practical significance.

As a preliminary result we show the following.

Let M be any positive integer and δ be any real number such that $0 < \delta < E/\sqrt{2}$. ($E\sqrt{2}$ is the side of the square which is the picture region; see Section 6.1.) Let d be the function defined as follows.

$$d(r, \phi) = \begin{cases} \sin(\pi|r|/\delta)\sin(M\phi) & \text{if } 0 \leq r \leq \delta, \\ 0 & \text{if } r > \delta, \\ d(-r, \phi - \pi) & \text{if } r < 0. \end{cases} \tag{4.3}$$

Then, for $0 \leq m < M$ and for all ℓ,

$$[\mathscr{R}d](\ell, m\pi/M) = 0. \tag{4.4}$$

In order to see the validity of this result, recall the definition of the Radon transform, as given by (1.4) of Chapter 6.

First consider the case when $\ell \neq 0$.

$$[\mathscr{R}d](\ell, m\pi/M) = \int_{-\infty}^{\infty} d\left(\sqrt{\ell^2 + z^2}, (m\pi/M) + \tan^{-1}(z/\ell)\right) \, dz$$

$$= \begin{cases} 0 & \text{if } \ell \geq \delta, \\ \int_{-\sqrt{\delta^2 - \ell^2}}^{\sqrt{\delta^2 - \ell^2}} \sin(\pi\sqrt{\ell^2 + z^2}/\delta)\sin(m\pi + M\tan^{-1}(z/\ell)) \, dz \\ \qquad \text{if } 0 < \ell < \delta. \end{cases} \tag{4.5}$$

It is easy to see that in the second case in (4.5), the integrand is an odd function of z (i.e., its value for $-z$ is minus its value for z), and so this integral also is equal to zero.

Finally, if $\ell = 0$, then using (4.3) we get

$$[\mathcal{R}d](0, m\pi/M) = \int_{-\infty}^{\infty} d(z, (m\pi/M) + \tfrac{1}{2}\pi)\,dz \qquad (4.6)$$

$$= \int_{-\delta}^{0} d(-z, (m\pi/M) - \tfrac{1}{2}\pi)\,dz$$

$$+ \int_{0}^{\delta} d(z, (m\pi/M) + \tfrac{1}{2}\pi)\,dz$$

$$= \int_{-\delta}^{0} \sin(\pi|z|/\delta)\sin(m\pi - \tfrac{1}{2}M\pi)\,dz$$

$$+ \int_{0}^{\delta} \sin(\pi|z|/\delta)\sin(m\pi + \tfrac{1}{2}M\pi)\,dz$$

$$= 0. \qquad (4.7)$$

Thus we have proved the validity of (4.4) for $0 \le m \le M$ and for all ℓ.
Now note that d is a continuous picture function and

$$d(\delta/2, \pi/2M) = 1. \qquad (4.8)$$

Furthermore, multiplication by a constant (scaling) and/or translation in the plane does not change the property of d expressed by (4.4). Hence, by choosing δ sufficiently small, we can define a continuous picture function e satisfying (4.1) and (4.2) as a sum of K scaled and translated versions of d.

At first sight, the result we have just proved seems to imply that reconstruction from a finite number of views is a hopeless task. This contradicts the already well-illustrated practical experience of successful reconstructions from a finite number of views.

The resolution of this apparent contradiction between theory and practice comes by investigating the nature of the function d defined by (4.3). We see that, for a large M, it is a highly oscillatory function: on a circle of radius $\delta/2$ it defines a harmonic function of ϕ of frequency $M/2\pi$ (or, equivalently, period $2\pi/M$). If we choose M so large that the objects we are interested in are unlikely to have regions with such oscillatory properties (and even if they do, we do not care to reproduce such fine oscillations), then there is a hope that algorithms may produce from the potential infinity of solutions the one which is similar to the sought after picture. In particular, if we demand that our reconstruction be similar to the original only after both the original and reconstruction have been blurred (say, by repeated applications of a smoothing matrix, see Section 12.3, or preferably by a corresponding continuous operation), addition of a function like d to f would not make any difference, since the blurred versions of f and $f + d$ are likely to be indistinguishable.

Similar arguments apply to other mathematical results showing the impossibility of reconstructing from a finite number of views; see the Notes and References at the end of this chapter.

16.5 ANALYSIS OF THE PHOTON STATISTICS

In this section we derive the unproved mathematical claims made in Section 3.1. regarding the nature of photon statistics.

First we show that the number of photons, which (a) are at a fixed energy $\bar{e}$, (b) reach the detector without having been absorbed or scattered, and (c) are counted by the detector, is a sample of a Poisson random variable with parameter $\lambda\rho\sigma$. (For definitions and notation see Section 3.1.)

The probability that exactly y photons at energy $\bar{e}$ are emitted by the source in one unit of time is

$$P_Y(y) = \exp(-\lambda)\lambda^y/y!. \tag{5.1}$$

[This is exactly (1.1) of Chapter 3.] The probability that one of these photons is counted by the detector without having been absorbed or scattered is $\rho\sigma$. Hence, the probability that x of the y photons are counted by the detector without having been absorbed or scattered is given by [see (2.3) of Chapter 1]

$$p_y(x) = \begin{cases} 0 & \text{if } x < 0 \text{ or } x > y, \\ (y!/(x!(y-x)!))(\rho\sigma)^x(1-\rho\sigma)^{y-x} & \text{if } 0 \le x \le y. \end{cases} \tag{5.2}$$

Hence the combined probability $p_X(x)$ that in one unit of time exactly x photons of energy $\bar{e}$ are counted by the detector without having been absorbed or scattered is

$$p_X(x) = \sum_{y=0}^{\infty} P_Y(y)p_y(x)$$

$$= \sum_{y=x}^{\infty} \exp(-\lambda)\frac{\lambda^y}{y!}\frac{y!}{x!(y-x)!}(\rho\sigma)^x(1-\rho\sigma)^{y-x}$$

$$= \exp(-\lambda)\frac{(\rho\sigma)^x}{x!}\sum_{y=x}^{\infty}\frac{1}{(y-x)!}\lambda^y(1-\rho\sigma)^{(y-x)}$$

$$= \exp(-\lambda)\frac{(\lambda\rho\sigma)^x}{x!}\sum_{t=0}^{\infty}\frac{\lambda^t(1-\rho\sigma)^t}{t!}$$

$$= \exp(-\lambda)\frac{(\lambda\rho\sigma)^x}{x!}\exp(\lambda-\lambda\rho\sigma)$$

$$= \exp(-\lambda\rho\sigma)\frac{(\lambda\rho\sigma)^x}{x!}, \tag{5.3}$$

where we have made use of the infinite expansion of $\exp(z)$ in powers of z. This shows, as required, that x is a sample of the Poisson random variable X with parameter $\lambda\rho\sigma$.

Next we derive (1.6) and (1.7) of Chapter 3. In order to do this we need to discuss the random variable which is the natural logarithm of the Poisson random variable (see Section 1.2). However, there is a basic difficulty here. The number zero is a possible sample of the Poisson variable, and the function ln is undefined for zero. For practical purposes, we usually deal with a Poisson random variable whose parameter λ is very large and, hence, the probability of zero as a sample [namely, $\exp(-\lambda)$] is very small. We may therefore introduce an altered Poisson distribution Z whose outcomes are all positive integers and such that $p_X(x)$ and $p_Z(x)$ are very similar for all positive integers x. A simple way of doing this is to define $p_Z(1) = p_X(0) + p_X(1)$. We refer to such a random variable Z as a *truncated Poisson random variable* with parameter λ. The following holds.

If Z_λ is a truncated random variable with a large parameter λ, and if $Y_\lambda = \ln Z_\lambda$, then

$$\mu_{Y_\lambda} \simeq \ln \lambda - 1/2\lambda, \tag{5.4}$$

and

$$V_{Y_\lambda} \simeq 1/\lambda. \tag{5.5}$$

The precise interpretation of this result is that there are constants c and Λ, such that for all $\lambda > \Lambda$, the absolute value of the differences between the two sides (5.4) and (5.5) are less than c/λ^2. The proof of this result is beyond the scope of this book.

Another result that we make use of is the following. If $X_1, \ldots, X_n$ are independent random variables, then

$$\mu_{X_1 + \cdots + X_n} = \mu_{X_1} + \cdots + \mu_{X_n}, \tag{5.6}$$

and

$$V_{X_1 + \cdots + X_n} = V_{X_1} + \cdots + V_{X_n}. \tag{5.7}$$

This is a standard result in probability theory, whose proof we do not repeat here.

Combining (5.1) of Chapter 2 with the discussion in Section 3.1, we see that the monochromatic ray sum m can be written as

$$m = -\ln \frac{(x_1/x_2)}{(x_3/x_4)} = -\ln x_1 + \ln x_2 + \ln x_3 - \ln x_4, \tag{5.8}$$

where x_1, x_2, x_3, and x_4 are samples from independent Poisson random variables X_1, X_2, X_3, and X_4 with parameters $\lambda_1 = \phi_d \lambda_a \rho_a \sigma_d$, $\lambda_2 = \phi_r \lambda_a \rho_r \sigma_r$, $\lambda_3 = \phi_d \lambda_c \rho_c \sigma_d$, and $\lambda_4 = \phi_r \lambda_c \rho_r \sigma_r$, respectively. Assuming that our photon counts are high enough that we may assume that these random variables are in fact truncated random variables Z_1, Z_2, Z_3, and Z_4, with the corresponding parameters, we find that m is a sample of a random variable M, where

$$M - -\ln Z_1 + \ln Z_2 + \ln Z_3 - \ln Z_4. \tag{5.9}$$

Since the variance of the negative of a random variable is clearly the same as the variance of the random variable ($V_X = V_{-X}$), we get from (5.4)–(5.7) that

$$\mu_M \simeq -\ln \frac{(\lambda_1/\lambda_2)}{(\lambda_3/\lambda_4)} - \frac{1}{2}\left(-\frac{1}{\lambda_1} + \frac{1}{\lambda_2} + \frac{1}{\lambda_3} - \frac{1}{\lambda_4}\right), \tag{5.10}$$

$$V_M \simeq \frac{1}{\lambda_1} + \frac{1}{\lambda_2} + \frac{1}{\lambda_3} + \frac{1}{\lambda_4}. \tag{5.11}$$

Rewriting (1.8) of Chapter 3 as

$$S = \frac{1}{\lambda_1} + \frac{1}{\lambda_2} + \frac{1}{\lambda_3} + \frac{1}{\lambda_4}, \tag{5.12}$$

we get (1.6) and (1.7) of Chapter 3 from (5.10) and (5.11), respectively.

16.6   THE INTEGRAL EXPRESSION FOR POLYCHROMATIC RAY SUMS

In this section we prove (2.1) of Chapter 3.

Assume that in the polychromatic x-ray beam, the number of photons of energy e which leave the source towards the detector during the calibration measurement and the actual measurement is approximately S_e. By (1.6) the number of photons at energy e counted by the detector during the calibration measurement is

$$T_e \simeq S_e \sigma_e \kappa_e \exp\left[-\int_0^D \mu_e^a(z)\, dz\right], \tag{6.1}$$

where σ_e is the detector efficiency at energy e and κ_e is used as the abbreviation

$$\kappa_e = \exp\left[-\int_z^0 \mu_e(z)\, dz\right]\exp\left[-\int_D^{Z_d} \mu_e(z)\, dz\right] \tag{6.2}$$

[for definition of $\mu_e(z)$ see Section 3.2].

Since C_p is the total number of photons (at any energy) detected during the calibration measurement, the detected spectrum during the calibration is

$$\tau_e = T_e/C_p. \tag{6.3}$$

Hence

$$p = -\ln A_p/C_p \simeq -\ln\left\{\left[\int_0^E S_e \sigma_e \kappa_e \exp\left[-\int_0^D \mu_e(z)\,dz\right] de/C_p\right]\right\}$$

$$\simeq -\ln\left\{\left[\int_0^E T_e \exp\left[-\int_0^D (\mu_e(z) - \mu_e^a)\,dz\right] de/C_p\right]\right\}, \quad (6.4)$$

which, in view of (6.3), provides us with (2.1) of Chapter 3.

We now discuss an alternative definition of CT numbers. Rather than using the relative linear attenuation at a fixed energy, one could use a weighted average of the relative linear attenuation over all energies, where the weighting is determined by the detected spectrum during calibration. This weighted average is defined precisely by

$$\mu(x, y) = \int_0^E \tau_e \mu_e(x, y)\,de. \quad (6.5)$$

This definition is motivated by CT scanners with a fixed length water bath. In such a situation the polychromatic ray sum provides a good approximation of the integral of $\mu(x, y)$ without any correction, and so one can use the polychromatic projection data in Radon's inversion formula to estimate $\mu(x, y)$.

However, in the same situation the function $\mu(x, y)$ is just about identical to the function $\mu_{\bar{e}}(x, y)$, provided $\bar{e}$ is what is called the *effective energy* of the spectrum τ_e for the reference material (in this case water) and is defined to be the energy $\bar{e}$ for which

$$\mu_{\bar{e}}^a = \int_0^E \tau_e \mu_e^a\,de. \quad (6.6)$$

Thus the function $\mu(x, y)$ of (6.5) is replaceable by the relative linear attenuation at the effective energy $\bar{e}$, bringing us back to our definition of a CT number.

16.7   PROOF OF THE REGULARIZATION THEOREM

In this section we prove the regularization theorem stated in Section 8.1. We first need to define what it means for a function ϕ to be reasonable at a point v.

A function ϕ is said to be *reasonable at a point v* if the following conditions are satisfied:

$$\phi(u) = 0 \qquad \text{if} \quad |u| \geq E, \quad (7.1)$$

$$\int_{-E}^E \phi(u)\,du \text{ exists}, \quad (7.2)$$

$$\lim_{\varepsilon \to 0} \int_\varepsilon^\infty \frac{|\phi(v - t) - \phi(v + t)|}{t}\,dt \text{ exists}. \quad (7.3)$$

(Here, and in the rest of this section all integrals can be interpreted as Riemann integrals.)

We first show that if ϕ is reasonable at the point v, then $[\mathscr{H}\phi](v)$, as defined by (1.7) of Chapter 8, exists.

$$
\begin{aligned}
[\mathscr{H}\phi](v) &= -\frac{1}{\pi}\lim_{\varepsilon\to 0}\left\{\int_{-\infty}^{v-\varepsilon}\frac{\phi(u)}{v-u}\,du + \int_{v+\varepsilon}^{\infty}\frac{\phi(u)}{v-u}\,du\right\} \\
&= -\frac{1}{\pi}\lim_{\varepsilon\to 0}\int_{\varepsilon}^{\infty}\frac{\phi(v-t)-\phi(v+t)}{t}\,dt,
\end{aligned}
\tag{7.4}
$$

which exists in view of (7.3). The last line in (7.4) is obtained by changes of variable $u = v - t$ and $u = v + t$, respectively, in the two integrals in the previous line.

It is an easily derivable consequence of what is known in analysis as the *Riemann–Lebesgue lemma for absolutely integrable functions* that

$$
\lim_{B\to\infty}\int_{-\infty}^{\infty}\phi(v-t)\frac{1-\cos 2\pi Bt}{t}\,dt = \int_{0}^{\infty}\frac{\phi(v-t)-\phi(v+t)}{t}\,dt,
\tag{7.5}
$$

which, combined with (7.4), gives us an alternative expression for $[\mathscr{H}\phi](v)$. We work on this further, to obtain an expression for $[\mathscr{H}\phi](v)$ which is particularly useful for proving the regularization theorem.

Let G_v be the function defined by

$$
G_v(U) = -2\int_{-\infty}^{\infty}\phi(u)\sin(2\pi(v-u)U)\,du.
\tag{7.6}
$$

Using (7.1) and (7.2) we get that, for any $B > 0$,

$$
\begin{aligned}
\int_{0}^{B}G_v(U)\,dU &= -2\int_{0}^{B}\left(\int_{-E}^{E}\phi(u)\sin(2\pi(v-u)U)\,du\right)dU \\
&= -2\int_{-E}^{E}\phi(u)\left(\int_{0}^{B}\sin(2\pi(v-u)U)\,dU\right)du \\
&= -\frac{1}{\pi}\int_{-\infty}^{\infty}\phi(u)\frac{1-\cos 2\pi B(v-u)}{(v-u)}\,du \\
&= -\frac{1}{\pi}\int_{-\infty}^{\infty}\phi(v-t)\frac{1-\cos 2\pi Bt}{t}\,dt,
\end{aligned}
\tag{7.7}
$$

where the last step is obtained by the change of variable $u - v - t$.

So, by (7.5), the limit as $B \to \infty$ of the left-hand side of (7.7) exists, and using (7.4) we get

$$
\int_{0}^{\infty}G_v(U)\,dU = [\mathscr{H}\phi](v).
\tag{7.8}
$$

The right-hand side of (7.8) is the same as the right-hand side of (1.9) of Chapter 8. What we now have to prove is that the left-hand sides are also equal. A step in this direction is the following. [We use (1.10) of Chapter 8.]

$$
\begin{aligned}
[\phi * \rho_A](v) &= \int_{-\infty}^{\infty} \rho_A(v - u)\phi(u)\,du \\
&= \int_{-E}^{E}\left[-2\int_0^{A/2} F_A(U)\sin(2\pi U(v - u))\,dU\right]\phi(u)\,du \\
&= \int_0^{A/2} F_A(U)\left[-2\int_{-\infty}^{\infty}\phi(u)\sin(2\pi(v - u)U)\,du\right]\,dU \\
&= \int_0^{A/2} F_A(U)G_v(U)\,dU.
\end{aligned}
\tag{7.9}
$$

What we have to show is that the right-hand side of (7.9) tends to the left-hand side of (7.8) as $A \to \infty$, i.e., that

$$
\lim_{A \to \infty} \psi_A(v) = 0,
\tag{7.10}
$$

where

$$
\begin{aligned}
\psi_A(v) &= \int_0^{\infty} G_v(U)\,dU - \int_0^{A/2} F_A(u)G_v(U)\,dU \\
&= \int_0^{A/2}[1 - F_A(U)]G_v(U)\,dU + \int_{A/2}^{\infty} G_v(U)\,dU.
\end{aligned}
\tag{7.11}
$$

Let ε be an arbitrary but fixed positive real number. There exists a real number $N(\varepsilon)$ such that, for any $C \geq N(\varepsilon)$,

$$
\int_C^{\infty} G_v(U)\,dU \leq \varepsilon.
\tag{7.12}
$$

Let $A > 2N(\varepsilon)$.

$$
\begin{aligned}
\psi_A(v) &= \int_0^{N(\varepsilon)}[1 - F_A(U)]G_v(U)\,dU + \int_{N(\varepsilon)}^{A/2}[1 - F_A(U)]G_v(U)\,dU \\
&\quad + \int_{A/2}^{\infty} G_v(U)\,dU.
\end{aligned}
\tag{7.13}
$$

By the statement of the regularization theorem, $0 \leq F_A(U) \leq 1$ and $F_A(U)$ is monotonically nonincreasing. It follows that $0 \leq [1 - F_A(U)] \leq 1$ and $1 - F_A(U)$ is monotonically nondecreasing. Furthermore $G_v(U)$ is continuous. Hence we can apply the second mean value theorem for Riemann integrals and obtain

$$\int_0^{N(\varepsilon)} [1 - F_A(U)]G_v(U)\, dU = [1 - F_A(N(\varepsilon))] \int_a^{N(\varepsilon)} G_v(U)\, dU, \quad (7.14)$$

for some a, $0 \le a \le N(\varepsilon)$, and

$$\int_{N(\varepsilon)}^{A/2} [1 - F_A(U)]G_v(U)\, dU = [1 - F_A(A/2)] \int_b^{A/2} G_v(U)\, dU, \quad (7.15)$$

for some b, $N(\varepsilon) \le b \le A/2$.

From (7.13), (7.14), and (7.15) we get

$$|\psi_A(v)| \le [1 - F_A(N(\varepsilon))] \left| \int_a^{N(\varepsilon)} G_v(U)\, dU \right|$$

$$+ [1 - F_A(A/2)] \left| \int_b^{A/2} G_v(U)\, dU \right|$$

$$+ \left| \int_{A/2}^{\infty} G_v(U)\, dU \right|$$

$$\le [1 - F_A(N(\varepsilon))] \left| \int_a^{N(\varepsilon)} G_v(U)\, dU \right| + 3\varepsilon \quad (7.16)$$

[recall (7.12)].

Note that $N(\varepsilon)$ does *not* depend on A. Hence $\int_a^{N(\varepsilon)} G_v(U)\, dU$ does not depend on A. According to the conditions of the regularization theorem $\lim_{A \to \infty} F_A(N(\varepsilon)) = 1$, and so the first term on the right-hand side of (7.16) converges to zero as A tends to infinity. Since ε was arbitrary, (7.10) holds and the proof of the regularization theorem is complete.

16.8   CONVERGENCE OF THE RELAXATION METHOD FOR INEQUALITIES

In this section we prove that the algorithm described in Chapter 11 by (2.4), (2.5), and (2.6) converges to an element of N, defined by (2.2) and (2.3) of Chapter 11.

Following Chapter 11, we assume that, for $1 \le i \le P$, $\|n_i\| \ne 0$. The notation of Section 11.2 is adopted without further reiteration.

Let k be a nonnegative integer such that $x^{(k)} \notin N_{i_k}$. Then

$$\|x^{(k+1)} - x^{(k)}\|^2 = \left\| \lambda^{(k)} \frac{q_{i_k} - \langle n_{i_k}, x^{(k)} \rangle}{\|n_{i_k}\|^2} n_{i_k} \right\|^2$$

$$= (\lambda^{(k)})^2 \frac{(q_{i_k} - \langle n_{i_k}, x^{(k)} \rangle)^2}{\|n_{i_k}\|^2}. \quad (8.1)$$

Let z be any vector in N. Using the positivity of $\lambda^{(k)}$ and the facts that $\langle n_{i_k}, z \rangle \le q_{i_k}$ and $\langle n_{i_k}, x^{(k)} \rangle > q_{i_k}$, we get that

$$-\lambda^{(k)} \frac{q_{i_k} - \langle n_{i_k}, x^{(k)} \rangle}{\|n_{i_k}\|^2} \langle n_{i_k}, z \rangle \le -\lambda^{(k)} \frac{q_{i_k} - \langle n_{i_k}, x^{(k)} \rangle}{\|n_{i_k}\|^2} q_{i_k}. \tag{8.2}$$

Combining the last two equations provides

$$\langle x^{(k+1)} - x^{(k)}, x^{(k)} - z \rangle = \lambda^{(k)} \frac{q_{i_k} - \langle n_{i_k}, x^{(k)} \rangle}{\|n_{i_k}\|^2} \langle n_{i_k}, x^{(k)} - z \rangle$$

$$\le \lambda^{(k)} \frac{q_{i_k} - \langle n_{i_k}, x^{(k)} \rangle}{\|n_{i_k}\|^2} (\langle n_{i_k}, x^{(k)} \rangle - q_{i_k})$$

$$= -\lambda^{(k)} \frac{(q_{i_k} - \langle n_{i_k}, x^{(k)} \rangle)^2}{\|n_{i_k}\|^2}$$

$$= -\frac{1}{\lambda^{(k)}} \|x^{(k+1)} - x^{(k)}\|^2. \tag{8.3}$$

From this we obtain that

$$\|x^{(k+1)} - z\|^2 = \|x^{(k+1)} - x^{(k)} + x^{(k)} - z\|^2$$
$$= \|x^{(k+1)} - x^{(k)}\|^2 + 2\langle x^{(k+1)} - x^{(k)}, x^{(k)} - z \rangle + \|x^{(k)} - z\|^2$$
$$\le (1 - (2/\lambda^{(k)}))\|x^{(k+1)} - x^{(k)}\|^2 + \|x^{(k)} - z\|^2. \tag{8.4}$$

Hence,

$$\|x^{(k+1)} - z\|^2 + ((2/\lambda^{(k)}) - 1)\|x^{(k+1)} - x^{(k)}\|^2 \le \|x^k - z\|^2. \tag{8.5}$$

We proved (8.5) under the assumption $x^{(k)} \notin N_{i_k}$. However, if $x^{(k)} \in N_{i_k}$, then $x^{(k+1)} = x^{(k)}$ and (8.5) is trivially satisfied.

From (2.6) of Chapter 11 we obtain that

$$\left(\frac{2}{\lambda^{(k)}} - 1\right) \ge \left(\frac{2}{\varepsilon_2} - 1\right) = \frac{2 - \varepsilon_2}{\varepsilon_2} > 0, \tag{8.6}$$

and so the sequence $\|x^{(k)} - z\|^2$, for $k = 0, 1, 2, \ldots$, is never increasing. Since it is bounded below, $\lim_{k \to \infty} (\|x^{(k)} - z\|^2)$ exists. Hence (8.5) and (8.6) imply that

$$\lim_{k \to \infty} \|x^{(k+1)} - x^{(k)}\|^2 = 0. \tag{8.7}$$

We also obtain that the sequence $x^{(0)}, x^{(1)}, x^{(2)}, \ldots$, is bounded.

Since the sequence $x^{(0)}, x^{(1)}, x^{(2)}, \ldots$, is bounded, there is at least one infinite subsequence which converges to some vector, y, say. We will show that y is in N and that y is independent of the subsequence which is used in its construction. This will complete the proof.

Consider an infinite subsequence of $x^{(0)}, x^{(1)}, x^{(2)}, \ldots$, which converges to a vector y. Let i be any integer, $1 \le i \le P$. We now show that $y \in N_i$, by proving that, for any $\varepsilon > 0$,

$$\langle n_i, y \rangle - q_i < \varepsilon. \tag{8.8}$$

Let

$$f = \min(1, \varepsilon_1)/\|n_i\| \tag{8.9}$$

For any $\varepsilon > 0$, there is an element $x^{(t)}$, say, in the infinite subsequence of $x^{(0)}, x^{(1)}, x^{(2)}, \ldots$, which converges to y, such that

$$\|y - x^{(t)}\| < (f/2P)\varepsilon. \tag{8.10}$$

Because of (8.7), this element $x^{(t)}$ can be chosen so that

$$\|x^{(s+1)} - x^{(s)}\| < (f/2P)\varepsilon,$$

for all $s \ge t$. There exists an s such that $t \le s < t + P$ and $i = i_s$. For this s,

$$\|y - x^{(s)}\| < P \frac{f}{2P} \varepsilon \le \frac{1}{2\|n_i\|} \varepsilon. \tag{8.11}$$

If $x^{(s)} \notin N_i$, then by (8.1)

$$\langle n_i, x^{(s)} \rangle - q_i = \frac{\|n_i\|}{\lambda^{(s)}} \|x^{(s+1)} - x^{(s)}\| < \frac{\|n_i\|}{\lambda^{(s)}} \frac{f}{2P} \varepsilon$$

$$\le \frac{\|n_i\|}{\lambda^{(s)}} \frac{\varepsilon_1}{\|n_i\|} \frac{\varepsilon}{2P} \le \frac{1}{2} \varepsilon. \tag{8.12}$$

If $x^{(s)} \in N_i$, then (8.12) is trivially true. Using (8.11) and (8.12), we get

$$\begin{aligned}
\langle n_i, y \rangle - q_i &= \langle n_i, y - x^{(s)} + x^{(s)} \rangle - q_i \\
&= \langle n_i, x^{(s)} \rangle - q_i + \langle n_i, y - x^{(s)} \rangle \\
&\le \tfrac{1}{2}\varepsilon + \|n_i\| \|y - x^{(s)}\| < \varepsilon,
\end{aligned} \tag{8.13}$$

proving (8.8). Since $y \in N_i$ for an arbitrary i, $1 \le i \le P$, we get that $y \in N$.

Suppose there exists another subsequence which converges to y^1. As above, we can show that $y^1 \in N$. Recalling that, for any $z \in N$,

$$\lim_{k \to \infty} (\|x^{(k)} - z\|^2)$$

exists, let

$$\alpha = \lim_{k \to \infty} (\|x^{(k)} - y\|^2 - \|x^{(k)} - y^1\|^2). \tag{8.14}$$

Using the subsequence which converges to y we get

$$\alpha = -\|y - y^1\|^2, \tag{8.15}$$

and using the other subsequence we get

$$\alpha = \|y^1 - y\|^2. \qquad (8.16)$$

Hence $\alpha = 0$ and $y = y^1$, completing our proof.

NOTES AND REFERENCES

Sections 16.1 and 16.2 are based on Herman (1979a).

Section 16.3 follows Radon (1917) very closely. The continuity of f is not necessary for the existence of the inverse Radon transforms. Inversion formulas and proofs exist for many large classes of functions; see, for example, Ludwig (1966), Smith *et al.* (1977), and Tuy (1979). Also, inversion of the Radon transform is possible (at least in principle) if the Radon transform is known only in parts of its domain, see, for example, Ein-Gal (1974), Nalciouglu *et al.* (1979), Lewitt (1979), Tuy (1979), and the references in those papers.

A much stronger version of the result in Section 16.4 exists. See, e.g., Theorem 4.3 of Smith *et al.* (1977). They summarize this result by saying "a finite set of radiographs tells us nothing at all." However, this is a somewhat extreme rephrasing of the precise mathematical statement. In particular, just assuming that all picture functions are bounded by the same value (a blatantly reasonable assumption in CT), allows one to give error estimates of the convolution method which are picture independent and converge to zero as the finite number of views increases; see, e.g., Davison and Grunbaum (1979). Resolution of such apparent contradictions can be given along the lines suggested at the end of Section 16.4. See also Katz (1978).

The mean and variance of the natural logarithm of a truncated Poisson distribution with a large parameter λ can be estimated by standard techniques of probability theory, as described, e.g., by Parzen (1960). A discussion in the framework of CT is given in Appendix B of Barrett *et al.* (1976), who provide some earlier references. The result expressed in (5.6) and (5.7) can be found, e.g., in Parzen (1960), as (4.4) in his Chapter 9.

Section 16.6 is based on Herman (1979a).

The results of mathematical analysis used in Section 16.7 can be found, for example, in Apostol (1957). The proof of the regularization theorem follows that given by Chang and Herman (1978).

The convergence of the relaxation methods for inequalities (under the general conditions stated in Section 11.2) follows from the results of Gubin *et al.* (1967). Our proof follows Herman, Lent, and Lutz (1975), which gives some additional relevant references.

For up-to-date information (at the time of writing) on mathematical matters related to CT, the reader should consult the proceedings of the conference on "Mathematical Aspects of Computerized Tomography," which was held at Oberwolfach, Germany, in February, 1980. The proceedings are edited by G. T. Herman and F. Natterer and are to be published by Springer Verlag. That book contains, in particular, an article by G. T. Herman and D. Webster entitled, "Surfaces of Organs in Discrete Three-Dimensional Space," which updates and puts on a rigorous mathematical foundation the contents of Chapter 15.

Another relevant recent mathematical development is the work of P. P. B. Eggermont, G. T. Herman, and A. Lent, who have published a single theorem (and proof) from which the convergence of rather different looking iterative procedures in Chapters 11, 12, and 14 all follow as straightforward corollaries. ("Iterative Algorithms for Large Partitioned Linear Systems, with Applications to Image Reconstruction," Technical Report No. MIPG40, Medical Image Processing Group, Department of Computer Science, State University of New York at Buffalo, Amherst, New York.)

References

Altschuler, M. D. (1979). Reconstruction of the global-scale three-dimensional solar corona. *In* "Image Reconstruction Implementation and Applications" (G. T. Herman, ed.), pp. 105-145. Springer Verlag, Berlin and New York.

Altschuler, M. D., and Perry, R. M. (1972). On determining the electron density distributions of the solar corona from K-coronameter data. *Sol. Phys.* **23**, 410-428.

Altschuler, M. D., and Herman, G. T. (1977). Fully-three-dimensional image reconstruction using series expansion methods. *In* "A Review of Information Processing in Medical Imaging" (A. B. Brill, *et al.*, eds.), pp. 124-142. Oak Ridge National Laboratory, Oak Ridge, Tennessee.

Altschuler, M. D., Censor, Y., Herman, G. T., Lent, A., Lewitt, R. M., Srihari, S., Tuy, H., and Udupa, J. (1979). Mathematical aspects of image reconstruction from projections. Tech. Rept. MIPG36, Medical Image Processing Group, Dept. of Computer Science, State University of New York at Buffalo, Amherst, New York.

Altschuler, M. D., Chang, T., and Chu, A. (1979). Rapid computer generation of three-dimensional phantoms and their cone-beam projections. *Proc. Soc. Photo-Opt. Instrum. Eng.* **173**, 287-290.

Altschuler, M. D., Censor, Y., Eggermont, P. P. B., Herman, G. T., Kuo, Y. H., Lewitt, R. M., McKay, M., Tuy, H., Udupa, J., Yau, M. M. (1980). Demonstration of a software package for the reconstruction of the dynamically changing structure of the human heart from cone-beam x-ray projections. *Proceedings of the Hawaii International Conference on System Sciences, 13th, Honolulu, Hawaii, 1980.*

Andrews, H. C., and Hunt, B. R. (1977). "Digital Image Restoration." Prentice-Hall, Englewood Cliffs, New Jersey.

Apostol, T. M. (1957). "Mathematical Analysis." Addison-Wesley, Reading, Massachusetts.

Artzy, E., and Herman, G. T. (1978). Boundary detection in three dimensions with a medical application. Tech. Rept. MIPG9, Medical Image Processing Group, Dept. of Computer Science, State University of New York at Buffalo, Amherst, New York.

Artzy, E. Elfving, T., and Herman, G. T. (1979). Quadratic optimization for image reconstruction II. *Comput. Graphics Image Processing.* **11**, 242-261.

Barrett, H. H., Gordon, S. K., and Hershel, R. S. (1976). Statistical limitations in transaxial tomography. *Comput. Biol. Med.* **6**, 307-323.

Barton, J. P. (1978). Feasibility of neutron radiography for large bundles of fast reactor fuel. Tech. Rept. IRT 6247-004, Instrumentation Research Technology Corporation, San Diego, California.

Bracewell, R. N. (1956). Strip integration in radio astronomy. *Aust. J. Phys.* **9**, 198–217.

Bracewell, R. N. (1977). Correction for collimator width (restoration) in reconstructive x-ray tomography. *J. Comput. Assisted Tomography* **1**, 6–15.

Bracewell, R. N. (1978). "The Fourier Transform and its Applications." 2nd ed, McGraw-Hill, New York.

Bracewell, R. N. (1979). Image reconstruction in radio astronomy. *In* "Image Reconstruction from Projections: Implementation and Applications (G. T. Herman, ed.), pp. 81–104. Springer-Verlag, Berlin and New York.

Bracewell, R. N., and Riddle, A. C. (1967). Inversion of fanbeam scans in radio astronomy. *Astrophys. J.* **150**, 427–434.

Bracewell, R. N., and Wernecke, S. J. (1975). Image reconstruction over a finite field of view. *J. Opt. Soc. Am.* **65**, 1342–1346.

Brigham, E. O. (1974). "The Fast Fourier Transform." Prentice-Hall, Englewood Cliffs, New Jersey.

Brooks, R. A., and DiChiro, G. (1976). Principles of computer assisted tomography (CAT) in radiographic and radioisotopic imaging. *Phys. Med. Biol.* **21**, 689–732.

Brooks, R. A., and Weiss, G. H. (1976). Interpolation problems in image reconstruction. *Proc. Soc. Photo-Opt. Instrum. Eng.* **96**, 313–319.

Budinger, T. F. (1960). Iceberg detection by radar. *In* "International Ice Observation and Ice Patrol Service in the North Atlantic," Coast Guard Bulletin No. 45, pp. 49–97. United States Government Printing Office, Washington, D.C.

Budinger, T. F., and Gullberg, G. T. (1975). Reconstruction by two-dimensional filtering of simple superposition of transverse section image. "Technical Digest: Image Processing for 2-D and 3-D Reconstruction from Projections: Theory and Practice in Medicine and Physical Sciences." Available from the Optical Society of America, Washington, D.C.

Budinger, T. F., Gullberg, G. T., and Huesman, R. H. (1979). Emission computed tomography, *In* "Image Reconstruction from Projections: Implementation and Applications" (G. T. Herman, ed.), pp. 147–246. Springer-Verlag, Berlin and New York.

Budinger, T. F., Yano, Y., Derenzo, S. E., Huesman, R. H., Cahoon, J. G., Moyer, B. R. Greenberg, W. L., and O'Brien, Jr., H. A. (1979). Myocardial uptake of Rubidium-82 using positron emission tomography. *J. Nucl. Med.* **20**, 603.

Butzer, P. L., and Nessel, R. J. (1971). "Fourier Analysis and Approximation," Vol. 1. Academic Press, New York.

Censor, Y., and Herman, G. T. (1979). Row-generation methods for feasibility and optimization problems involving sparse matrices and their applications. *In* "Sparse Matrix Proceedings 1978" (I. S. Duff and G. W. Stewart, eds.), pp. 197–219. SIAM, Philadelphia, Pennsylvania.

Chang, T. (1979). Attenuation correction and incomplete projection in single photon emission computed tomography. *IEEE Trans. Nucl. Sci.* **NS-26**, 2780–2789.

Chang, T., and Herman, G. T. (1978). Filter selection for the fan beam convolution algorithm. Tech. Rept. No. MIPG6, Medical Image Processing Group, Department of Computer Science, State University of New York at Buffalo, Amherst, New York.

Chen, A. C. M., Berninger, W. H., Redington, R. W., Godbarsen, R., and Barrett, P. (1976). Five-second fan beam CT scanner. *Proc. of Soc. Photo-Opt. Instrum. Eng.* **96**, 294–298.

Chesler, D. A., and Riederer, S. J. (1975). Ripple suppression during reconstruction in transverse tomography. *Phys Med. Biol.* **20**, 632–636.

Christensen, E. E., Curry, T. S., III, and Nunnally, J. (1973). "An Introduction to the Physics of Diagnostic Radiology." Lea and Febiger, Philadelphia, Pennsylvania.

Colsher, J. G. (1977). Iterative 3-D image reconstruction from tomographic projections. *Comput. Graphics Image Processing* **6**, 513–537.

Cormack, A. M. (1963). Representation of a function by its line integrals, with some radiological applications. *J. Appl. Phys.* **34**, 2722–2727.

Courant, R., and Hilbert, D. (1953). "Methods of Mathematical Physics," Vol. I, Wiley (Interscience), New York.

Crowther, R. A., DeRosier, D. J., and Klug, A. (1970). The reconstruction of a three-dimensional structure from projections and its application to electron microscopy. *Proc. R. Soc. London,* **A317**, 319–340.

Davis, P. J., and Rabinowitz, P. (1967). "Numerical Integration." Ginn (Blaisdell), Boston, Massachusetts.

Davison, E., and Grunbaum, F. A. (1979). Convolution algorithms for arbitrary projection angles. *IEEE Trans. Nucl. Sci.* **NS-26**, 2670–2673.

Denton, R. V., Friedlander, B., and Rockmore, A. J. (1979). Direct three-dimensional image reconstruction from divergent rays. *IEEE Trans. Nucl. Sci.* **NS-26**, 4695–4703.

Dreike, P., and Boyd, D. P. (1976). Convolution reconstruction of fan beam projections. *Comput. Graphics Image Processing* **5**, 459–469.

Edelheit, L. S., Herman, G. T., and Lakshminarayanan, A. V. (1977). Reconstruction of objects from diverging x-rays. *Med. Phys.* **4**, 226–231.

Ein-Gal, M. (1974). The shadow transform: an approach to cross-sectional imaging. Tech. Rept. No. 6851–1, Center for Systems Research, Stanford University, Stanford, California.

Elfving, T. (1978). A method for computing the maximum entropy solution of a linear system. Tech. Rept. LiTh-MAT-R-1978-4, Dept. of Mathematics, Linkoping University, Linkoping, Sweden.

Evans, R. D. (1955). "The Atomic Nucleus." McGraw–Hill, New York.

Fuchs, H., Kedem, Z. M., and Uselton, S. P. (1977). Optimal surface reconstruction from planar contours. *Commun. A.C.M.* **20**, 693–702.

Gilbert, B. K., Chu, A., Atkins, D. E., Schwarzlander, E. E., and Ritman, E. L. (1979). Ultra high speed transaxial image reconstruction of the heart, lung and circulation via numerical approximation methods and optimized processor architecture. *Comput. Biomed. Res.* **12**, 17–38.

Gilbert, P. (1972). Iterative methods for the three-dimensional reconstruction of an object from projections. *J. Theor. Biol.* **36**, 105–117.

Glenn, W. V., Johnston, R. J., Morton, P. E., and Dwyer, S. J. (1975). Image generation and display techniques for CT scan data. *Invest. Radiol.* **10**, 403–416.

Glover, G., and Pelc, N. (1979). The nonlinear partial volume artifact. *J. Comput. Assisted Tomography* **3**, 573–574.

Gordon, R. (1974). A tutorial on ART (Algebraic Reconstruction Techniques). *IEEE Trans. Nucl. Sci.* **NS-21**, 78–93.

Gordon, R., and Herman, G. T. (1974). Three-dimensional reconstruction from projections: a review of algorithms. *In* "International Review of Cytology," Vol. 38 (G. H. Bourne and J. F. Danielli, eds.), pp. 111–151. Academic Press, New York.

Gordon, R., Bender, R., and Herman, G. T. (1970). Algebraic Reconstruction Techniques (ART) for three-dimensional electron microscopy and x-ray photography. *J. Theor. Biol.* **29**, 471–481.

Greenleaf, J. F., Tu, J. S. and Wood, E. H. (1970). Computer generated three-dimensional oscilloscopic images and associated techniques for display and study of the spatial distribution of pulmonary blood flow. *IEEE Trans. Nucl. Sci.* **NS-17**, 353–359.

Gubin, L. G., Polyak, B. T., and Raik, E. V. (1967). The method of projections for finding a common point of convex sets. *USSR Comput. Math. Math. Phys.* **7**, 1–24.

Gullberg, G. T. (1977). Fan beam and parallel beam projection and back-projection operators. Tech. Rept. LBL-5604, Lawrence Berkeley Laboratory, University of California, Berkeley, California.

Gullberg, G. T. (1979). The reconstruction of fan-beam data by filtering back-projection. *Comput. Graphics Image Processing* **10**, 30–47.

Halmos, P. R. (1958). "Finite Dimensional Vector Spaces," 2nd ed. Van Nostrand–Reinhold, Princeton, New Jersey.

Hamaker, C., and Solmon, D. C. (1978). The angles between the null spaces of x-rays. *J. Math. Anal. Appl.* **62**, 1–23.

Hanson, K. M. (1979). Proton Computed tomography. *In* "Computer Aided Tomography and Ultrasonics in Medicine" (J. Raviv, J. F. Greenleaf, and G. T. Herman, eds.), pp. 97–106. North-Holland Publ. Amsterdam.

Harris, L. D., Robb, R. A., Johnson, S. A., and Khalafalla, S. (1978). Stereo display of computed tomographic data. *In* "Challenges and Prospects for Advanced Medical Systems" (H. E. Emlet, Jr., ed.), pp. 127–135. Miami Symposia Specialists, Inc., Miami, Florida.

Herman, G. T. (1972). Two direct methods for reconstructing pictures from their projections: a comparative study. *Comput. Graphics Image Processing* **1**, 123–144.

Herman, G. T. (1973). Reconstruction of binary patterns from a few projections. *In* "International Computing Symposium 1973" (A. Gunther, B. Levrat, and H. Lipps, eds.), pp. 371–379. North-Holland Publ. Amsterdam.

Herman, G. T. (1975). A relaxation method for reconstructing objects from noisy x-rays. *Math. Programming* **8**, 1–19.

Herman, G. T. (1978). An introduction to some basic mathematical concepts in computed tomography. *In* "Roentgen-Video Techniques for Dynamic Studies of Structure and Function of the Heart and Circulation" (P. H. Heintzen and T. M. Bursch, eds.), pp. 253–260. Thieme, Stuttgart.

Herman, G. T. (1979a). Correction for beam hardening in computed tomography. *Phys. Med. Biol.* **24**, 81–106.

Herman, G. T. (1979b). Demonstration of beam hardening correction in computerized reconstruction of head cross-section. *J. Comput. Assisted Tomography*, **3**, 373–378.

Herman, G. T., ed. (1979c). "Image Reconstruction from Projections: Implementation and Applications". Springer-Verlag, Berlin and New York.

Herman, G. T. (1979d). On modifications to the algebraic reconstruction techniques. *Comput. Biol. and Med.* **9**, 271–276.

Herman, G. T. (1979e). Representation of 3-D surfaces by a large number of simple surface elements. Tech. Rept. MIPG26, Medical Image Processing Group, Dept. of Computer Science, State University of New York at Buffalo, Amherst, New York.

Herman, G. T. (1980). Principles of reconstructing algorithms. *In* "Radiology of Skull and Brain," Vol. 5 (G. Potts and T. H. Newton, eds.), C. V. Mosby, St. Louis, Missouri.

Herman, G. T., and Lent, A. (1976a). Iterative reconstruction algorithms. *Comput. Biol. and Med.* **6**, 273–294.

Herman, G. T., and Lent, A. (1976b). Quadratic optimization for image reconstruction I. *Comput. Graphics Image Processing* **5**, 319–332.

Herman, G. T., and Lent, A. (1978). A family of iterative quadratic optimization algorithms for pairs of inequalities with application in diagnostic radiology. *Math. Programming Study* **9**, 15–29.

Herman, G. T., and Liu, H. K. (1977). Display of three-dimensional information in computed tomography. *J. Comput. Assisted Tomography* **1**, 155–160.

Herman, G. T., and Liu, H. K. (1979). Three-dimensional display of human organs from computed tomograms. *Comput. Graphics Image Processing* **9**, 1–21.

Herman, G. T., and Lung, H. P. (1979). Reconstruction from divergent beams: a comparison of algorithms with and without rebinning. *Proc. Seventh New England (Northeast) Bioengineering Conference, Troy, New York*, (L. T. Ostrander, ed.), pp. 351–354. Institute of Electrical and Electronic Engineers, New York.

Herman, G. T., and Naparstek, A. (1978). Fast image reconstruction based on a Radon inversion formula appropriate for rapidly collected data. *SIAM J. Appl. Math.* **33**, 511–533.

Herman, G. T., and Rowland, S. W. (1973). Three methods for reconstructing objects from x-rays: a comparative study. *Comput. Graphics Image Processing* **2**, 151–178.

Herman, G. T., and Rowland, S. W. (1978). SNARK77: a programming system for image reconstruction from projections. Tech. Rept. No. 130, Dept. of Computer Science, State University of New York at Buffalo, Amherst, New York.

Herman, G. T., and Simmons, R. G. (1979). Illustration of a beam hardening correction method in computerized tomography. *Proc. Soc. Photo-Opt. Instrum. Eng.* **173**, 264–270.

Herman, G. T., Hurwitz, H., and Lent, A. (1978). A storage efficient algorithm for finding the regularized solution of a large inconsistent system of equations. Tech. Rept. MIPG14, Medical Image Processing Group, Dept. of Computer Science, State University of New York at Buffalo, Amherst, New York.

Herman, G. T., Hurwitz, H., Lent, A., and Lung, H. P. (1979). On the Bayesian approach to image reconstruction. *Inf. Control*, **42**, 60–71.

Herman, G. T., Lakshminarayanan, A. V., and Rowland, S. W. (1975). The Reconstruction of objects from shadowgraphs with high contrast. *Pattern Recognition* **7**, 157–165.

Herman, G. T., Lent, A., and Lutz, P. H. (1975). Iterative relaxation methods for image reconstruction. *ACM'75, Proc. Ann. Conf. Minneapolis, Minnesota*, pp. 169–174.

Herman, G. T., Lent, A., and Lutz, P. H. (1978). Relaxation methods for image reconstruction. *Comm. A.C.M.* **21**, 152–158.

Herman, G. T., Rowland, S. W., and Yau, M. M. (1979). A comparative study of the use of linear and modified cubic spline interpolation for image reconstruction. *IEEE Trans. Nucl. Sci.* **NS-26**, 2879–2894.

Hinderling, T., Ruegsegger, P., Anliker, M., and Diteschi, C. (1979). Computed tomography reconstruction from hollow projections: an application to in vivo evaluation of artificial hip joints. *J. Comput. Assisted Tomography* **3**, 52–57.

Hounsfield, G. N. (1972). A method and apparatus for examination of a body by radiation such as X or gamma radiation. Patent Specification 1283915, The Patent Office, London, England.

Hounsfield, G. N. (1973). Computerized transverse axial scanning tomography: Part I, description of the system. *Br. J. Radiol.* **46**, 1016–1022.

Huang, S. C., Phelps, M. E. and Hoffman, E. J. (1977). Effect of out-of-field objects in transaxial reconstruction tomography *In* "Reconstruction Tomography in Diagnostic Radiology and Nuclear Medicine" (M. M. Ter Pogossian *et al.*, eds.), pp. 185–198. Univ. Park Press, Baltimore, Maryland.

Huesman, R. H., Gullberg, G. T., Greenberg, W. L., and Budinger, T. F. (1977). "RECLBL Users Manual – Donner Algorithms for Reconstruction Tomography". Lawrence Berkeley Laboratory Publication PUB214, Berkeley, California.

Hurwitz, H., Jr., and Rumbaugh, J. E. (1977). Comparison of point response function and Bayesian criteria in image reconstruction. Rept. No. 76CRD207 General Electric Corporate Research and Development, Schenectady, New York.

Joseph, P. M., and Spital, R. D. (1978). A method for correcting bone induced artifacts in computed tomography scanners. *J. Comput. Assisted Tomography* **2**, 100–108.

Kaczmarz, S. (1937). Angenaehrte Aufloesung von Systemen linearer Gleichungen. *Bull. Int. Acad. Pol. Sci. Lett. A.*, 355–357.

Katz, M. B. (1978). "Questions of Uniqueness and Resolution in Reconstruction from Projections." Springer-Verlag, Berlin and New York.

Kolmogorov, A. N., and Fomin, S. V. (1957, 1961). "Elements of the Theory of Functions and Functional Analysis" Vol. 1 (1957); Vol. 2 (1961). Graylock Press, Baltimore, Maryland.

Kowalski, G. (1977). Fast 3-D scanning systems using a limited tilting angle. *Appl. Opt.* **16**, 1686–1690.

Kuhl, D. E., and Edwards, R. Q. (1963). Image separation radioisotope scanning. *Radiology* **80**, 653–662.

Lai, C., Shook, J. W., and Lauterbur, P. C. (1979). Microprocessor-controlled reorientation of magnetic field gradients for NMR zeugmatographic imaging. *Chem. Biomed. Environ. Instrum.* **9**, 1–27.

Lakshminarayanan, A. V. (1975). Reconstruction from divergent ray data. Tech. Rept. No. 92, Dept. Computer Science, State University of New York at Buffalo, Amherst, New York.

Lakshminarayanan, A. V., and Lent, A. (1979). Methods of least squares and SIRT in reconstruction. *J. Theor. Biol.* **76**, 267–295.

Lauterbur, P. C. (1979). Medical imaging by nuclear magnetic resonance zeugmatography. *IEEE Trans. Nucl. Sci.* **NS-26**, 2808–2811.

Ledley, R. S., and Park, C. M. (1977). Molded picture representation of whole body organs generated from CT scan sequences. *Proc. 1st Annual Symposium of Computer Applications in Medical Care, Washington, D.C.*, pp. 363–367.

Ledley, R. S., DiChiro, G., Luessenhop, A. J. and Twigg, H. L. (1974). Computerized transaxial X-ray tomography of the human body. *Science* **186**, 207–212.

Lent, A. (1977). A convergent algorithm for maximum entropy image restoration, with a medical x-ray application. *In* "Image Analysis and Evaluation" (R. Shaw, ed.), pp. 249–257. Society of Photographic Scientists and Engineers, Washington, D.C.

Lent, A., and Censor, Y. (1980). Extensions of Hildreth's row generation method for quadratic programming. *SIAM J. Control Optimization.* To appear.

Levine, R. D., and Tribus, M., eds. (1979). "The Maximum Entropy Formalism." MIT Press, Cambridge, Massachusetts.

Lewitt, R. M. (1979). Processing of incomplete measurement data in computed tomography. *Med. Phys.* **6**, 412–417.

Lewitt, R. M., and Bates, R. H. T. (1978). Image reconstruction from projections: III projection completion methods (theory). *Optik* **50**, 189–204.

Liu, H. K. (1977). Two and three-dimensional boundary detection. *Comput. Graphics Image Processing* **6**, 123–134.

Ludwig, D. (1966). The Radon transform on Euclidean Space. *Commun. Pure Appl. Math.* **19**, 49–81.

Luenberger, D. G. (1969). "Optimization by Vector Space Methods." Wiley, New York.

Lutz, P. H. (1975). Fourier image reconstruction incorporating three simple interpolation techniques. Tech. Rep. 104, Dept. of Computer Science, State University of New York at Buffalo, Amherst, New York.

Macovski, A., Alvarez, R. E., Chan, J. L.-H., Stonestrom, J. P., and Zatz, L. M. (1976). Energy dependent reconstruction in x-ray computerized tomography. *Comput. Biol. Med.* **6**, 325–336.

Marr, R. B. (1974). On the reconstruction of a function on a circular domain from a sampling of its line integrals. *J. Math. Anal. Appl.* **45**, 357–374.

Mazziotta, J. C. and Huang, H. K. (1976). THREAD (Three-dimensional reconstruction and display) with biomedical applications in neuron ultrastructure and computerized tomography. *Am. Fed. Information Processing Soc.*, **45**, 241–250.

Mersereau, R. M. (1976). Direct Fourier transform techniques in 3-D image reconstruction. *Comput. Biol. Med.* **6**, 247–258.

Metz, C. E., Starr, S. J., and Lusted, L. B. (1976). Quantitative evaluation of visual detection performance in medicine: ROC analysis and determination of diagnostic benefits. *In* "Medical Images: Formation, Perception and Measurement" (G. A. Hay, ed.), pp. 220–241. The Institute of Physics, London and Wiley, New York.

Minerbo, G. (1979a). MENT: A maximum entropy algorithm for reconstructing a source from projection data. *Comput. Graphics Image Processing* **10**, 48–68.

Minerbo, G. (1979b). Convolutional reconstruction from cone-beam projection data. *IEEE Trans. Nucl. Sci.* **NS-26**, 2682–2684.

Minerbo, G. N., and Sanderson, J. G. (1977). Reconstruction of a source from a few (2 or 3) projections. Tech. Rept. LA-6747-MS, Los Alamos Scientific Laboratory of the University of California, Los Alamos, New Mexico.

Moore, W. E., and Garmire, G. P. (1975). The X-ray structure of the Vela supernova remnant. *The Astrophys. J.* **199**, 680–690.

Nalciouglu, O., Cho, Z. H., and Lou, R. Y. (1979). Limited field of view reconstruction in computerized tomography. *IEEE Trans. Nucl. Sci.* **NS-26**, 546–551.

Oldendorf, W. H. (1961). Isolated flying-spot detection of radiodensity discontinuities; displaying the internal structural pattern of a complex object. *IRE Trans. Bio–Med. Electron.* **BME-8**, 68–72.

Oppenheim, B. E. (1977). Reconstruction tomography from incomplete projections *In* "Reconstruction Tomography in Diagnostic Radiology and Nuclear Medicine" (M. M. Ter-Pogossian, *et al.*, eds.), pp. 155–183. Univ. Park Press, Baltimore, Maryland.

Parzen, E. (1960). "Modern Probability Theory and Its Applications." Wiley, New York.

Pavkovich, J. (1979). Apparatus and method for reconstructing data. U.S. Patent 4,149,248, Patent Office, Washington, D.C.

Perry, R. M., Altschuler, M. D. and Altschuler, B. R. (1975). Medical image reconstruction: multiangular section roentgenography by computer. NCAR Tech. Note NCAR-TN/STR108, High Altitude Observatory, National Center for Atmospheric Research, Boulder, Colorado.

Phelps, M. E., Hoffman, E. J., and Ter-Pogossian, M. M. (1975). Attenuation coefficients of various body tissues, fluids, and lesions at photon energies of 18 to 136 keV. *Radiology* **117**, 573–583.

Rabiner, L. R., and Gold, B. (1975). "Theory and Application of Digital Signal Processing." Prentice-Hall, Englewood Cliffs, New Jersey.

Radon, J. (1917). Uber die Bestimmung von Funktionen durch ihre Integralwerte langs gewisser Mannigfaltigkeiten. *Ber. Verh. Saechs. Akad. Wiss., Leipzig, Math. Phys. Kl.* **69**, 262–277.

Radulovic, P. T., and Vest, C. M. (1976). Determination of three-dimensional temperature fields by holographic interferometry. Tech. Rept. INTFL-7601, Interferometry Laboratory, Dept. of Electric Engineering, The University of Michigan, Ann Arbor, Michigan.

Ralston, A., and Meek, C. L., eds. (1976). "Encyclopedia of Computer Science." Petrocelli/Charter, New York.

Ralston, A., and Rabinowitz, P. (1978). "A First Course in Numerical Analysis," 2nd ed. McGraw-Hill, New York.

Ramachandran, G. N., and Lakshminarayanan, A. V. (1971). Three-dimensional reconstruction from radiographs and electron micrographs: application of convolutions instead of Fourier transforms: *Proc. Nat. Acad. Sci. U.S.* **68**, 2236–2240.

Raviv, J., Greenleaf, J. F., and Herman, G. T., eds. (1979). "Computer Aided Tomography and Ultrasonics in Medicine." North-Holland Publ., Amsterdam.

Ritman, E. L., Robb, R. A., Johnson, S. A., Chevalier, P. A., Gilbert, B. K., Greenleaf, J. F., Sturm, R. E., and Wood, E. H. (1978). Quantitative imaging of the structure and function of the heart, lungs and circulation. *Mayo Clinic Proc.* **53**, 3–11.

Robb, R. A., Harris, L. D., and Ritman, E. L. (1976). Computerized x-ray reconstruction tomography in stereometric analysis of cardiovascular dynamics. *Proc. Soc. Photo-Opt. Instrum. Eng.* **89**, 69–82.

Rockmore, A. J., and Macovski, A. (1977). A maximum likelihood approach to image reconstruction. *Proc. Joint Automatic Control Conference*, San Francisco, California, pp. 782–786.

Rowland, S. W. (1979). Computer implementation of image reconstruction formulas. *In* "Image Reconstruction from Projections: Implementation and Applications" (G. T. Herman, ed.), pp. 9–80. Springer-Verlag, Berlin and New York.

Sage, A. P., and Melsa, J. L. (1971). "Estimation Theory with Application to Communications and Control." McGraw-Hill, New York.

Shepp, L. A., and Logan, B. F. (1974). The Fourier reconstruction of a head section. *IEEE Trans. Nucl. Sci.* **NS-21**, 21–43.

Shepp, L. A., and Stein, J. A. (1977). Simulated reconstruction artifacts in computerized tomography. *In* "Reconstruction Tomography in Diagnostic Radiology and Nuclear Medicine" (M. M. Ter-Pogossian *et al.*, eds.), pp. 33–48. Univ. Park Press, Baltimore, Maryland.

Smith, K. T., Solmon, D. C., and Wagner, S. L. (1977). Practical and mathematical aspects of the problem of reconstructing objects from radiographs. *Bull. Am. Math. Soc.* **83**, 1227–1270.

Smith, K. T., Solmon, D. C., Wagner, S. L., and Hamaker, C. (1978). Mathematical aspects of divergent beam radiography. *Proc. Nat. Acad. Sci. USA* **75**, 2055–2058.

Smith, P. R., Aebi, U., Josephs, R., and Kessel, M. (1976). Studies of the structure of the T4 bacteriophage tail sheath. I. The recovery of three-dimensional information from the extended sheath. *J. Mol. Biol.* **106**, 243–275.

Smith, P. R., Peters, T. M., and Bates, R. H. T. (1973). Image reconstruction from a finite number of projections. *J. Phys.* **A6**, 361–382.

Stonestrom, J. P., and Macovski, A. (1976). Scatter considerations in fan beam computerized tomographic systems. *IEEE Trans. Nucl. Sci.* **NS-23**, 1453–1458.

Strohbehn, J. W., Carter, H. Y., Curran, B. H., and Sternick, E. S. (1979). Image enhancement of conventional transverse-axial tomograms. *IEEE Trans. Biom. Eng.* **BME-26**, 253–262.

Stuck, B. W. (1977). A new proposal for estimating the spatial concentration of certain types of air pollutants. *J. Opt. Soc. Am.* **67**, 668–678.

Tanaka, E. and Iinuma, T. A. (1975). Correction functions for optimizing the reconstructed image in transverse section scan. *Phys. Med. Biol.* **20**, 789–798.

Taylor, J. H. (1967). Two-dimensional brightness distribution of radio sources from linear occultation observations. *Astrophys. J.* **150**, 421–426.

Tretiak, O. J. (1975). The point-spread function for the convolution algorithm. "Technical Digest: Image Processing for 2-D and 3-D Reconstruction from Projections: Theory and Practice in Medicine and Physical Sciences." Available from the Optical Society of America, Washington, D.C.

Tuy, H. (1979). "Reconstruction of a Three-Dimensional Object from X-ray Projections taken from an Incomplete Range of Views." Masters Thesis, Department of Computer Science, State University of New York at Buffalo, Amherst, New York.

Wee, W. G., and Prakash, A. (1978). Evaluation of Fourier reconstruction techniques in relation to the total number of ray-sums. *Proc. IEEE Comput. Soc. Conf. Pattern Recognition Image Processing*, Chicago, Illinois, pp. 200–204.

Weiss, H. P., and Stein, J. A. (1978). The effect of interpolation in CT image reconstruction. *Proc. IEEE Comput. Soc. Conf. Pattern Recognition Image Processing Chicago, Illinois*, p. 193.

Wood, E. H. (1977). New vistas for the study of structural and functional dynamics of the heart, lungs, and circulation by noninvasive numerical tomographic vivisection. *Circulation* **56**, 506–520.

Wood, E. H., Kinsey, J. H., Robb, R. A., Gilbert, B. K., Harris, L. D., and Ritman, E. L. (1979). Applications of high temporal resolution computerized tomography to physiology and medicine. *In*: "Image Reconstruction from Projections: Implementation and Applications" (G. T. Herman, ed.), pp. 247–279. Springer-Verlag, Berlin and New York.

Wood, S. L., Morf, M., and Macovski, A. (1977). Stochastic methods applied to medical image reconstruction. *Proc. IEEE Conf. Decision and Control, New Orleans, Louisiana*, pp. 35–41.

Young, D. M. (1971). "Iterative Solution of Large Linear Systems." Academic Press, New York.

Author Index

Numbers in italics refer to pages on which the complete references are listed.

A

Aebi, U., 25, *304*
Altschuler, B. R., 236, *303*
Altschuler, M. D., 24, 236, 259, 276, *297, 303*
Alvarez, R. E., 53, *302*
Andrews, H. C., 107, *297*
Anliker, M., 259, *301*
Apostol, T. M., 146, 236, 295, *297*
Artzy, E., 221, 276, *297*
Atkins, D. E., 179, 259, *299*

B

Barrett, H. H., 295, *297*
Barrett, P., 89, *298*
Barton, J. P., 25, *297*
Bates, R. H. T., 160, 236, *302, 304*
Bender, R., 107, 204, *299*
Berninger, W. H., 89, *298*
Boyd, D. P., 179, *299*
Bracewell, R. N., 24, 54, 145, 146, 159, 259, *298*
Brigham, E. O., 160, *298*
Brooks, R. A., 54, 116, *298*
Budinger, T. F., 24, 160, *298, 301*
Butzer, P. L., 107, *298*

C

Cahoon, J. G., 24, *298*
Carter, H. Y., 39, *304*
Censor, Y., 204, 259, 276, *297, 298, 302*
Chan, J. L.-H., 53, *302*
Chang, T., 146, 179, 259, 295, *297, 298*
Chen, A. C. M., 89, *298*
Chesler, D. A., 145, *298*
Chevalier, P. A., 54, *303*
Cho, Z. H., 295, *303*
Christensen, E. E., *298*
Chu, A., 179, 259, *297, 299*
Colsher, J. G., 259, *298*
Cormack, A. M., 24, 236, *299*
Courant, R., 236, *299*
Crowther, R. A., 159, *299*
Curran, B. H., 39, *304*
Curry, T. S., III, *298*

D

Davis, P. J., 116, *299*
Davison, E., 295, *299*
Denton, R. V., 259, *299*
Derenzo, S. E., 24, *298*
DeRosier, D. J., 159, *299*
DiChiro, G., 24, 54, *298, 302*

Subject Index

A

Actual measurement, 33
Additive normalization, 112
Algebraic reconstruction techniques (ART), 180–205
  additive, 189–193
  ART4, 192–193
  continuous, 205
  multiplicative, 205
Algorithm, 36, 39, 265
  for boundary detection, 265
  reconstruction, 36–38, 90–100, 204
  storage efficient, 181
Aliasing, 136
Amplitude, 130, 148
Annular harmonic decomposition, 222–228, 236
A priori probability density function, 102
Argument of complex number, 130
ART (*see* Algebraic reconstruction techniques)
Artifacts, 45–50, 54, 67–88, 217
  beam hardening, 45–47
  motion, 49
  scatter, 49–50
Astrophysics, 4

B

Backprojection, 96, 108–117
  continuous, 108–110
  discrete, 114–116
  method, 108–117
  operator, 96

Bandlimited functions, 131, 149
Bandwidth, 124, 131, 149
  of bandlimited function, 131, 149
  of window, 124
Basis, 98, 224–225, 228, 238–239
  objects, 238–239
  pictures, 98, 224–235, 236, 228
Bayesian estimate, 103, 107, 189, 204–205, 251–253, 259
Beam hardening, 35, 45–47, 53, 76–83
Bilinear interpolation, 154–155
Binomial, 21
  probability law, 21
  random variable, 21
Boundary, 262
  detection, 262–266, 276
Brightness, 268

C

Calibration measurement, 33
Chebyshev
  polynomials of second kind, 229, 236
  semi-iteration, 221
Complex numbers, 130
  argument, 130
  modulus, 130
Complimentary matrix, 205
Computerized tomography, 1, 24, 296
  emission, 14, 24
  x-ray, 8, 24
Cone beam, 250
Confidence, 22
Conjugate gradient method, 221

Computer Science and Applied Mathematics

A SERIES OF MONOGRAPHS AND TEXTBOOKS

Editor
Werner Rheinboldt
University of Pittsburgh

ARNOLD O. ALLEN. Probability, Statistics, and Queueing Theory: With Computer Science Applications

ELLIOTT I. ORGANICK, ALEXANDRA I. FORSYTHE, AND ROBERT P. PLUMMER. Programming Language Structures

ALBERT NIJENHUIS AND HERBERT S. WILF. Combinatorial Algorithms, Second Edition

AZRIEL ROSENFELD. Picture Languages, Formal Models for Picture Recognition

ISAAC FRIED. Numerical Solution of Differential Equations

ABRAHAM BERMAN AND ROBERT J. PLEMMONS. Nonnegative Matrices in the Mathematical Sciences

BERNARD KOLMAN AND ROBERT E. BECK. Elementary Linear Programming with Applications

CLIVE L. DYM AND ELIZABETH S. IVEY. Principles of Mathematical Modeling

ERNEST L. HALL. Computer Image Processing and Recognition

ALLEN B. TUCKER, JR. Text Processing: Algorithms, Languages, and Applications

MARTIN CHARLES GOLUMBIC. Algorithmic Graph Theory and Perfect Graphs

GABOR T. HERMAN. Image Reconstruction from Projections: The Fundamentals of Computerized Tomography

WEBB MILLER AND CELIA WRATHALL. Software for Roundoff Analysis of Matrix Algorithms

ULRICH W. KULISCH AND WILLARD L. MIRANKER. Computer Arithmetic in Theory and Practice

LOUIS A. HAGEMAN AND DAVID M. YOUNG. Applied Iterative Methods

I. GOHBERG, P. LANCASTER AND L. RODMAN. Matrix Polynomials.

AZRIEL ROSENFELD AND AVINASH C. KAK. Digital Picture Processing, Second Edition, Vol. 1, Vol. 2

DIMITRI P. BERTSEKAS. Constrained Optimization and Lagrange Multiplier Methods

JAMES S. VANDERGRAFT. Introduction to Numerical Computations, Second Edition

FRANÇOISE CHATELIN. Spectral Approximation of Linear Operators

GÖTZ ALEFELD AND JÜRGEN HERZBERGER. Introduction to Interval Computations. Translated by Jon Rokne

In preparation

LEONARD UHR. Algorithm-Structured Computer Arrays and Networks: Architectures and Processes for Images, Percepts, Models, Information

ROBERT KORFHAGE. Discrete Computational Structures, Second Edition

O. AXELSSON AND V. A. BARKER. Finite Element Solution of Boundary Value Problems: Theory and Computation

MARTIN D. DAVIS AND ELAINE J. WEYUKER. Computability, Complexity, and Languages: Fundamentals of Theoretical Computer Science

PHILIP J. DAVIS AND PHILIP RABINOWITZ. Methods of Numerical Integration, Second Edition